Neonatal Tumours

Springer
London
Berlin
Heidelberg
New York
Barcelona
Budapest
Hong Kong
Milan
Paris
Santa Clara
Singapore
Tokyo

Prem Puri (Ed.)
With assistance from Rajendra Surana

Neonatal Tumours

With 54 Figures

Springer

Prem Puri MS, FACS
Consultant Paediatric Surgeon
Our Lady's Hospital for Sick Children
National Children's Hospital
The Children's Hospital, Dublin
and Director of Research
Children's Research Centre
Our Lady's Hospital for Sick Children
Dublin, Ireland

ISBN-13:978-1-4471-3030-7

British Library Cataloguing in Publication Data
Neonatal Tumours
I. Puri, Prem II. Surana, Rajendra
618.92994
ISBN-13:978-1-4471-3030-7 e-ISBN-13:978-1-4471-3028-4
DOI: 10.1007/978-1-4471-3028-4

Library of Congress Cataloging-in-Publication Data
A catalog record for this book is available from the Library of Congress

Softcover reprint of the hardcover 1st edition 1996

Typesetting: EXPO Holdings, Malaysia

28/3830-543210 Printed on acid-free paper

Preface

Neonatal tumours comprise 2% of paediatric tumours. Although uncommon, these tumours form an interesting group for a number of reasons. There are differences in type, incidence, natural history and response to therapy from those of apparently similar tumours seen in older children. Until recently, genetic factors have been implicated in many congenital tumours, but during the last few years, the effect of the environment on the pathogenesis of these tumours has been gaining much attention. Neonatal tumours, because of their short exposure to environmental factors, offer new avenues to the understanding of the pathogenesis of these tumours.

This book is intended for those who have a clinical responsibility for newborn babies. It provides an authoritative, comprehensive and complete account of the various tumours that can be found in the neonate. It reviews the epidemiology of neonatal tumours, the genetic association and clinical features of tumours, their recognition and management. It is designed to cover the entire spectrum of neonatal tumours. Although emphasis is placed on relatively common tumours, a chapter on rare tumours is also included. The book is specifically designed for oncologists, paediatric surgeons, neonatologists, trainees in paediatric surgery and oncology, and paediatricians seeking more detailed information on the subject of neonatal tumours

I am grateful to all my colleagues who have contributed chapters to this book, to Ms Ann Brennan for secretarial help and to the staff of Springer for their help during the preparation and publication stages. I am thankful to the Children's Centre, Our Lady's Hospital for Sick Children, for their support.

Prem Puri

Contents

Contributors

C.C. BAILEY, FRCP
Professor and Consultant Paediatric Oncologist,
St James's University Hospital,
Beckett Street,
Leeds LS9 7TF,
UK

JEHUDA A. BAR-MAOR, MD, FACS, FAAP
Professor and Head of Department of Paediatric Surgery,
Rambam Medical Center, Bat-Galim,
Haifa 31096,
Israel

PETER FREY, MD, BSc, PD, FMH (Paed Surg)
Chirurgie Pediatrique,
Centre Hospitalier Universitaire Vaudois,
CH-1011 Lausanne,
Switzerland

JEAN GAUDIN, MD
Chirurgie Pediatrique,
Hopital Saint Louis,
La Rochelle,
France

JAY GROSFELD, MD
Professor and Chairman, Department of Surgery, Indiana University School of Medicine,
Surgeon-in-Chief, James Whitcomb Riley Hospital for Sick Children,
702 Barnhill Drive,
Indianapolis, Indiana 46202-5200,
USA

KOICHI ISHIMOTO, MD, PhD
Assistant Professor of Paediatrics,
Juntendo University, School of Medicine,
2-1-1 Hongo, Bunkyo-ku,
Tokyo 113, Japan

V. KALIDASAN, MCh
Senior Registrar,
Children's Research Centre,
Our Lady's Hospital for Sick Children,
Crumlin,
Dublin 12, Ireland

JACOB C. LANGER, MD
Division of Pediatric Surgery,
Room 5W-12,
St Louis Children's Hospital
One Children' Place
St Louis, MO 63110, USA

TAKESHI MIYANO, MD, PhD
Professor and Head,
Department of Paediatric Surgery,
Juntendo University, School of Medicine,
2-1-1 Hongo, Bunkyo-ku,
Tokyo 113, Japan

S.W. MOORE, MB, ChB FRCS (Ed), MD (UCT)
Professor of Surgery,
Head, Department of Paediatric Surgery,
University of Stellenbosch,
Faculty of Medicine,
Tygerberg 7505,
South Africa

GEORGE NINAN, FRCSI
Consultant Paediatric Surgeon,
Royal Aberdeen Children's Hospital,
Cornhill Road,
Aberdeen AB9 2ZG,
UK

MICHAEL O'KEEFE, FRCS
The Children's Hospital,
Temple Street,
Dublin 1, Ireland

JACK PLASCHKES, MD, FRCS (Eng)
Consultant Paediatric Surgeon,
Department of Paediatric Surgery,
University Children's Hospital,
Freiburgstrasse,
CH3010 Bern, Switzerland

PREM PURI, MS, FACS
Consultant Paediatric Surgeon
Our Lady's Hospital for Sick Children,
National Children's Hospital and
The Children's Hospital, Dublin and
Director of Research,
Children's Research Centre,
Our Lady's Hospital for Sick Children,
Crumlin,
Dublin 12, Ireland

RAJENDRA SURANA, MS, FRCSI
Senior Research Fellow,
Children's Research Centre,
Our Lady's Hospital for Sick Children,
Crumlin,
Dublin 12, Ireland

YECHIEL SWEED, MD
Consultant Paediatric Surgeon,
Rambam Medical Center, Bat-Galim 1,
Haifa 31096,
Israel

Epidemiology of Neonatal Tumours

Jack Plaschkes

1

Introduction

Epidemiology is a method of investigating diseases to find causal relationships between disease and environmental factors. The same methodology has been used to pinpoint hereditary and other links. The classic clear simplified distinction between genetic and environmental factors does not always correspond to reality, as the complexity of molecular genetics has shown. The concept of ecogenetics, "the genetic predisposition to environmental factors", has also blurred this distinction[1].

The systematic study of tumours in children clearly demonstrates that the incidence, types of tumour, natural history and response to therapy are quite different from those seen in adults. Most tumours are of an embryonal type (sarcomas) – often classified as "blastomas" – rather than epithelial (carcinomas). The natural history and response to therapy are often age related and more favourable in newborns than in older children and adults. Nevertheless, in spite of their differences, these tumours have served as ideal models to provide basic knowledge on carcinogenesis (two-hit mutation theory, chromosomal aberrations, oncogenes, proto-oncogenes, genomic imprinting, amplifications of specific proteins, etc.)[2]. Environmental factors per se are not very prominent[3].

The little detailed knowledge available on neonatal tumours also indicates that there are differences in type, incidence and natural history from those of apparently similar tumours seen in older children. In particular, the course is more often benign – the classic examples being neuroblastoma with spontaneous regression[4,5], the Wilms' tumour complex[6] (including mesoblastic nephroma)[7,8] and some of the fibrous tumours indistinguishable by histology alone from fibrosarcoma[9–13].

The fetal period is much shorter and therefore much easier to study than the lifespan of an individual, and there is a clear cut-off time for possible oncogenic factors. This is reason enough to devote more intensive effort to a search for such causes.

A newer and interesting field is the investigation of the effect of the environment, e.g. occupation, on the gametes of the parents before conception. The father is now being included in environmental studies, and not only the mother during pregnancy, as was previously the case. Genomic imprinting has shown that alleles from mother and father are not necessarily identical in their effect[14]. It is likely that the routine use of ultrasonography during pregnancy may offer new insights into these interesting concepts.

Neonatal tumours are uncommon, comprising 0.5%–2% of all paediatric tumours[15]. Not surprisingly, therefore, they have not been the subject of much research, and systematic hard information is extremely sparse. Although interest is increasing there have as yet been only isolated conferences devoted to this topic[16].

Definitions

Neonatal versus congenital

For most purposes the "neonatal" period is defined as the first 28 days of life. Strictly speaking, "congenital" tumours should include only those diagnosed at birth, and which must therefore have arisen during fetal life, but it has been said that two-thirds will be found within the first week of life[17], and presumably some or most of those discovered later will also have been present in the fetus. The question therefore arises as to whether the 28 day period is appropriate. Clearly with the present state of knowledge the decision is an arbitrary one, but routine use of prenatal ultrasonography may help to clarify matters.

There have been various definitions of neonatal tumours. Some authors have adhered to the classic 28 days; others consider 3 or 6 months or even a year a reasonable cut-off time. The usual 28 day definition was selected mainly because of the various phases of adaptation and maturation of the neonate and probably has no relevance to oncogenesis.

Clinical tumour versus neoplasia

A malignant tumour has the potential for uncontrolled invasive, almost always exponential, growth and metastatic spread, leading, if untreated, to the death of the host. This trait can usually be determined on histological examination.

It is a special feature of many tumours in newborns that a clear distinction between histological malignancy and clinical outcome cannot in all instances be made decisively. Some tumours that would by all criteria appear to be malignant can regress spontaneously, e.g. 4-S neuroblastoma[4,5]; others are clearly benign but because of their size and location can be life threatening, e.g. haemangioendotheliomas (mesenchymal hamartomas) of the liver[18,19]. Yet others, initially benign, can undergo malignant transformation – the best clinical example being sacrococcygeal teratoma[9]. An intermediate group has some malignant characteristics, such as infiltrative growth, but do not metastasize; for example, fibrous tumours or fibromatoses are often indistinguishable from fibrosarcoma[6].

There is also the fascinating group of so-called "in situ" tumours discovered as an incidental finding in autopsies of stillbirths or on routine ultrasonography during pregnancy. Screening programmes for neuroblastoma have clearly shown that tumours discovered under such circumstances cannot be directly compared to those diagnosed later.

Many benign tumours are hamartomas but have been included by pathologists and surgeons in some reviews of neonatal tumours. Understanding the complex relationship between malformations, teratogenesis and oncogenesis should provide a valuable source of information.

Historical background

Credit for the first systematic study of neonatal tumours should go to the pathologists. Wells was the first to collect and classify a large series – of 255 neonatal tumours[20]. In his estimate only about 60 of the 255 cases could be considered malignant tumours. These 60 included mainly embryonal tumours, neuroblastomas and sarcomas, with very few true carcinomas. Willis speculates on the unique position of neonatal tumours, as is evident in the title of his book *The borderland of embryology and pathology*[21]. Both authors were concerned mainly with autopsies on fetuses and stillbirths. Dehner[22], Berry[23] and Satge (personal communication), all pathologists, have also extensively reviewed neonatal tumours. Isolated case reports were published before this and also appeared in early textbooks of paediatrics and in some of the first textbooks on cancer in children[11,24,25]. Much valuable epidemiological information can be gleaned from this material.

The relatively benign course of congenital and infantile neuroblastoma under the age of 1 year, in contrast to the very poor prognosis in older children, was noted in the 1960s, and since then similar unique behaviour has been reported of other congenital tumours, particularly soft-tissue "sarcomas"[26]. Renal tumours previously considered mostly as Wilms' tumours are now separated and called "mesoblastic nephroma"[11].

Incidence

Several methods of ascertaining the incidence of tumours in children are in use (Table 1.1). Hospital activity analysis is one; establishment of regional or national tumour registries is another.

Table 1.1 Published series of "neonatal" tumours since 1980

Date	Author	Country	Time span	No. of cases	Per year	Source
1982	Gale et al.[27]	USA (Philadelphia)	Not given	22	?	Hospital series
1985	Isaacs[28]	USA (Los Angeles)	1958–1982	110	110/25 = 4.4	Pathology review
1986	Pinter and Hock[29]	Hungary	1975–1987	141 (including infants)	141/12 = 11.8	Hospital series
1987	Campbell et al.[30]	Canada (Toronto)	1922–1982	102	102/60 = 1.7	Hospital series
1988	Davis et al.[31]	Scotland (Glasgow)	1955–1986	51	51/32 = 1.6	Hospital series
1989	Crom et al.[32]	USA (Memphis)	1962–1988	34	34/16 = 2.1	Hospital series
1989	Plaschkes and Dubler[33]	Switzerland (Bern)	1973–1987	39	39/15 = 2.6	Hospital series
1990	Mur[34]	Argentina	1967–1990	51	51/23 = 2.2	Hospital series
1992	Werb et al.[35]	Australia (Melbourne)	1939–1989	46	46/50 = 0.9	Autopsies
1992	Brch et al.[36]	Denmark (Copenhagen)	1943–1985	76	76/42 = 1.8	National cancer registry
1992	Teinturier et al.[80]	France (Paris)	1975–1986	75	75/10 = 7.5	Hospital series
1994	Parkes et al.[81]	UK (Birmingham)	1960–1989	149(+21 leukemia)	149/30 = 5	Population-based registry
1995	Moore and Kaschula[37]	South Africa	1957–1991	60	60/34 = 1.8	Hospital series

Table 1.2

Country	Author	Incidence	Source
UK	Barson[39]	70 per million live births	National Survey by Pathologists (GB)[a]
UK	Oxford Children's Cancer Group[40]	17 per million live births	Cancer Registry
UK	Manchester Children's Tumour Registry[41]	121.29 per 10^6 child years	Tumour Registry, population based[b]
USA	Bader and Miller[42]	36.4 per 10^6 child years	Third National Cancer Survey (USA)
Switzerland	Plaschkes and Dubler[33]	93 per million live births	Hospital activity analysis
Hungary	Pinter and Hock[29]	100.5 per million live births	Hospital activity analysis[c]
Denmark	Brch et al.[36]	23 per million live births	Danish Cancer Registry (ICD)

[a] Benign–malignant.
[b] Neonates and infants less than 1 year of age (including lymphoma and leukaemia).
[c] Under 3 months of age, malignant and lifethreatening benign tumours.

Mortality registers have also been used, but improvements in treatment results give very incomplete figures. To use any of these figures for a meaningful study of causal factors a standard nomenclature is also essential. The International Classification of Disease (ICD) and the Manual of Tumour Nomenclature and Coding (MOTNAC) are not particularly adapted to children, and many "home-made" systems are in use. There is no general agreement on nomenclature of neonatal tumours, but a serious attempt has been made recently by the group from the Manchester Children's Tumour Registry for tumours in children[39]. In view of these discrepancies, it is surprising that the range of incidence shown in Table 1.2 is not greater. The incidence in various reports varies from 17 per million live births to 121 per million child years. Probably the most accurate figure is that from the population-based Manchester Children's Tumour Registry, which estimates a number of 121.29 per 10^6 child years but includes all infants under 1 year of age and leukaemias and lymphomas. A comparison of the various tumour types shows the differences in incidence in older children and in various countries. Overall, the incidence reported is highest in Japanese children and lowest in black children in the USA[41].

Distribution of tumours

In the various series, including many isolated case reports, a number of hospital series and a few comprehensive reviews, the distribution of the various types of neonatal tumour is fairly constant but different from that found in older children. In a survey by pathologists of 285 tumours occurring within the first month of life, teratomas (24%) and neuroblastomas (23%) were the most common, followed by soft-tissue sarcomas (8%), renal tumours (7%) and brain tumours (6%)[39]. Liver tumours, malignant and benign, are not uncommon. Many others tend to be one-off rarities, but therefore possibly of great theoretical interest.

Table 1.3 International Society for Paediatric Oncology (SIOP) tumour registry 1987–1991

Diagnosis	No. of cases
Neuroblastoma	85
Teratoma	24
Rhabdomyosarcoma	13
Retinoblastoma	10
Mesoblastic nephroma	8
Hepatoblastoma	6
Undifferentiated sarcoma	5
Histiocytosis	4
Fibromatosis	3
Haemangiopericytoma	3
Renal (unclassified)	3
Yolk sac tumour	3
Brain tumour	2
Choriocarcinoma	2
Fibrosarcoma	2
Liver tumours	2
Prospective neuroectodermal tumour (PNET)	2
Angiofibroma	1
Arterioventricular malformations	1
Embryonal tumours	1
Ependymoblastoma	1
Glioma grade III–IV	1
Infantile myofibromatosis	1
Juvenile xanthogranuloma	1
Leiomyosarcoma	1
Lymphosarcoma	1
Melanoma	1
Neurofibroma	1
Oligodendroglioma	1
Rhabdoid tumour	1
Testicular carcinoma	1
Wilms' tumour	1
Total	192

True carcinomas as found in adults make up only 1%–2%[43].

Age and sex

Fifty to seventy-five per cent of the tumours are diagnosed by 1 week to 1 month of age. In most cases the male to female ratio is virtually equal except retinoblastoma (male preponderance) and teratoma (female preponderance).

Table 1.3 shows the distribution of 192 cases collected from 12 countries by the International Society for Paediatric Oncology over 4 years from 1987 to 1991 (personal communication). On the whole, these data are similar to those of other series as far as the more common diagnoses are concerned. There were 33 different types of tumour. Overall, 34% presented with metastatic disease, 62% had surgery, 19% radiotherapy, 44% chemotherapy, and 41% were treated according to a protocol. More than half (53%) are alive and disease free, 15% are dead from tumour, and in 2% death was caused by treatment. Most neonatal tumours have better outcome than those in older children, but brain tumours and rhabdomyosarcomas appear to have a worse prognosis.

Table 1.4 Diagnosis of primary cancer in the first 3 months of life

Diagnosis	No. of cases
Neuroblastoma	44
Acute lymphoblastic leukaemia	12
Retinoblastoma	
Unilateral	8
Bilateral	14
Acute non-lymphoblastic leukaemia	6
Wilms' tumour	
Unilateral	5
Bilateral	1
Hepatoblastoma	4
Rhabdomyosarcoma	3
Infantile fibrosarcoma	3
Embryonal carcinoma	2
Choroid plexus carcinoma	2
Astrocytoma	2
Sarcoma (not otherwise specified)	1
Melanoma	1
Teratoma	1
Sacrococcygeal	1
Brain	1
Glioblastoma	1
Rhabdoid tumour	1

In another retrospective series (personal communication) from St Jude's Research Hospital, Memphis, the distribution of 112 cases in the first 3 months of life was as shown in Table 1.4. Excluding leukaemia, the most common tumours in order of frequency were neuroblastoma, retinoblastoma and Wilms' tumour.

Binding conclusions should not be made from these series because of their different study designs. However, they do serve to illustrate the distribution and frequency of tumours, and may provide insights for future research.

Mortality rate

The reported mortality rate from neonatal tumours varies from 6.24 to 7.6 per million live births[42,44]. In the third National Cancer Survey, 50% of deaths occurred within 1 week of birth[44]. One must be aware in interpreting these figures that by definition only deaths in the first 28 days of life are included. In some of the series reported, deaths caused by treatment are relatively high. The special problems of chemotherapy[45] and radiotherapy[46] in the neonate have to be considered.

Aetiology and carcinogenesis

The causes and progression of carcinogenesis or spontaneous regression in neonatal tumours are unknown. Some parallels with what is known about tumours in older children have been assumed, and the only cell biology studies of any significance in newborns are those in stage 4-S neuroblastoma, which is one of the commonest and best studied of the well known neonatal tumours with atypical behaviour[47].

To explain the tendency to regression, Bolande coined the concept of a period of "oncological grace" in the first few weeks of life[48,49]. There is no experimental evidence to support this attractive theory. It would imply that host factors are different in this early period and particularly active in surveillance.

The debate as to whether neonatal tumours arise because of a local failure in the arrest of growth during embryogenesis or de novo because of other causes (what causes the "switch off" or "switch on") remains unresolved. A fundamental understanding of this process on the genetic level could have far-reaching implications in the study of cancer. Paediatric tumours have served as ideal models in this respect[2], in particular in the study of oncogenes, proto-oncogenes and other changes at the level of the genome[50]. In the future neonatal tumours should also be investigated similarly.

Environmental factors should play a far smaller role in neonatal tumours than in adults' tumours. If they have any relevance at all, their influence must be restricted to the short and therefore more easily studied intrauterine period and the transplacental route. This opens up a wide field of study concerning maternal habits. Recently, rather unexpectedly, parental occupation has been found to be related to the occurrence of some paediatric tumours. An example is the possible association of brain tumours with occupational exposure to heavy metals[51], but this has not been studied in neonatal tumours. So far, direct environmental agents are largely unidentified.

Parents and neonatal tumours

Pregnancy and transplacental transfer

Events during pregnancy could be of key significance in neonatal tumours, and have aroused particular interest. The distinction between environmental and genetic factors is being eroded, and both environmental and genetic influences can be transmitted by both parents to their offspring. Those of known or possible relevance in neonatal tumours are discussed briefly below.

Tumours in the mother

Only very occasionally has transplacental spread of a tumour in the mother been observed[52]. A number of reports record the transfer of a melanoma to the fetus[53], and choriocarcinoma occurring at different sites, e.g. the eye and brain have also been recorded[54]. The assumption is that choriocarcinoma originates in the placenta, but this has not always been confirmed[55]. It is also assumed that seeding of tumours is more frequent than the incidence of neonatal tumours would suggest; but that the fetus rejects the "foreign" tumour cells.

An unusual reverse event describing the effects of catecholamines on a mother carrying a fetus with neuroblastoma has been described[56]. A fascinating and conceptionally quite different association between a tumour in the mother and her child is found in the Li-Fraumeni syndrome, where there is a greater risk of breast cancer in a mother who has given birth to a child with rhabdomyosarcoma, and in her relatives.

Drugs taken during pregnancy

Adenocarcinoma of the cervix in young girls whose mothers took oestrogens during pregnancy is well known, but has not yet been reported as early as the neonatal period. There are no reports of definite associations between any congenital tumours and the use of drugs except possibly the occurrence of neuroblastoma in fetal hydantoin syndrome[57]. Sacrococcygeal teratoma associated with maternal intake of acetazolamide has been reported[58]. Other indirect influences are only conjectural (see also Environmental exposure of parents, below).

Infections during pregnancy

No clear association between infections during pregnancy and neonatal tumours is known (unlike the association between infection and malformations), although an association has been reported in the origin of germ cell tumours[59]. In particular, the role of viruses is not clear – at least as a single factor – but may be of significance in a multistep process: the Epstein–Barr virus has been found in many cancers but is rarely implicated directly; the hepatitis B virus has been associated with hepatocellular carcinoma in young children, and transplacental infection has been postulated.

Pregnancy outcome after childhood cancer

It is estimated that, by the year 2000, one in 200 persons aged 20 or more will have been cured of cancer[60]. There is no evidence that offspring of mothers who have had a childhood cancer are more susceptible to cancer[61]. Cohort studies on nearly 4000 such offspring have been published[62,63]. This implies that the effect of cancer treatment on the genetic constitution of the mother is not very significant. Low birth weight and increased risk of abortion have been associated with pregnancies in cancer survivors, but it is not known whether these are independent variables[62].

Environmental exposure of parents

There is active debate on the roles of environmental exposure and the habits of parents in causing neoplasms in children. A powerful stimulus to the debate was concern about the increased risk of leukaemia in children born to mothers living near nuclear reactors[63]. These mothers were originally the main focus of investigation, but there are also findings implicating the fathers[64]. Many investigations now extend to occupational exposure. The factors at present under active investigation in paediatric tumours include electromagnetic fields[65], radon[66], metals in industry[52,67], vitamin K given to neonates[68], pesticides, nitrous compounds (in cured meat, and vegetables) and rubber pacifiers[69].

Congenital malformation and tumours (birth defects)

The association between malformations and tumours has been known for some time and has given rise to various theories[70]. There is evidence to suggest that a single insult or genetic error can be both teratogenic and carcinogenic[71,72]. A defect at the level of DNA transmission or replication could be responsible for both.

Many malformation syndromes are associated with specific tumours, e.g. hemihypertrophy with Wilms' tumour, hepatoblastoma and Beckwith–Wiedemann syndrome with aniridia, and hepatoblastoma with familial adenomatous polyposis. There are also tumour malformations (hamartomas and teratomas) in which a malignancy can arise, e.g. germ cell tumour in sacrococcygeal teratoma, or melanoma in basal cell naevus syndrome. The clinical significance of tumours associated with malformation syndromes lies in the possibility of screening at birth for these tumours in children with such malformation stigmata. However, one must be wary of making treatment decisions based on what is known of similar tumours discovered at a later age, as the natural history can be quite different. For example, many neuroblastomas discovered by screening can regress spontaneously, making the prognosis more favourable.

In both the malformation syndromes and the tumour malformations, knowledge of the genetics involved is already vast and is increasing exponentially. Research on the "two-hit" mutation theory, chromosomal aberrations (deletions and translocations), ploidy, loss of heterozygosity, the p53 gene and proteins, and oncogenes, proto-oncogenes and gene amplification (e.g. N-*myc*) have moved from the research laboratory into clinical application, leading to improvements in diagnosis and more differentiated treatment. Such research in neonatal tumours is largely lacking, but more concerted studies can be expected to produce similar benefits.

In situ tumours

Before the ultrasound era, pathologists identified in stillbirths what they called "in situ" tumours in various tissues in a much higher incidence than found later on. They therefore assumed that there must be some spontaneous regression[73,74].

Growth factors

The angiogenic factors – mainly basic fibroblastic growth factor (BFGF) and its inhibitors[75] – are also known to have a role in tumour genesis, and are particularly amenable to experimental investigation. Other growth factors, such as growth hormone (GH), platelet derived growth factor (PDGF), insulin-like growth factor and other cytokines (G-CSF, etc.), which are mostly naturally occurring, could be very important in this age group, where all tissue is growing rapidly[76,77].

Adult types of tumour (carcinoma) in neonates

Almost all types of carcinoma found in adults have also been described in children and neonates, but because they are even more rare than the embryonal tumours very little except descriptive information is available. Nevertheless, the trend to a different natural history is also seen. For example, thyroid carcinoma has different causes (mostly radiation) and a better prognosis. The same may be true for carcinoma of the breast and of the pancreas. Closer detailed examination reveals not only a better prognosis but also differences in morphology.

Clinical implications and conclusion

The reasons for giving neonatal tumours more systematic attention are manifold:

1. Universal use of ultrasonography during pregnancy will increasingly bring to light tumours whose natural history and correct management is largely unknown.
2. More knowledge of their biological behaviour and prognosis could help to reduce unnecessary treatment (surgery, chemotherapy and radiotherapy) with their particularly deleterious late effects in this age group[45,46,78,79].
3. Molecular genetic information derived from these tumours identify risk factors and provide models for carcinogenesis in general.
4. Environmental factors (apparent or hidden) and transmission via the parents are easier to study in this age group with a clearly defined exposure time.
5. A pragmatic approach applicable to all these tumours may be the answer for clinical purposes until more specific information becomes available. Such a system could be as follows:
   - I Clearly malignant by all usual criteria but:
     - (a) Behave as in older children
     - (b) Behave better than expected
     - (c) Behave worse than expected
     - (d) Unpredictable or unknown behaviour
   - II Semimalignant – invasive growth but no metastatic potential
   - III Clearly benign but:
     - (a) Life threatening because of size and location
     - (b) Known tendency to malignant transformation
   - IV Extreme rarities, e.g. malignant carcinomas similar to adult tumours

From all the evidence to date it is clear that the natural history of neonatal tumours is different (mostly better) than that of comparable tumours in older children. The basis of this behaviour is largely unknown, and hard epidemiological and aetiological data in this age group are lacking. Because of the rarity of these tumours it should be clear that such data can only be realized by international cooperation in clearly defined clinical studies and research projects.

References

1. Mulvihill JJ (1986) Clinical ecogenetics – cancer in families. N Engl J Med 312: 1569–1570.
2. Israel MA (1989) Pediatric oncology; model tumours of unparalleled import. J Natl Cancer Inst 81: 404–408.

3. Buckley JD (1992) The aetiology of cancer in the very young. Br J Cancer 66 (Suppl XVIII): S8–S12.
4. Evans AR (1965) Congenital neuroblastoma. J Clin Pathol 18: 54–62.
5. Nietschke R, Humphrey GB, Sexauer CHL et al. (1986) Neuroblastoma: therapy for infants with good prognosis. Med Pediatr Oncol 11: 154–158.
6. Hrabovsky E, Othersen H, Delorimier A et al. (1986) Wilms' tumor in the neonate: a report from the National Wilms' Tumor Study. J Pediatr Surg 21: 383–387.
7. Beckwith JB, Weeks DA (1986) Congenital mesoblastic nephroma. Arch Pathol Lab Med 110: 98–99.
8. Walterhouse D (1990) Mesoblastic nephroma. Med Pediatr Oncol 18: 64–67.
9. Plaschkes J (1974) Congenital fibromatosis: localized and generalized forms. J Pediatr Surg 9: 95–100.
10. Wiswell TE, Davis J, Cunningham BE et al. (1988) Infantile myofibromatosis: the most common fibrous tumor of infancy. J Pediatr Surg 23: 314–318.
11. Salloum E, Flamant F, Caillaud JM et al. (1990) Diagnostic and therapeutic problems of soft tissue tumors other than rhabdomyosarcoma in infants under 1 year of age: a clinicopathological study of 34 cases treated at the Institut Gustave-Roussy. Med Pediatr Oncol 18: 37–43.
12. Madden NP, Spicer RD, Allibone EB, Lewis I II (1992) Spontaneous regression of neonatal fibrosarcoma. Br J Cancer 66: 372–375.
13. Batcup G (1992) Cancer in the very young child – pitfalls and problems for the pathologist. Br J Cancer 66 (Suppl XVIII): S5–S7.
14. Reik W, Surani MA (1989) Genomic imprinting and embryonal tumours. Nature 338: 112–113.
15. McWhirter WR, Stiller CA, Lennox EL (1981) Carcinomas in childhood. A registry based study of incidence and survival. Cancer 61: 2242–2246.
16. Cancer in the very young (1992) Proceedings of Conference at St James Hospital, Leeds, September 1990. Br J Cancer 66 (Suppl XVIII).
17. Favara EB (1981) Origins of Cancer in the Neonate. Am J Pediatr Hematol Oncol 3: 187–193.
18. Alkalay AL, Puri AR, Pomerance JJ (1985) Mesenchymal hamartomas of the liver responsive to cyclophosphamide therapeutic approaches. J Pediatr Surg 20: 125–129.
19. Barto S, Schultz MJ, Bollman R, Specht U (1992) Prenatally diagnosed hamartoma of the liver. Zentralbl Pathol 138: 141–144.
20. Wells HG (1940) Occurrence and significance of congenital malignant neoplasms. Arch Pathol 30: 535–601.
21. Willis RA (1962) The borderland of embryology and pathology. Butterworths, London.
22. Dehner LP (1981) Neoplasms of the fetus and neonate. In: Naye L, Kissane JM, Kaufmann N, eds, Monographs in pathology – prenatal diseases, Williams and Wilkins, Baltimore.
23. Berry PJ (1987) Congenital tumours. In: Keeling JW, ed. Fetal and neonatal pathology. Springer-Verlag, Berlin, pp 229–247.
24. Jones PG, Campbell PE (1976) Tumours in infancy and childhood. Blackwell Scientific, Oxford.
25. Schweissguth O (1979) Tumeurs solides de l'enfant. Flammarion, Paris.
26. Kaufmann SI, Stout AP (1965) Congenital mesenchymal tumours. Cancer 18: 460–476.
27. Gale GB, D'Angio GJ, Uri A, Chatten J, Koop CE (1982) Cancer in neonates: the experience of the Children's Hospital Philadelphia. Pediatrics 70: 409–413.
28. Isaacs H (1985) Perinatal (congenital and neonatal) neoplasms: a report of 110 cases. Pediatr Pathol 3: 165–216.
29. Pinter A, Hock A (1986) Cancer in neonates and infants, national survey of 141 patients. In: Thomasson B, Holscheider AM, eds. 26th Congress of the Scandinavian Association of Paediatric Surgeons, Stockholm, 22–24 May. Supplement. Hippokrates Verlag, Stuttgart, pp 180–184.
30. Campbell AN, Chan HSL, O'Brien A, Smith CR, Becker LE (1987) Malignant tumours in the neonate. Arch Dis Child 62: 19–23.
31. Davis CF, Carachi R, Young DG (1988) Neonatal tumours: Glasgow 1955–86. Arch Dis Child 63: 1075–1078.
32. Crom DB, Wilimas JA, Green AA, Pratt CB, Jenkins JJ III, Behm FG (1989) Malignancy in the neonate. Med Pediatr Oncol 17: 101–104.
33. Plaschkes J, Dubler M (1989) Neoplasmen beim Neugeborenen. Dissertation, Medical Faculty, University of Bern, Switzerland.
34. Mur N (1990) Neonatal malignant tumours: a retrospective experience. Paper presented at Cancer in the very young, Conference, St James University Hospital, Leeds.
35. Werb P, Scurry J, Oestoer A, Fortune Attwood M (1992) Survey of congenital tumours in perinatal necropsies. Pathology 24: 247–253.
36. Brch K, Jacobsen T, Olsen JH, Hirsch F, Hertz H (1992) Neonatal cancer in Denmark 1943–1985. Pediatr Hematol Oncol 9: 209–216.
37. Moore SW, Kaschula R (1995) The outcome of solid tumours in the neonatal period. Ped Surg Int, in press.
38. Birch JM, Marsden HB (1987) A classification scheme of childhood cancer. Int J Cancer 40: 620.
39. Barson AJ (1978) Congenital neoplasia: the Society's experience. Arch Dis Child 53: 436 (abstract).
40. Broadbent VA (1986) Malignant disease in the neonate. In: Robertson N, ed. Textbook of neonatology. Churchill Livingstone, Edinburgh, pp 689–695.
41. Birch JM, Blair V (1992) The epidemiology of infant cancers. Br J Cancer 66 (Suppl XVIII): S52–S54.
42. Bader JL, Miller RW (1979) US cancer incidence and mortality in the first year of life. Am J Dis Child 133: 157–159.
43. Satge D, Philippe E, Ruppe M et al. (1988) Les carcinomes neonatals. Revue de la littérature à propos d'un cas. Bull Cancer 75: 373–384.
44. Fraumeni JF, Miller RW (1969) Cancer deaths in the newborn. Am J Dis Child 117: 186–189.
45. Siegel SE, Moran RG (1981) Problems in the chemotherapy of cancer in the neonate. Am J Pediatr Hematol Oncol 3: 287–296.
46. Littmann P, D'Angio GJ (1981) Radiation therapy in the neonate. Am J Pediatr Hematol Oncol 3: 279–285.
47. Kemshead JT, Patel K, Phimister B (1992) Neuroblastoma in the very young child – biological consideration. Br J Cancer 66 (Suppl XVIII): 102–105.
48. Bolande RP (1971) Benignity of neonatal tumours and concept of cancer regression in early life. Arch Dis Child 122: 12–14.
49. Laury WS, Bolande RP (1972) Benignity of neonatal tumours. Am J Dis Child 123: 85–86.
50. Malcolm S (1988) Oncogenes in childhood malignancy. Arch Dis Child 63: 1099–1103.
51. Wilkins, Sinks (1990) Brain tumour risk and paternal exposure to heavy metals. Am J Epidemiol 132: 275.
52. Potter EL, Schoenmann M (1970) Metastasis of maternal cancer to the placenta and fetus. Cancer 25: 380–388.
53. Prose NS, Laude TA, Hielman ER, Coren C (1987) Congenital malignant melanoma. Pediatrics 79: 967–970.
54. Chandra SA, Gilbert EF, Viseskul C (1987) Neonatal intracranial choriocarcinoma. Arch Pathol Lab Med 114: 1079–1082.
55. Kalifa C, Brule F, Barliff P, Carlland JM, Schweissguth O (1981) Metastases chez un nourrisson d'un choriocarcinome placentaire. Arch Fr Pediatr 38: 351–352.

56. Voute PA, Wadmann SK, Van Putten WJ (1970) Congenital neuroblastoma, symptoms in the mother during pregnancy. Clin Pediatr 9: 206.
57. Sherman S, Roizen N (1976) Fetal hydantoin syndrome and neuroblastoma. Lancet ii: 517.
58. Worsham GF, Beckmann EN, Mitchell EH (1978) Sacrococcygeal teratoma in a neonate associated with maternal use of acetazolamide. JAMA 240: 251–252.
59. Birch JM, Marsden HB, Swindell R (1982) Pre-natal factors in the origin of germ cell tumours of childhood. Carcinogenesis 3: 75–80.
60. Rosenstock JG (1983) Neoplasia: the mother and the neonate. Semin Perinatol 7: 226–235.
61. Hawkins MM (1994) Pregnancy outcome and offspring after childhood cancer. Br Med J 309: 1037.
62. Smith RA, Hawkins MM (1989) Pregnancies and childhood cancer. Br J Obstet Gynaecol 96: 378–380.
63. Gardner MJ, Hall AJ, Downes S, Terrel JD (1987) Follow-up study of children born to mothers resident in Seascale (West Cumbria). Br Med J 295: 822–827.
64. Down R, Evans HJ, Darby SC (1994) Paternal exposure. Native 367: 678–680.
65. Draper G (1993) Electromagnetic fields and childhood cancer. Br Med J 307: 884–886.
66. Henslow DL, Enlough JP, Richardson RB (1990) Radon as a causative factor in the induction of myeloid leukaemia and other cancers. Lancet 335: 1008–1012.
67. Bunin GR, Petrakova A, Meadows AT et al. Occupation of parents of children with retinoblastoma. A report from the Children's Cancer Study Group. Cancer Res 50: 7129–7133.
68. Klebanoff MA, Read JS, Mills JL, Shiomo PH (1993) The risk of childhood cancer after exposure to vitamin K. N Engl J Med 329: 905–908.
69. Bunin GR, Kuijten RR, Buckley JD, Rorke LB, Meadows AT (1993) Relation between maternal diet and subsequent neuroectodermal tumours in young children. N Engl J Med 329: 536.
70. Warkany J (1975) Congenital malformations – tumors. Year Book Medical, Chicago.
71. Pelfrene AF (1976) Malformations et cancers congenitaux: une probléme de cancerogenese transplantaire. Rev Pediatr 12: 562–564.
72. Bolande RP (1987) Concepts derived from human teratogenesis and oncogenesis in early life. J Histochem Cytochem 32: 874–884.
73. Shanklin DR, Sotela-Avila C (1969) In situ tumours in fetusus, newborns and young infants. Biol Neonate 14: 286–316.
74. Backwith JB, Perrin EV (1963) In situ neuroblastoma. A contribution to the natural history of neural crest tumours. Am J Pathol 43: 1089–1104.
75. Folkman J (1990) What is the evidence that tumours are angiogen dependent? J Natl Cancer Inst 82: 4–6.
76. Gashier (1992) Platelet derived growth factor (PDGF): Wilms' tumour. Proc Natl Acad Sci USA 89: 10984.
77. Olshan AF (1986) Wilms' tumour and fetal growth factors. Cancer Genet Cytogenet 21: 303–305.
78. Pastore G, Antonelli R, Fine W (1982) Late effect of treatment of cancer in infancy. Med Pediatr Oncol 10: 369–375.
79. Meadows AT, Gallagher JA, Bunin GR (1992) Late effects of early childhood cancer therapy. Br J Cancer 66 (Suppl XVIII): S92–S94.
80. Teinturier C et al. (1992) Tumours solides malignes néonatales. Apropos de 75 cas. Arch Fr Pediatr 49: 187–92.
81. Parkes SE et al. (1994) Neonatal tumours. A thirty-year population-based study. Med Pediatr Oncol 22: 309–317.

Genetic and Clinical Associations of Neonatal Tumours

2

S.W. Moore

Introduction

In the majority of series, cancer is the second most common cause of death in both children and adults. Neonatal tumours comprise 2% of childhood malignancies, with an incidence of one in every 12 500 or 27 500 live births in the UK and USA, respectively[1]. The death rate from malignancy occurring in the neonatal period has been reported as being 6.26 per million live births[2,3]. The prevalence, sites of origin and pathological nature of these tumours vary from unit to unit[4–8]. An increasing awareness of the genetic implications of inheritance for certain congenital tumours[9–16] makes further study of these tumours worthwhile.

Genetic factors have been implicated in both non-hereditary and hereditary forms of malignancy in children and adults[15]. At least two methods of transmission have been recorded: the inheritance of damaged genes (which immediately results in tumorigenesis) and the occurrence of genetic disorders (which later result in the development of cancer). Further study of the genetic constitution of individual cells of malignant tumours has afforded valuable clues about the pathogenesis of malignancy. Familial clustering of malignancy is not uncommon, and investigation may provide opportunities for early diagnosis and effective treatment as well as being of potential value in future cancer prevention.

Identification of the nature of these genetic associations may be of importance in understanding the molecular basis of specific tumours. With the technological advances made in molecular biology over the past decade, there has been a sharp increase in the number of associated genetic defects reported in malignancies affecting children and adults. In tumours such as breast carcinoma in adults, the race to identify the specific gene is still on.

Current evidence indicates that many forms of childhood cancer arise from largely genetic influences. Much current research addresses the genetic influences on malignant tumours in the older child and adult. As genetic mutations associated with malignancy in children mostly occur spontaneously, tumours occurring in the neonatal period provide a unique opportunity to study the familial and genetic associations. This is partly because of minimal interactions between the neonate and the environment during the development of the tumour. As a result, modern genetic surveillance techniques could offer opportunities for prevention of tumours in children, in contrast to the possibilities for prevention of most malignancies encountered in older patients.

Despite the considerable advances made in recombinant DNA technology, several potential problem areas have been identified in the epidemiology of neonatal tumours. These include a paucity of available data on familial occurrence, on genetic associations and on the future risks of these uncommon tumours. There appear to be four broad groups of patients with an inherited predisposition to cancer. Ponder[13] has suggested that these are the recessive syndromes of defective DNA repair, inherited cancer syndromes (e.g. retinoblastoma, familial polyposis, multiple endocrine [MEN] syndromes), familial clustering without a clear predisposition, and an inherited predisposition to cancer without familial clustering.

Pathogenesis of neonatal tumours: the two-hit theory

It has long been suspected that the loss of genetic material may be important in determining the susceptibility of an individual to the development of cancer. Current data suggest that alterations in genes that regulate cell growth in extracellular matrices and intracellular communication may play a role in the development of malignancy in childhood. In addition, several alternative genetic mechanisms may be involved in this process. For example, oncogenes may be activated as a result of chromosomal defects, point mutations or gene amplification.

Chromosomal abnormalities such as a deletion may result in a susceptibility to cancer in a particular patient and may be inherited by other family members. Genetic mutations predisposing to malignant disease include the Wilms' tumour 1 gene (*WT1*), where an 11p13 chromosomal defect is often typical, and the neurofibromatosis type 1 gene, which is not uncommon in certain tumours. Amplification of the N-*myc* and N-*ras* oncogenes have been observed in neuroblastoma. The N-*myc* amplification has been shown to be associated with the more severe form of malignancy.

In an attempt to understand the pathogenesis of neonatal retinoblastomas, Knudson[17] extrapolated statistical data and proposed that retinoblastoma resulted from a combination of a prezygotic (germinal) mutation and a postzygotic (somatic) event. This suggestion, that retinoblastoma can be initiated by two events, is the "two-hit" theory. Comings[18] further suggested that both of these events could apply to mutations of the *RB1* gene.

Briefly, the two-hit hypothesis holds that the rate-limiting step in the development of malignancy depends on the two genetic events involved. The initial mutation would either be inherited or result from a spontaneous genetic event. Although the gene is transmitted in a recessive form, inheritance tends to follow a dominant pattern. Heterozygous defects in the retinoblastoma tumour suppressor gene thus result in only one further allele of the gene needing to be inactivated. The effect of this mutation on the tumour suppressor gene activity results in a loss of regulation, and the tumour develops as a result of abnormal cell growth.

These hypotheses have since been validated for retinoblastoma[19], but also hold true for other tumour types arising from genetic mutations (e.g. Wilms' tumour). They may therefore provide a basis for understanding tumour pathogenesis in the neonatal period, including defects in chromosomal breakage syndromes and disorders of sexual differentiation as well as the observation that the mutations in the relevant tumour suppressor genes appear to be more likely to arise from paternal than maternal chromosomes. This latter observation suggests some form of genomic imprinting[15].

Genetic associations of malignancy

The first genetic abnormality to be associated with malignancy was the Philadelphia or PH1 chromosome[20]. The fusion of the *bcr* and *c-abl* genes on the Ph chromosome demonstrates the creation of fusion genes from chromosomal breakage. This abnormality, found on the affected cells of patients with chronic myeloid leukaemia (CML) implicated genetic mechanisms and opened new areas of diagnosis and prognosis.

The application of recombinant DNA technology has led to new horizons in the pathogenesis of malignancy. At least three main cytogenetic changes have been associated with tumour development: deletions of specific chromosomal alleles, translocations (or inversions) and the amplification of specific domains. Most mutations associated with malignancy in the neonate are inherited from parents or occur spontaneously as the result of a mutational event that occurs de novo. As a result, the chances are higher that the majority of cancers arising from these defects will be preventable. This is in contrast to tumours in which genetic–environmental interactions (e.g. smoking) form the basis of the development of cancer.

Focusing on the genetic influences will probably yield further insights into the influences of genetic mutations and other genetic abnormalities in the development of such tumours. On the other hand, the identification of a genetic association of a specific tumour may be hampered if precise genetic mechanisms are not recognized by the genetic testing methods used. Paediatric malignancies falling into this category may be distinguished by an increase in familial occurrence or an increased risk in monozygotic twins. Alternatively, the identification of an association between a specific malignancy and a set of alleles at a specific locus may be demonstrated. This may not be exclusive to a particular tumour, however, and may be associated with the pathogenesis of other types of tumour in patients with the defect. Examples of these are the associations between leukaemia, lymphomas, central nervous system neoplasms and soft-tissue tumours. Further identification and characterization of chromosomal defects associated with the development of paediatric cancer may be of considerable importance. The further evaluation of clinical associations and syndromes associated with specific tumour types may therefore be of considerable importance as they may indicate which areas require closer scrutiny.

Mendelian single-gene related syndromes

A number of Mendelian single-gene malignancy-related syndromes have been described, including:

1. *Chromosome breakage syndromes:*
   Bloom's syndrome
   Fanconi's anaemia
   Ataxia–telangiectasia
   Xeroderma pigmentosum
2. *Neurocristopathies:*
   Neurofibromatosis
   Tuberous sclerosis
   Turcot's syndrome
   Multiple mucosal neuroma syndrome
   Basal cell naevus syndrome
3. *Metabolic disorders:*
   Tyrosinaemia (hereditary)
   α_1 Antitrypsin deficiency
   Glycogenolysis (type 1)
4. *Immune deficiency disorders:*
   Sex-linked lymphoproliferative syndrome
   Wiskott–Aldritch syndrome
   Severe combined immunodeficiency
   Bruton's agammaglobulinaemia

These may be autosomal dominant, recessive or X-linked. In addition, certain disorders of sexual differentiation may be associated with cancer in children.

Autosomal dominant syndromes include familial colonic polyposis, neurofibromatosis and the naevoid basal cell carcinoma syndrome. Although extremely interesting from a genetic point of view (because they allow affected individuals in family groups to be traced), these tumours do not normally present in the neonatal period and are mentioned for completeness only.

Autosomal recessive syndromes include xeroderma pigmentosum, Fanconi's anaemia, Bloom's syndrome and ataxia–telangiectasia. Bloom's syndrome is a rare autosomal recessive condition, which includes a sensitivity to ultraviolet light, growth retardation and immunodeficiency as well as a higher rate of associated malignancy at an earlier age[21]. The majority of the tumours occurring in Bloom's syndrome are leukaemias and gastrointestinal malignancies. Fanconi's anaemia is also linked to leukaemia and liver tumours. Similar to the findings in the autosomal dominant inheritance group, tumours associated with an autosomal recessive familial inheritance occur later, suggesting some degree of genetic–environmental influence to initiate the malignant process. Tumours associated with the largely immunodeficient X-linked recessive syndromes also occur mainly outside the neonatal period. In the X-linked lymphoproliferative syndrome, the Epstein–Barr virus has been suggested as a possible pathogenetic factor[22].

Other associations between a genetic influence and neoplasia occur. Some of these have been identified but others are not yet known. Of particular interest are the fragile chromosomal defects. Certain fragile sites can be transmitted through families. A high percentage of the inheritable and constitutive fragile sites have been mapped to genetic sites associated with human cancer[23]. These chromosomal rearrangements have been associated with malignancy in at least six of the 16 inheritable fragile chromosome sites, and have been identified in other non-inherited fragile chromosome sites[23]. As a result of the chromosome fragility in these cases, deletions and chromosomal fragments may occur. Should the fragile sites break close to a proto-oncogene location, the activation of the oncogene may result in the malignant transformation of the cells.

There is an increased risk of leukaemia and other tumours in patients with Down's syndrome[24]. In the neonatal period, leukaemoid reactions may confuse the issue[25]. Adrenal cortical tumours are rarely encountered in the newborn but may be seen in association with Beckwith–Wiedemann syndrome[26]. A report of spontaneous regression of these lesions has been reported in neonates[26]. In addition, gonadal tumours have an increased incidence in several disorders in sexual differentiation.

Abnormalities of the neurofibromatosis 1 gene (*NF1*) has been identified in patients with von Recklinghausen's disease[27,28]. Although a family history may be observed in the group of neurocristopathies associated with neural crest abnormalities, the tumours tend to appear at a later age. Examples of this are phaeochromocytoma, von Recklinghausen's disease, Sturge–Weber syndrome, tuberose sclerosis and von Hippel–Landau disease, as well as the MEN II tumour syndrome. Although a mutational hotspot has been associated with several tumours[29], Imamura et al.[30] were unable to identify any specific abnormalities associated with the *NF1* gene in specimens from 50 patients with neuroblastoma.

Tumour suppressor genes

Current evidence supports at least six known tumour suppressor genes. In each case they give rise to a different spectrum of human cancer and are thought to regulate tumour growth by the control of cellular proliferation.

These tumour suppressor genes include the retinoblastoma gene *RB* (chromosome 13q), the Wilms' tumour *WT1* gene (11p), the neurofibromatosis gene *NF1* (17q) and the *p53* tumour suppressor gene (17p). There is also considerable evidence of other genes that are deleted in carcinoma of the colon (18q), and the *APC* gene in familial polyposis coli (5q)[19].

Retinoblastoma

Knudson's work[17] in 1971 was based on an analysis of the age of presentation of hereditary as opposed to non-hereditary cases. His hypothesis that these tumours resulted from two separate genetic events was extended to suggest that these events could be mutations of the same *RB1* gene. It has further been shown that 90%–95% of individuals with the *RB1* gene will develop a retinal tumour. Multiple tumours affecting both eyes occur in the majority of patients. The genetic association with retinoblastoma was linked with chromosome 13q14 and a homozygous loss of function of both alleles at the *RB1* locus identified.

In hereditary cases there is a germline mutation of the *RB1* gene. Current evidence suggests that the remaining *RB1* allele is mostly lost because there is a lack of heterogeneity in these cases. In patients with hereditary disease it appears that the chromosome 13 which is retained in the tumour cells comes from the affected parent. The occurrence of two somatic mutations within the same cell could give rise to non-hereditary forms. In addition to the *RB1* mutation, a small number of these patients (5%) have additional associated genetic disturbances (deletions or translocations at 13q14).

The cloning of the *RB1* gene[31] provided an association with osteosarcoma as well as retinoblastoma. This was later confirmed in a child with hereditary retinoblastoma and a balanced 1 : 13 translocation[32]. It was also reported in a germline mutation without deletion in the lymphocytes of an affected child[33].

In addition to the risk of retinoblastoma, approximately 10% of patients with *RB1* mutations have a relatively high risk of developing other tumours, such as osteogenic sarcomas, fibrosarcomas and melanomas, in early adult life. The risk of a second tumour is enhanced (approximately 35%) if radiotherapy has been administered in the treatment of the initial tumour. Mutations of the *RB1* gene in osteosarcomas tend to involve the parental allele, which is not the case in patients with retinoblastoma.

Although the deletion of the *RB1* gene is specific to particular tumours, unstable *RB1* mRNA may be detected in many tissues[34]. A further mechanism therefore appears to control the rate of transcription of *RB1* mRNA.

The reasons for the tissue specificity of malignancy are as yet unclear. Cell differentiation and growth are largely determined by microenvironmental factors. The role of growth factors, and oncogenes such as *c-fos*, may be of importance and require further investigation.

Current data suggest that the *RB1* gene product ($p110^{RB1}$) is important in the control of cell differentiation, maturation and proliferation[35,36]. The additional finding that normally proliferating cells express $p110^{RB1}$ suggests that the *RB1* gene product plays an important role in the regulation of the cell cycle[36]. It probably has an important role to play in transcriptional regulation in its phosphorylation state. In addition, the inhibition of the normal function of $p110^{RB1}$ may be related to the way in which DNA viruses affect tumour growth. Further evidence indicates that viral proteins bind to and inhibit $p110^{RB1}$, leading to a blocking of phosphorylation[36–39]. The reasons for the observed tissue specificity and the loss of regulation of cellular proliferation remain unclear.

Wilms' tumour

A number of syndromes have been associated with Wilms' tumour[40]:

1. Aniridia (0.75%–1%)
2. Hemihypertrophy (3.3%)
3. Beckwith–Wiedemann syndrome (3.7%)
4. Musculoskeletal abnormalities (2.9%)
5. Genitourinary abnormalities (5.2%)
6. Denys–Drash syndrome:
   - Nephroblastoma
   - Male pseudohermaphroditism
   - Glomerulonephritis
   - Nephrotic syndrome
   - Renal failure
7. WAGR syndrome (11p13 deletion)
   - Nephroblastoma
   - Aniridia
   - Genitourinary anomalies
   - Mental retardation
8. Klippel–Trenaunay–Weber syndrome
9. Other associated tumours
   - Hepatoblastoma (6%–10% of Wilms' tumours)
   - Adrenocortical carcinoma

In addition to these associations, a familial association of the order of 1%–2.4% with a slight female preponderance has been reported, particularly in multicentric and bilateral tumours[41,42]. There appears to be autosomal dominant inheritance with incomplete penetration[43].

Genetic deletions in children suffering from the uncommon association between aniridia, urogenital malformations and mental retardation (WAGR syndrome) were initially shown to involve chromosome 11 (band p13). The further molecular identification of the *WT1* gene[44] has helped to validate the Knudson model for Wilms' tumour[45]. The subsequent identification of a loss of heterozygosity within 11p13 suggested a tumour suppressive role for the gene[46]. The further demonstration of the expression of the *WT1* gene in selected tissues (kidney, testes, ovary, spleen, mesothelium) during embryogenesis[47], as well as the selective expression of the gene to the nephron pathway[48], suggests that mutation or deletion of the *WT1* gene would result in proliferation or alternatively stimulate the development of epithelial components from these cells. Kreidberg et al.[49] have shown extensive urogenital abnormalities in the offspring of an animal model without the *WT1* gene.

It would appear that the *WT1* gene acts as a tumour suppressor gene and that deletion results in the development of Wilms' tumour[50]. It may be that the *WT1* gene inhibits the genes involved in cellular proliferation (*ERGI* and insulin-like growth factor *IGF2*)[51,52].

There are additional associations between Wilms' tumour, WAGR syndrome and Denys–Drash syndrome[53]. The latter includes features of intersex disorders, nephropathy and Wilms' tumour. Although initially described only in males with pseudohermaphroditism[53–55], this syndrome has been extended to include female children with ambiguous genitalia, nephropathy and Wilms' tumour[56–58]. An observed constant association with genetic mutations located at chromosome 11p13 (*WT1* or Wilms' tumour gene) and Denys–Drash syndrome indicates a possible molecular marker for this syndrome. The exact site of the point mutation, which was identified in the majority of cases, was located on the *WT1* exon 9, which affects the amino acid residue 394 arginine[40]. Ten exons then encode for a protein with a predicted molecular weight of 45–49 000 at this site.

There is also an association between other tumours, such as hepatoblastomas or adrenocortical carcinoma, and Wilms' tumour, which may coexist in 6%–10% of patients.

Against this hypothesis is the fact that deletions or mutations are identifiable in only 5%–10% of tumours. As many as 50% of patients show reduced or virtually absent function at the *WT1* site[41]. Based on current evidence, it would appear that the genetic factors involved in Wilms' tumour are much more complex than those involved in other tumours, such as retinoblastoma. In addition to the *WT1* gene at 11p13, there is evidence for a second genetic locus at 11p15 (the *WT2* site) as well as at 16q and an unidentified familial locus[40–41]. Familial Wilms' tumour does not, however, appear to map to the 11th chromosome[59,60]. The *WT2* site has been associated with the Beckwith–Wiedemann syndrome, but it is not yet clear whether the same gene or two adjacent loci are involved.

Genetic abnormalities may be of a more subtle nature and not as easily identified by current testing methods. A functional difference between the maternally and paternally derived alleles[12,41] imply that other mechanisms such as genomic imprinting also apply to Wilms' tumour[61]. This function does not appear to be situated at the *WT1* gene site. The *WT2* locus has been suggested as a possible alternative.

Neonatal Wilms' tumour is known to be associated with nephroblastomatosis in the kidneys. Although this may represent stage 1 of a two-hit process as described by Knudson, it is not clear whether the oncogenic mechanism always relates to the two-hit theory. Other genetic or environmental factors may contribute to the early development of these tumours.

Neuroblastoma

Neuroblastoma is the most common neonatal tumour in most series and remains one of the commonest tumours of childhood. It is a biologically unique tumour with a high rate of spontaneous remission or maturation to more benign forms such as ganglioneuroma.

Neuroblastoma is occasionally associated with profuse watery diarrhoea, which probably results from an abnormal increase in vasoactive intestinal polypeptide (VIP)[62]. It is also associated with the myoclonus–opsoclonus syndrome, which generally occurs in older children and is usually noted where a thoracic neuroblastoma is associated with polymyoclonic cerebellar ataxia and an abnormal gait.

Genetic studies have demonstrated chromosomal abnormalities in up to 80% of cases of neuroblastoma[63]. These include amplification of the N-*myc* proto-oncogene, deletion of chromosome 1 and an abnormal DNA content of the tumour cells. These have been identified as being of prognostic significance. Where present, the defect is most frequently found to be on chromosomes 1 and 17, the most consistent being a deletion on the short arm of chromosome 1 (1p36.1– 1p36.3)[64]. Additional chromosomal abnormalities have been identified[65] at 4p, 6q, 9q, 10q, 11q, 12q, 13q, 14q, 16q, 22p and 22q. In addition, other genetic mechanisms (e.g. N-*myc*, tumour suppressor genes) probably play a role in the growth and aggressiveness of the tumour[66]. In this context, it is interesting to note that mutations of the tumour suppressor *p53* gene are mostly absent in neuroblastoma[67], although present in other tumours of childhood[68]. In a recent study, *p53* gene mutations (17p13) were identified in only two of 20 cases investigated, confirming the low frequency of these mutations in neuroblastoma[69]. A recent report of high levels of *TRK* gene, which correlated with a good clinical outcome, is of considerable prognostic interest. The *TRK* gene encodes a high affinity for nerve growth factor receptor (NGFR), suggesting other avenues of research[70].

The proportion of nuclei in each of the cell cycles is a measure of the rate of multiplication of the tumour. Aneuploidy is defined as a G0 : G1 ratio of greater than one compared with normal cells. Although aneuploidy is considered to be generally associated with poor prognosis, in children a diploid DNA content is associated with a poorer outcome in neuroblastoma and lymphoblastic leukaemia. In addition, the cellular DNA content is of prognostic significance in children less than 1 year of age[71]. If the ratio of DNA content compared with normal cells is greater than 1, the tumour has a good prognosis. A DNA index of 1 is associated with a worse prognosis[70], which includes a poor drug response and a decrease in tumour-free survival time. This is in contrast to other tumours in adults, where diploid cells have a more favourable prognosis. Hyperdiploidy in a child less than 1 year of age is associated with a better prognosis, possibly due to an increased sensitivity to chemotherapy and radiotherapy.

Oncogene amplification has been described in neuroblastoma cells. The oncogenes N-*myc* and N-*ras* have been reported as being increased in neuroblastomas. Amplification of the N-*myc* oncogene (usually found on chromosome 2) has been associated with a more advanced form of the malignancy and is a poor prognostic sign[70]. Tumours with diploid cell lines are more likely to have amplification of N-*myc*[72].

The proto-oncogene N-*myc* may be identified in a number of tissues during early development. Additional copies of N-*myc* were described in neuroblastoma, making it the first clinically relevant oncogene to be described. In this context, N-*myc* amplification is generally accepted as indicating a poorer prognosis. It is also identified in other neuroectodermal tumours[73,74] and in approximately 10% of retinoblastomas[75,76]. In the latter, tumour induction by the retinoblastoma gene mutation was shown to be independent of N-*myc* overexpression. N-*myc* was further shown not to be expressed in osteogenic tumours that demonstrate *RB1*. The oncogene N-*myc* does not undergo change, is stable and does not progress in malignant tumours[77]. Identification of the N-*myc* copy number may identify patients for whom more aggressive therapy is appropriate, as it is associated with an increased tendency to invade adjacent structures[78].

Other recognized associations with N-*myc* amplification include the fetal hydantoin–alcohol syndrome[79] and other chromosomal abnormalities in neuroblastoma, which include double minutes (dms) and homogeneous staining regions (HSRs). The latter may represent amplification of the cellular genes.

Teratomas

Teratomas are thought to arise from the primordial germ cells as the result of an early event. A genetic tendency towards spontaneous gonadal teratomas is seen in a specific strain of experimental mice (strain 129)[80]. There also appears to be a genetic predisposition to develop a presacral mass in association with anorectal, sacral and urogenital abnormalities[81]. This genetic association has been shown to be of a Mendelian dominant nature[82]. Patients with an imperforate anus and a hemisacrum have a high incidence of presacral masses, many of which are teratomas, which may occasionally be malignant[82].

Soft-tissue tumours

The observed preferential retention of parental alleles in certain embryonal tumours such as Wilms' tumour[83] and rhabdomyosarcoma[84] suggest a possible role for genomic imprinting in these tumours.

A specific chromosomal translocation involving chromosomes 2 and chromosomes 13 have been associated with alveolar rhabdomyosarcomas (t[2;13][q35;q14])[85,86].

More recently, the human *Pax 3* gene has been shown to map to the breakpoint region on chromosome 2. The breakpoint is described as being in the 3′ region. A consistent rearrangement of the 5′ portion of the *Pax 3* gene on chromosome 2q35 has been identified and may act as a new transcription factor for these tumours[87]. Although *p53* mutations have been shown to be infrequent in childhood fibrous tumours[88], there remains a relatively high occurrence in association with rhabdomyosarcomas.

Rhabdomyosarcoma cell lines express the specific gene of muscle differentiation, *MYOD*, which characteristically marks these tumours[89]. Studies that focus on the specific biological features of myogenesis have demonstrated genetic control for each step[90].

Hepatoblastoma

Although relatively little is known about the molecular basis of hepatoblastomas in infancy, it has been postulated that the mechanism of tumorigenesis is similar to that of Wilms' tumour and rhabdomysarcoma[91]. This may be due to a common action on the *IGF2* locus. Current evidence suggests that this does not result from a relaxation of paternal imprinting as in the other examples quoted[91].

Loss of heterozygosity at 11p15 has been reported in two patients with hepatoblastoma[74]. The common association with Beckwith–Wiedemann syndrome further suggests a loss of heterozygosity in these tumours[92]. Hepatocellular carcinoma does not usually occur in the neonatal period.

Other tumours

Other genetic aberrations associated with tumours (such as the loss of heterozygosity on chromosome 5q in identifying the gene for familial polyposis coli, defects in tumour suppressive genes on 17q (*p53*), the *RET* proto-oncogene in multiple endocrine neoplasia and 18q (DCC) in carcinoma of the colon, and translocation of the end of the long arm of chromosome 8 with chromosome 14 or an alteration in *c-myc* regulation or p53[93] (in Burkitt's lymphoma) are interesting associations with paediatric tumours which are not particularly associated with the neonatal period.

The *p53* tumour suppressor gene

p53 is a tumour suppressor gene located on the short arm of chromosome 17[94,95], initially thought to be a cellular proto-oncogene related to the SV40 T-antigen[96]. Its phosphoprotein structure binds DNA and it is thought to act as a tumour suppressor gene. p53 point mutations and allelic deletions have been demonstrated in a wide variety of tumours, which include those of the lung, thyroid, gastrointestinal tract and breast[97]. These chromosomal abnormalities are thought to inactivate the tumour suppressor action of *p53*, allowing abnormal cellular proliferation. *p53* is thought to act as a "molecular policeman" to protect the integrity of the genetic system. Under normal circumstances replication of DNA is arrested if DNA is damaged, and *p53* is then thought to switch off cell division and allow the genetic system time to effect repair.

Although *p53* mutations play an important role in the pathogenesis of adult cancers, little is known about its role in tumours that are present at birth or arise shortly thereafter. It has been suggested that *p53* has a greater role to play in tumours occurring later in life. Overexpression of the *p53* oncoprotein results in the arrest of the cell cycle in the G1 phase. Where cells lack *p53* because of a mutation there is loss of control of the cell cycle, resulting in tumorigenesis.

Inherited *p53* mutations have been described in association with the Li–Fraumeni syndrome. The risk of tumours in these patients is considered high and may well find expression in the neonatal period. This association was, however, observed in only two of the eight cases reported by Santibanez-Koref et al.[99], and was thought to be related to a genetic hotspot related to the *p53* gene[99,100]. *p53* has also been shown to play a role in Ewing's sarcoma, but not in neuroblastoma[69]. This is an interesting finding because the known trisomy of the long arm of chromosome 17 (and the associated monosomy of the short arm) in neuroblastoma is close to the position of the *p53* at 17p13.

In cells in which mutation has occurred or there is damage to the host by viral DNA, these and other mechanisms may result in inactivation of the normal *p53* mechanism. Certain tumours probably occur where there is deletion of *p53* by certain DNA viruses[101,102]. This can be explained by the model advanced by Lane, in which *p53* is removed to make way for viral DNA replication in the cell nucleus[96]. This is also a possible explanation of the genetic bases of fibroblasts in the Li–Fraumeni syndrome[103] and the high incidence of tumours in *p53* null 1 mice[104]. The role of *p53* in neonatal tumours is not yet clear.

Familial associations of neonatal tumours: a prospective clinical study

In addition to the genetic predispositions associated with neonatal tumours, a study of the familial associations is important to ascertain whether certain families are at risk for the development of malignant tumours in their offspring. To determine this relationship, we recently undertook a prospective study to evaluate the family histories of patients to identify any genetic links or familial patterns of inheritance.

Survivors of neonatal tumours presenting to the Red Cross War Memorial Children's Hospital from January 1957 to July 1990 and the Children's Tumour Registry Tygerberg Hospital in 1991–1993 were interviewed. The protocol included an enquiry into antenatal history, prenatal drugs, complications of pregnancy, gestational age at birth, birth weight, associated congenital anomalies, and family history of malignancy or other anomalies.

Of the 52 survivors of 75 neonatal tumours 38 responded to interview. There was a relative with cancer in 40%. Chromosomal abnormalities were identified in three patients; one had a chromosome 21 abnormality and one trisomy 13, and in the other a distinctive familial translocation pattern was located on chromosome 9 in a girl with neuroblastoma. The same abnormality was present in her mother and her maternal grandmother (p13–q34: p21–p24), but was absent in her father and grandfather. Review of the banding pattern in this family suggested that the translocation was balanced and that no large deletion had occurred.

Autosomal dominant transmission patterns were notably absent, and the incidence of associated congenital abnormalities low. Although no significant differences were identified in the overall incidence of tumours within the families interviewed, tumours were three times more common in the maternal family, suggesting some form of maternal imprinting. Immediate family members were affected in only four instances; one sibling had leukaemia, a parent developed carcinoma of the stomach, and breast carcinoma developed in two mothers of children with immature sacrococcygeal teratomas, a four-generation familial history of breast carcinoma being present in one case. Although the association between familial carcinoma of the breast and other malignancies is well established[105,106], in three of these four instances the pattern of tumours suggested a Li–Fraumeni type association[100,107].

The overall lack of increased malignancy in the families of patients with neonatal tumours agrees with the findings of Li et al.[108], who could not demonstrate any inherited effects of childhood tumours or tumour therapy in 107 pregnancies among survivors of childhood neoplasms. In addition, in at least one other series[6] no significant family history has previously been reported. Current data suggest a difference in maternally and paternally derived autosomal genes for particular tumours[109,110]. Although loss of a chromosome segment of a specific chromosome pair (heterozygosity) may be involved in the pathogenesis of certain tumours[65,110], a specific chromosome from one of the parents appears to be given preference in particular situations[109,110]. Examples of this are the loss of a maternally derived gene on chromosome 11 in sporadic Wilms' tumour and the successive loss of function of both alleles of *RB* (retinoblastoma susceptibility gene) in the development of retinoblastoma as well as certain sarcomas such as osteosarcoma[110]. Genetic processes other than chromosome anomalies may also be involved in the familial transmission of a tendency to develop certain tumours[111].

Conclusions

Recognition of specific cancer-prone syndromes has implications for clinical management. The chromosomal arrangement of the parental chromosomes is of importance in ascertaining the presence or absence of a balanced chromosomal rearrangement.

The examples given by Knudson and the ataxia–telangiectasia syndromes have historically shown that a thorough study of the associations with cancer are the most promising method of studying the causes of abnormal proliferation of cells in cancer.

We need to continue to identify these genetic associations and investigate further the cancer-producing genes to identify the genetic alleles associated with cancer. In addition, we need to investigate families with a genetic susceptibility to malignant tumours to identify specific genetic loci, which may or may not be related to a specific allele.

Further investigation along these lines will add to a growing body of knowledge, which in turn will lead to a greater understanding of the cellular events that result in the pathogenesis of malignancy.

References

1. Bader JL, Miller RW (1979) US Cancer incidence and mortality in the first year of life. Am J Dis Child 133: 157–159.
2. Anderson DH (1951) Tumours of infancy and childhood. Cancer 4: 890–906.
3. Fraumeni JF, Millar RW (1969) Cancer deaths in the newborn. Am J Dis Child 117: 186–189.
4. Barson AJ (1978) Congenital neoplasia: the Society's experience. Arch Dis Child 53: 436 (abstract).
5. Campbell AN, Chan HSL, O'Brien A, Smith CR, Becker C (1987) Malignant tumours in the neonate. Arch Dis Child 62: 19–23.
6. Crom DB, Wilimas JA, Green AA, Pratt CB, Jenkins JJ, Behm FG (1979) Malignancy in the neonate. Med Pediatr Oncol 17: 101–104.
7. David CF, Carachi R, Young DG (1988) Neonatal tumours in Glasgow 1955–1986. Arch Dis Child 63: 1075–1078.
8. Gale GB, D'Angio GJ, Uri A, Chatten J, Koop CE (1982) Cancer in the neonate: the experience of the Children's Hospital in Philadelphia. Pediatrics 70: 409–413.
9. Arthur DC (1986) Genetics and cytogenetics in pediatric cancer. Cancer 58: 534–540.
10. Swift M, Reitnauer PJ, Rao KW (1986) Hereditary and other antecedent conditions of childhood neoplasia. In: Finegold MJ, Bennington JL, eds. Pathology and neoplasia in children and adolescents. WB Saunders, Philadelphia, pp 1–17.
11. Miller RW (1966) Relation between cancer and congenital defects in man. N Engl J Med 275: 87–93.
12. Ponder B (1989) Is imprinting to blame? Nature 340: 264.
13. Ponder BAJ (1990) Inherited predisposition to cancer. Trends Genet 6: 213–218.
14. Vogelstein B, Kinzler KW (1993) The multistep nature of cancer. Trends Genet 4: 138–141.
15. Bishop JM (1991) Molecular themes in oncogenesis. Cell 64: 235–248.
16. Brodeur GM (1987) The involvement of oncogenes and suppressor genes in human neoplasia. Adv Pediatr 34: 1–44.
17. Knudson AG Jr (1971) Mutation and cancer: statistical study of retinoblastoma. Proc Natl Acad Sci USA 68: 820–823.
18. Comings DE (1973) A general theory of carcinogenesis. Proc Natl Acad Sci USA 70: 3324–3328.
19. Malcolm S (1988) Oncogenes in malignancy. Arch Dis Child 63: 1079–1103.
20. Nowell PC, Hungerford DA (1960) A minute chromosome in human chronic granulocytic leukaemia. Science 132: 147.
21. German J, Passarge E (1989) Bloom's syndrome. XII. Report from the registry for 1987. Clin Genet 35: 57–69.
22. Purtilo DT, Sakamoto K, Barnabei V. et al. (1982) Epstein–Barr virus-induced diseases in boys with the X-linked lymphoproliferative syndrome (XLP). Am J Med 73: 49–56.
23. Yunis JJ, Soreng AL (1984) Constitutive fragile sites and cancer. Science 226: 1199–1204.
24. Holland WW, Doll R, Carter CO (1962) The mortality of leukaemia and other cancers among patients with Down's syndrome (Mongols) and among their parents. Br J Cancer 16: 177–186.
25. Weinberg AG, Schiller G, Windmiller J (1982) Neonatal leukaemia reaction: an isolated manifestation of mosaic trisomy 21. Am J Dis Child 136: 310–311.
26. Saracco S, Abramowsky C, Taylor S et al. (1988) Spontaneously regressing adrenocortical carcinoma in a newborn: a case report with DNA ploidy analysis. Cancer 62: 507–511.
27. Viscochil D, Buchberg A, Xu G et al. (1990) Deletions and a translocation interrupt a cloned gene at the neurofibromatosis type 1 locus. Cell 62: 187–192.
28. Cawthon R, Weiss R, Xu G et al. (1990) A major segment of the neurofibromatosis type I gene: cDNA sequence, genomic structure and point mutations. Cell 62: 193–201.
29. Li Y, Bollag G, Clark R et al. (1992) Somatic mutation in the neurofibromatosis gene in human tumours. Cell 69: 275–281.
30. Imamura J, Bartram C, Berthold F, Harms D, Nakamura H, Koeffler H (1993) Mutation of the p53 gene and its relationship to N-*myc* amplification. Cancer Res 5: 4053–4058.
31. Friend SH, Bernards R, Rogelj S et al. (1986) A human DNA segment with properties of the gene that predisposes to retinoblastoma and osteogenic sarcoma. Nature 323: 643–646.
32. Mitchell CD, Cowell JK (1989) Predisposition to retinoblastoma due to a translocation within the 4.7R locus. Oncogene 4: 253–257.
33. Dunn JM, Philips RA, Becker AJ et al. (1988) Identification of germline and somatic mutations affecting the retinoblastoma gene. Science 241: 1797–1800.
34. Goddard AD, Balakier H, Canton M et al. (1988) Infrequent genomic arrangement and normal expression of the putative RB1 gene in retinoblastoma tumours. Mol Cell Biol 8: 2082–2088.
35. Gallie BL, Dunn JM, Chan HSL, Hamel PA, Philips RA (1991) The genetics of retinoblastoma. Pediatr Clin North Am 38: 299–315.
36. Hamel PA, Gallie BI, Philips RA (1992) The retinoblastoma protein and cell cycle regulation. Trends Genet 8: 180–185.
37. Whyte P, Buchkovich KJ, Horowitz JM et al. (1988) Association between oncogene and anti-oncogene: the E1A proteins bind to retinoblastoma gene product. Nature 334: 124–129.
38. de Caprio JA, Ludlow JW, Figge J et al. (1988) SV40 large tumour antigen forms a specific complex with the product of the retinoblastoma susceptibility gene. Cell 54: 275–283.
39. Dyson N, Howley PM, Munger K et al. (1989) The human papillovirus-16 E7 oncoprotein is able to bind to the retinoblastoma gene product. Science 242: 934–937.
40. Riccardi V, Sujansky E, Smith A, Francke U (1978) Chromosomal imbalance in the aniridia–Wilms' tumour association: 11p interstitial deletion. Pediatrics 61: 604–610.
41. Coppes MJ, Campbell CE, Williams BRG (1993) The role of WT1 in Wilms' tumorigenesis. FASEB J 7: 886–895.
42. Coppes MJ, Williams BRG (1994) The molecular genetics of Wilms' tumour. Cancer Inv 12: 57–65.
43. Matsunaga E (1981) Genetics of Wilms' tumour. Hum Genet 57: 231–246.
44. Knudson A, Strong L (1972) Mutation and cancer: a model for Wilms' tumour of the kidney. J Natl Cancer Inst 48: 313–324.
45. Orkin S, Goldman D, Sallan S (1984) Development of homozygosity for chromosome 11p markers in Wilms' tumour. Nature 309: 172–174.
46. Call K, Glaser T, Ito C et al. (1990) Isolation and characterization of a zinc finger polypeptide gene at the human chromosome 11 Wilms' tumour locus. Cell 60: 509–520.
47. Pritchard-Jones K, Fleming S, Davidson D et al. (1990) The candidate Wilms' tumour gene is involved in genito-urinary development. Nature 346: 194–197.
48. Hastie ND, Blickmore N, Pritchard-Jones K, Porteus DJ, van Heyningen V (1989) Wilms' tumour: a developmental approach. Int Symp Princess Takamatsu Cancer Fund 20: 45–50.
49. Kreidberg JA, Sariola H, Loring J et al. (1993) WT1 is required for early kidney development. Cell 74: 697–691.
50. Madden S, Cook D, Morris J, Gashler A, Sukhtame V, Rauscher F III (1991) Transcriptional repression mediated by the WT1 Wilms' tumour gene product. Science 253: 1330–1333.

51. Yun K, Fidler A, Eccles M, Reeve A (1993) Insulin-like growth factor II and WT1 transcript localisation in human fetal kidney and Wilms' tumour. Cancer Res 53: 5166–5171.
52. Denys P, Malvaux P, Van den Berghe H, Tanghe W, Proesmans W (1967) Association d'un syndrome anatomo-pathologique de pseudohermaphroditism masculin, d'une tumeur de Wilms d'une nephropathie parenchymateuse et d'un mosaicism XX/XY. Arch Fr Pediatr 24: 729–739.
53. Drash A, Sherman F, Hartmann W, Blizzard RM (1970) A syndrome of pseudohermaphroditism, Wilms' tumour, hypertension and degenerative renal disease. J Pediatr 76: 585–593.
54. Goldman SM, Garfinkel DJ, Oh KS, Dorst JP (1981) The Drash syndrome, male pseudohermaphroditism, nephritis and Wilms' tumour. Pediatr Radiol 141: 87–91.
55. Thorner P, McGraw M, Weitzman S, Balfe WW, Klein M Baumal R (1984) Wilms' tumour and glomerular disease. Occurrence with features of membranoproliferative glomerulonephritis and secondary focal, segmental glomerulosclerosis. Pathol Lab Med 108: 141–146.
56. Eddy AA, Mauer SM (1985) Pseudohermaphroditism, glomerulopathy, and Wilms' tumour (Drash syndrome): frequency in end stage renal failure. J Pediatr 106: 584–587.
57. Habib R, Liorat C, Grubler MC et al. (1985) The nephropathy associated with male pseudohermaphroditism and Wilms' tumour (Drash syndrome): a distinctive glomerular lesion – report of 10 cases. Clin Nephrol 24: 269–278.
58. Coppes MJ, Huff V, Pelletier J (1993) Denys–Drash syndrome: relating a clinical disorder to genetic alteration in the tumour suppressor gene WT1. J Pediatr 123: 673–678.
59. Strong LC, Compton DA, Chao L et al. (1988) Lack of linkage of familial Wilms' tumour to chromosome band 11p13. Nature 336: 337–338.
60. Grundy P, Koufos A, Morgan K et al. (1988) Familial predisposition of Wilms' tumour does not map to the short arm of chromosome 11. Nature 336: 374–376.
61. Wilkins RJ (1988) Genomic imprinting and carcinogenesis. Lancet i: 329–330.
62. Kaplan SJ, Holbrook T, McDaniel HG, Buntain WL, Crist WM (1980) Vasoactive intestinal peptide secreting tumours of childhood. Am J Dis Child 134: 21–24.
63. Smith EI, Castleberry RP (1990) Neuroblastoma. Curr Probl Surg 578–620.
64. Cowell J, Rupniak H (1983) Chromosome analysis of human neuroblastoma line TR14 showing double minutes and an aberration involving chromosome 1. Cancer Genet Cytogenet 9: 273–280.
65. Woods WG, Lemieux B, Tuchman M (1992) Neuroblastoma represents distinct clinical–biologic entities: a review and perspective from the Quebec Neuroblastoma screening project. Pediatrics 89: 114–118.
66. Philips WS, Stafford PW, Duvol-Arnold B, Ghosh BC (1991) Neuroblastoma and the clinical significance of N-*myc* amplification. Surg Gynecol Obstet 172: 73–80.
67. Hosoi G, Hara J, Okamura T et al. (1994) Low frequency of the p53 gene mutations in neuroblastoma. Cancer 73: 3087–3093.
68. Vogan K, Bernstein M, Leclerc J et al. (1993) Absence of p53 gene mutations in primary neuroblastomas. Cancer Res 53: 5269–5273.
69. Komoro H, Hayashi Y, Kawamura M et al. (1993) Mutations of the P53 gene are involved in Ewing's sarcomas but not in neuroblastomas. Cancer Res 53: 5284–5288.
70. Brodeur GM, Seeger RC, Schwab M et al. (1984) Amplification of N-*myc* in untreated human neuroblastomas correlates with advanced disease state. Science 224: 1121–1124.
71. Look AT, Hayes FA, Nitschke R et al. (1984) Cellular DNA content as a predictor of response to chemotherapy in infants with irresectable neuroblastoma. N Engl J Med 311: 231–235.
72. Look AT, Hayes FA, Shuster JJ et al. (1991) Clinical relevance of tumour cell ploidy and N-*myc* amplification in childhood neuroblastoma: a pediatric oncology group study. J Clin Oncol 9: 581–591.
73. Kohl NZ, Kanda N, Schreck RR et al. (1983) Transposition and amplification of oncogene related sequences in human neuroblastomas. Cell 35: 359–367.
74. Schwab M, Ellison J, Busch M et al. (1984) Enhanced expression of the human gene N-*myc* consequent to amplification of DNA may contribute to malignant progression of neuroblastoma. Proc Natl Acad Sci USA 81: 4940–4944.
75. Lee WH, Murphree AL, Benedict WF (1984) Expression and amplification of the N-*myc* gene in primary retinoblastoma. Nature 309: 458–460.
76. Squire J, Goddard AD, Canton M et al. (1986) Tumour induction by the retinoblastoma mutation is independent of N-*myc* expression. Nature 322: 555–557.
77. Brodeur GM, Hayes FA, Green AA et al. (1987) Consistent N-*myc* copy number in simultaneous or consecutive neuroblastoma samples from sixty individual patients. Cancer Res 47: 4728–4753.
78. Nakagawara A, Ikeda K, Yokoyama T, Tsuda T, Higashi K (1988) Surgical aspects of N-*myc* amplification in neuroblastoma. Surgery 104: 34–40.
79. Seeler RA, Israel JN, Royal JE, Kaye CI, Rao S, Abdulaban M (1979) Ganglioneuroblastoma and fetal hydantoin-alcohol syndromes. Pediatrics 63: 524–527.
80. Ilmensee K, Stevens LC (1979) Teratomas and chimeras. Sci Am 240: 87–98.
81. Keen WW, Coplin WMC (1906) Sacrococcygeal tumour (teratoma). Surg Gynecol Obstet 3: 661–671.
82. Ashcraft K, Holder TM (1974) Hereditary presacral teratoma. J Pediatr Surg 9: 691–697.
83. Schroeder W, Cahn L-Y, Dao D et al. (1987) Nonrandom loss of maternal chromosome 11 alleles in Wilms' tumours. Am J Hum Genet 40: 413–420.
84. Scrable H, Cavanee W, Ghavimi F, Lovell M, Morgan K, Sapienza C (1989) A model for embryonal rhabdomyosarcoma tumorigenesis that involves genome imprinting. Proc Natl Acad Sci USA 86: 7480–7484.
85. Douglass E, Valentine M, Etubanas E et al. (1987) A specific chromosomal abnormality in rhabdomyosarcoma. Cytogenet Cell Genet 45: 148–155.
86. Wang Wuu J, Soukup S, Ballard E, Gotwals B, Lampkin B (1988) Chromosomal analysis of sixteen human rhabdomyosarcomas. Cancer Res 48: 983–987.
87. Barr F, Galli N, Holick J, Biegel J, Rovera G, Emmanuel B (1993) Rearrangement of the Pax 3 paired box gene in the pediatric solid tumour alveolar rhabdomyosarcoma. Nature Genet 3: 113–117.
88. Boman F, Peters J, Ragge N, Triche T (1993) Infrequent mutation of the p53 gene in fibrous tumors of infancy and childhood. Med Pediatr Oncol 21: 583.
89. Helman LJ, Thiele CJ (1991) New insights into the causes of cancer. Pediatr Clin North Am 38: 201–221.
90. Houghton PJ, Shapiro DN, Houghton JA (1991) Rhabdomyosarcoma: from the laboratory to the clinic. Pediatr Clin North Am 38: 349–364.
91. Davies S (1993) Maintenance of genomic imprinting at the IgF2 locus in hepatoblastoma. Cancer Res 53: 4781–4783.
92. Koufos A, Hansen M, Copland N, Jenkins N, Lambkin B, Cavenee W (1985) Loss of heterozygosity in three embryonal tumours suggests a common pathogenetic mechanism. Nature 316: 330–334.
93. O'Connor P, Jackman J, Jondle D, Bhatia K, Magrath I, Kohn K (1993) Role of p53 tumour suppressor gene in cell cycle arrest and radiosensitivity of Burkitt's lymphoma cell lines.

Cancer Res 53: 4776–4780.
94. Levine A, Momand J, Finlay C (1991) The p53 suppressor gene. Nature 351: 453–456.
95. Levine A (1992) The p53 tumour suppressor gene. N Engl J Med 326: 1350–1352.
96. Lane D, Crawford L (1979) T antigen is bound to a host protein in SV40 transformed cells. Nature 278: 261–263.
97. Holstein M, Sidransky D, Vogelstein B, Harris C (1991) p53 mutations in human cancers. Science 253: 49–53.
98. Felix C, Kappel C, Mitsudomi T et al. (1992) Frequency and diversity of p53 mutations in childhood rhabdomyosarcomas. Cancer Res 52: 2243–2247.
99. Santibanez-Koref M, Birch J, Hartley A et al. (1991) p53 germline mutations in Li-Fraumeni syndrome. Lancet 338: 1490–1491.
100. Mailkin D, Li F, Strong L et al. (1990) Germ line p53 mutations in a familial syndrome of breast cancer, sarcomas and other neoplasms. Science 250: 1233–1238.
101. Sarnow P, Ho Y, Williams J, Levine A (1982) Adenovirus E1b-58 kd tumour antigen and SV 40 large tumour antigen are physically associated with the same 54 kd cellular protein in transformed cells. Cell 28: 387–394.
102. Werness BA, Levine AJ, Howley PM (1990) Association of human papillomavirus types 16 and 18 E6 proteins with p53. Science 248: 76–79.
103. Bischoff FZ, Yim SO, Pathak S et al. (1990) Spontaneous abnormalities in normal fibroblasts from patients with Li-Fraumeni cancer syndrome: aneuploidy and immortalization. Cancer Res 50: 7979–7984.
104. Donehower L, Harvey M, Slagle B et al. (1992) Mice deficient for p53 are developmentally normal but susceptible to spontaneous tumours. Nature 358: 215–221.
105. Andrieu N, Demanais F, Martinez M (1988) Genetic analysis of human breast cancer: implications for family study design. Genet Epidemiol 5: 225–233.
106. Lindblom A, Skoog L, Rotstein S, Werelius B, Larsson C, Nordenskjold M (1993) Loss of heterozygosity in familial breast carcinomas. Cancer Res 53: 4356–4361.
107. Srivastava S, Zou Z, Pirollo K, Blattner W, Chang E (1990) Germ line transmission of a cancer prone family with Li-Fraumeni syndrome. Nature 348: 747–749.
108. Li FP, Cassady JR, Jaffe N (1975) Risk of second tumours in survivors of childhood cancer. Cancer 35: 1230–1235.
109. Hall J (1990) Genomic imprinting. Arch Dis Child 65: 1013–1016.
110. Toguchida J, Ishizaki K, Sasaki MS et al. (1989) Preferential mutation of paternally derived RB gene as the initial event in sporadic osteosarcoma. Nature 338: 156–158.
111. Reik W, Surani MA (1987) Genomic imprinting and embryonal tumours. Nature 338: 248–251.

Mass Screening for Neuroblastoma

Takeshi Miyano and Koichi Ishimoto

3

Introduction

Neuroblastoma is the most common solid tumour in infancy. The introduction of multimodality therapy has improved treatment, but the prognosis of advanced neuroblastoma remains dismal. In 1974, Sawada and colleagues started experimental screening for neuroblastoma at 6 months of age using the vanillylmandelic acid (VMA) spot test[1,2]. The excellent results of treatment in these patients led to the introduction in 1985 of a nationwide mass screening programme in Japan[3,4]. The idea of mass screening infants at 6 months is largely based on the following three findings:

1. Over 90% of children with neuroblastoma excrete increased quantities of catecholamine metabolites, which can be measured in random urine samples obtained from diapers: it is therefore possible to screen and detect these tumours before symptoms become manifest.
2. Children who present before 1 year of age have a better outlook than older children.
3. Patients with localized disease fare better than those with advanced disease.

Thus, one might assume that diagnosing neuroblastoma in children less than 1 year old whose disease is not advanced would lead to a decrease in mortality rate. Indeed, by the end of 1990, the mass screening programme had detected 598 patients with neuroblastoma and 580 patients (97%) were still alive[5]. These figures seem to suggest that mass screening for neuroblastoma is improving the outlook of this disease.

However, recent studies indicate that there are at least two types of neuroblastoma, based on biological and clinical findings[6–8]. One group of patients is usually diagnosed before 1 year of age, has localized disease and presents with tumours that are responsive to therapy. The other group presents after 1 year of age, with advanced tumours that are refractory to therapy. It appears that the Japanese mass screening system may be biased towards detecting patients of the former group[9–13], and these findings have thrown some doubt over the success of the mass screening programme.

Biology and epidemiology of tumours detected by mass screening

Basic research in tumour biology has enabled paediatric oncologists to treat neuroblastoma based on the biological findings of the disease. Poor prognosis can now confidently be identified with certain biological characteristics, including amplification of the N-*myc* oncogene[6,14], diploid or tetraploid chromosome mode[7,8,10] (or non-aneuploid DNA content[15–17]), low expression of Ha-*ras p21*[18] and unfavourable histology[19]. Good prognosis is associated with single N-*myc* oncogene, triploid chromosome mode (or aneuploid DNA content), high expression of Ha-*ras p21* or *Trk-A* transcript[20], and favourable histology.

The growing biological data gathered from mass screening show that tumours detected by the programme (mass-screened positive tumours) nearly always show no N-*myc* amplification, but about 80% have triploid chromosome mode and favourable histology. The first important findings were reported in 1987 by Kaneko et al.[7], who studied the karyotypes of eight tumour samples obtained from patients detected by mass screening. They reported that five of the samples had near-triploid chromosome mode, and that this karyotype was rarely found before the introduction of mass screening. Since then, they have enrolled another 31 cases in their ongoing study[10]. Among the 39 positive mass-screened tumours, 37 were determined by their ploidy patterns: 28 (76%) showed near-triploid or hyper-tetraploid mode, and nine (24%) near-diploid or near-tetraploid status. No N-*myc* amplification was found. They also reported that patients with near-triploid tumours, either detected by mass screening or presenting clinically, have a better prognosis than those with near-diploid or near-tetraploid tumours.

Hayashi et al.[8] analysed 41 cases detected by mass screening, and reported that all had near-triploid or hyperdiploid karyotype without N-*myc* amplification. Nakagawara et al.[21] also reported that, in 30 screen detected patients, no cases had N-*myc* gene amplification.

Hachitanda et al.[22] recently analysed 100 neuroblastoma cases diagnosed through a mass screening programme, and evaluated their characteristics according to Shimada histological classification (100 cases), N-*myc* oncogene status (58 cases), DNA ploidy pattern (31 cases) and serum ferritin level (27 cases). In this study, 93% (93 of 100) had favourable histology, 100% (58 of 58) non-amplified N-*myc* gene, 81% (25 of 31) a favourable ploidy pattern, and 96% (26 of 27) normal serum ferritin levels. A total of 13 cases were associated with one or two poor risk factors: six had unfavourable histology, five an unfavourable ploidy pattern, one unfavourable histology and unfavourable ploidy pattern, and one an elevated ferritin level.

Kusafuka et al.[23] observed a higher proportion of unfavourable neuroblastomas in the screen detected patients. In their study, although no cases with N-*myc* amplification (0 of 41) were observed, 25% (18 of 73) had unfavourable ploidy pattern and 40% (28 of 70) lower expression of Ha-*ras p21*. They also indicated a significant correlation between these two unfavourable prognostic factors and, of 70 cases in which both factors were evaluated, 14 (20%) had both, and 38 (54%), including 35 cases with early clinical stage, revealed favourable biological status with regard to both DNA aneuploidy and expression of Ha-*ras p21*.

We had very few epidemiological statistics for mass-screened infants in Japan. Nevertheless, nationwide data have revealed a dramatic increase in the incidence of neuroblastoma since mass screening employing high-performance liquid chromatography (HPLC) was introduced (1 per 5 000)[5]. This has led us to suspect that some detected tumours may regress spontaneously or not present clinically later. Bessho et al.,[24] analysing data from the Japan Children's Cancer Registry (JCCR), reported that mass screening nearly doubled the number of neuroblastoma cases under 1 year of age to 121 in 238 (50.8%) after mass screening was commenced. They noted, however, that when only clinically presenting cases were counted (that is, when neuroblastoma cases detected by mass screening are excluded from the total number of neuroblastoma cases) this figure decreases to 42 in 159 (26.4%). Significantly, this figure is almost the same as the number of cases under 1 year of age (25%) registered with the JCCR before mass screening commenced. Their findings suggest that mass screening is picking up a unique type of tumour, which can be treated successfully because of its non-aggressive behaviour or which would probably regress spontaneously had it not been detected by mass screening and immediately treated.

On the other hand, some encouraging results have been reported. Nishi et al.[25] demonstrated that there is a significant reduction in the incidence of neuroblastoma diagnosed between the ages of 1 and 4 years, by about one-third of the number of cases encountered in the prescreening period in Sapporo City. Sawada et al.[5,26] also reported a significant increase in patients diagnosed before 1 year of age and, at the same time, a decrease in patients aged 1–4 years after the introduction of the mass screening program. These authors believe that the decreased incidences of neuroblastoma in patients aged 1–4 years may be due to early detection of tumours by screening.

It is well known that some neuroblastomas, especially stage IV-S tumours, can regress spontaneously[27]. Furthermore, the frequency of "occult" in situ neuroblastomas has been reported to be much greater than that of neuroblastomas diagnosed by clinical symptoms[28]. It is difficult to say whether mass screening is picking up these occult tumours, because few patients with neuroblastoma detected by mass screening have simply been observed without undergoing therapy involving surgical removal[29,30]. In one instance, however, we were able to follow a case for 3 years without intervening surgically[29]. This patient tested positive at the time of mass screening. However, owing to a miscommunication, the results of the test went unreported for another 4 months. When the patient was examined for the first time at 10 months of age, a localized tumour was found in the retroperitoneum. The parents refused therapy and the patient has been under careful observation for the last 3 years, during which the tumour has decreased somewhat in size.

Nakagawara et al.[21] reported two similar cases, which were not re-examined for 13 and 17 months after initial screening because of difficulties in communication between the examination centre and the parents. The values of urinary VMA and homovanillic acid (HVA) had not changed much between initial screening and re-examination (33.8 μg/mg creatinine and 23.1 μg/mg creatinine at initial screening, and 36.0 μg/mg creatinine and 18.7 μg/mg creatinine after 13 months for one case; 48.0 μg/mg creatinine and 69.7 μg/mg creatinine at screening and 43.2 μg/mg creatinine and 77.6 μg/mg creatinine after 17 months for the other). These two cases were successfully treated. Considering these observations, it is possible that some cases detected at screening may have potential to regress spontaneously or remain stable, and it seems very likely that the increased incidence of neuroblastoma may result from the detection of this group of occult neuroblastomas, which may not manifest clinically at later life. Further investigations such as follow-up studies of the natural course of selected cases with early-stage neuroblastoma that are not receiving treatment will be helpful in the future.

From these biological and epidemiological findings, it seems that approximately 20% of the tumours detected by mass screening had one or more unfavourable prognostic factor(s) and would have developed to clinically aggressive tumours had they not been detected; there may be an advantage in detecting these tumours early by screening. However, a number of the screen-detected neuroblastomas had favourable prognostic features, and the detection and subsequent treatment of these neuroblastomas appears unlikely to lead to a reduction in the mortality rate of this disease.

Neuroblastomas not detected by mass screening

Neuroblastoma is a heterogeneous tumour, which can be divided into three biologically different groups[31]. The first group consists of tumours showing no amplification of N-*myc*. These tumours either regress or are treated successfully. Tumours of the second group also show no amplification of N-*myc* at the time of diagnosis, but eventually progress. The third group consists of tumours with N-*myc* amplification; progression in tumour growth is rapid after diagnosis. Our ongoing clinical studies have yielded 13 neuroblastoma cases not detected by mass screening but which later presented clinically (mass-screened negative tumours)[12,29]. These patients represent the second and third groups of tumours. The clinical characteristics of these patients are shown in Table 3.1. The age at diagnosis ranged from 10 months to 3 years 11 months (mean 2 years 3

Table 3.1 Clinical characteristics of mass-screened negative cases

Patient	Age	Testing method	VMA	HVA	Primary site	Stage
1	2 years 11 months	VMA spot	–	+	Adrenal	IV
2	3 years 11 months	VMA spot	+	+	Mediastinum	IV
3	3 years 11 months	VMA spot	+	+	Mediastinum	IV
4	2 years 4 months	VMA spot	–	+	Retroperitoneum	III
5	10 months	VMA spot	–	–	Adrenal	IV
6	3 years 7 months	VMA spot	+	+	Adrenal	IV
7	1 year 10 months	VMA spot	–	+	Adrenal	IV
8	1 year 2 months	HPLC	–	+	Adrenal	IV
9	2 years 2 months	HPLC	–	+	Adrenal	IV
10	1 year 2 months	HPLC	+	+	Mediastinum	II
11	1 year 6 months	HPLC	–	+	Adrenal	IV
12	1 year 11 months	HPLC	–	+	Retroperitoneum	IV
13	2 years 0 months	HPLC	+	+	Mediastinum	IV

HPLC, high-performance liquid chromatography; HVA, homovanillic acid at presentation; VMA, vanillylmandelic acid at presentation.

months). Seven of the patients underwent the VMA spot test and the other six HPLC. The results for all were negative. The urinary VMA levels at presentation in eight of the 13 patients were normal. All patients except one were in advanced stages and eight patients have already died of tumour progression. Two of the other five patients, despite receiving chemotherapy, have relapsed. The cytogenetic and N-*myc* oncogene findings for 11 of the patients are shown in Table 3.2. The advanced tumours analysed cytogenetically showed diploid or tetraploid chromosome mode, frequently associated with structural abnormalities such as 1p–, double minutes (DM) and/or homogeneous staining regions (HSRs), whereas the stage II tumour showed triploid chromosome mode. N-*myc* oncogene analysis revealed amplification in seven of 11 tumours. The stage II tumour showed no amplification of N-*myc*. The findings for these mass-screened negative cases clearly indicate aggressive clinical and biological features, which are strikingly different from those of mass-screened positive cases.

Table 3.2 Biological analysis of mass-screened negative cases

Patient	Mode	Chromosome structural abnormalities	N-*myc* copy number
1	Diploid	1p–, DM, marker chromosome	60
2	Diploid	1q+, marker chromosome	1
3	Diploid	None	1
4	Not tested	Not tested	4
5	Tetraploid	1p–, DM	15
6	Tetraploid	None	1
7	Diploid	DM, homogeneously staining regions	32
8	Diploid	1p–, DM	30
9	Diploid	1p–, DM	20
10	Triploid	None	1
11	Tetraploid	1p–, DM	14

Cases 12 and 13 were not tested.
DM, double minutes.

Nakagawara et al.[13] have reported 17 mass-screened negative cases with similar features. All their cases presented with advanced tumours. Ten showed N-*myc* amplification associated with immature catecholamine metabolism. These authors also emphasized the biological differences between mass-screened positive patients with generally good prognosis and negative cases with poor prognosis. Improving the prognosis of patients with mass-screened negative tumours may be possible by measuring catecholamine metabolites at a later time, such as 1–2 years of age.

Why are aggressive neuroblastomas missed by mass screening?

We think that there may be two answers to this question. The first concerns the method of testing the urine samples. In seven of our 13 patients (Table 3.1), the urine VMA spot test was employed. This is a qualitative test and is known to lack accuracy. In addition, four of these seven patients had VMA non-producing tumours, which cannot be detected by this test. When quantitative HPLC testing measuring both VMA nd HVA levels was introduced in almost all the testing sites, it appeared that this problem would be solved. However, this is not the case, as can be seen from Table 3.1. Six of the 13 mass-screened negative cases had HPLC testing, indicating that there may also be false negatives with this procedure.

The other answer is likely to be related to the biological heterogeneity of the tumour. As discussed above there are different types of neuroblastoma based on the cytogenetics, oncogenetics and clinical behaviour. It has also been found that these different types of tumour remain consistent and do not change their biological characteristic over time. From a cytogenetic standpoint, this means that triploid tumours are not likely to progress to diploid or tetraploid tumours[8,9] and N-*myc* copy number in a given tumour will remain consistent at any site and during the whole course of the disease[32,33]. Because of differences in the biological characteristics, it will be safe to assume that there will be differences in the clinical behaviour, including the pattern of catecholamine metabolite excretion. What we are now beginning to recognize, therefore, is that these aggressive tumours either do not exist at the time of mass screening or are too small to produce urinary catecholamine levels high enough to be detected.

Does mass screening reduce the mortality rate of neuroblastoma?

A critical determinant of the social and medical utility of any nationwide mass screening program for neuroblastoma is the overall mortality rate.

Because there are no population-based control studies in Japan regarding the overall mortality rate for neuroblastoma, investigators have so far had to conduct studies concerning only survival rates among the screened population. The survival curves reported by Sawada et al. during a 27 year period showed that the rate jumped from 17.1% before mass screening (1962–1974) to 54.8% during the experimental mass screening period (1974–1982) and to 85.2% after mass screening commenced (1983–1988)[34]. Nishi et al.[35] have also reported their treatment results for Sapporo City, in which the 48 month survival rates improved significantly from 21.3% to 87.5% after mass screening started. However, these survival rates are likely to reflect not only the contribution of mass screening but also two other factors: one is the recent advances in the treatment of neuroblastomas; the other, and more important, factor is the existence of a neuroblastoma population consisting of cases which, had they not been detected by mass screening, would not have presented clinically later in childhood. This "increase" in survival rate does not necessarily imply a correlative decrease in the overall mortality rate. We therefore feel that there is not a correspondingly dramatic decrease in the overall mortality rate as a result of mass screening.

Recently, in North America, Quebec Genetic Medicine, in collaboration with the University of Minnesota, has established the Quebec Neuroblastoma Screening Study[36], which conducted a two-step screening programme: at 3 weeks of age and at 6 months. Infants screened included all those born during a 5 year period (more than 450 000 infants) from 1 May 1989 to 30 April 1994, and they will be observed for a minimum of 3 years. Although these results are still preliminary[37], by 28 August 1993 a total of 32 infants (15 patients screened at 3 weeks, 17 at 6 months) had been identified as having neuroblastoma, and 47 additional children in the birth cohort had been diagnosed clinically with neuroblastoma (17 prior to screening at 3 weeks of age, 12 with negative results at 3 week screening, 14 with negative results at both screenings, and four not screened). The results obtained from the Quebec province will be compared with those of several concurrent population-based non-screened control groups[38]. This should help to clarify whether mass screening leads to a reduction in the mortality rate, as well as giving data on the incidence, clinical staging and survival rates of neuroblastoma.

References

1. Sawada T, Todo S, Fujita S, Iino S, Imashuku S, Kusunoki T (1982) Mass screening for neuroblastoma in infancy. Am J Dis Child 136: 710–712.
2. Sawada T, Kidowaki T, Sakamoto I et al. (1984) Neuroblastoma: mass screening for early detection and its prognosis. Cancer 53: 2731–2735.
3. Sawada T, Hirayama M, Nakata et al. (1984) Mass screening for neuroblastoma in infants in Japan. Interim report of a mass screening study group. Lancet ii: 271–273.
4. Sawada T (1986) Outcome of 25 neuroblastomas revealed by mass screening. Lancet i: 377.
5. Sawada T, Kawakatsu H, Matsumura T, Kizaki Z, Shikata T, Sugimoto T, members of the Screening Study Group (1994) Recent results of neuroblastoma mass screening in Japan. In: Sawada T, Matsumura T, Kizaki Z, eds. Proceedings of the 3rd International Symposium on Neuroblastoma Screening, Kyoto, 1993. Department of Pediatrics, Kyoto Prefectural University of Medicine, Kyoto, pp. 101–106.
6. Seeger RC, Brodeur GM, Sather H et al. (1985) Association of multiple copies of the N-*myc* oncogene with rapid progression of neuroblastoma. N Engl J Med 313: 1111–1116.
7. Kaneko, Y, Kanda N, Maseki N et al. (1987) Different karyotypic patterns in early and advanced stage neuroblastoma. Cancer Res 47: 311–318.
8. Hayashi Y, Hanada R, Yamamoto K (1992) Biology of neuroblastomas in Japan found by screening. Am J Pediatr Hematol Oncol 14: 342–347.
9. Kaneko Y, Maseki N, Sakurai M et al. (1988) Chromosomes and screening for neuroblastoma. Lancet i: 174–175.
10. Kaneko Y, Kanda N, Maseki N et al. (1990) Current urinary mass screening for catecholamine metabolites at 6 months of age may be detecting only a small portion of high-risk neuroblastomas: a chromosome and N-*myc* amplification study. J Clin Oncol 8: 2005–2013.
11. Hayashi Y, Inaba T, Hanada R, Yamamoto K (1988) Chromosome findings and prognosis in 15 patients with neuroblastoma found by mass screening. J Pediatr 112: 567–571.
12. Ishimoto K, Kiyokawa N, Fujita H et al. (1991) biological analysis of neuroblastoma in mass screened negative cases. In: Evans AE, ed. Advances in neuroblastoma research 3. Wiley-Liss, New York, pp 603–608.
13. Nakagawara A, Zaizen Y, Suita S (1991). Genomic and metabolic aspects of neuroblastomas in children under one year of age. In: Evans AE, ed. Advances in neuroblastoma research 3. Wiley-Liss, New York, pp. 115–125.
14. Tsuda T, Obara M, Hirano H et al. (1987) Analysis of N-*myc* amplification in relation to disease stage and histologic types in human neuroblastomas. Cancer 60: 820–826.
15. Look AT, Hayes FA, Nitschke R, McWilliams NB, Green AA (1984) Cellular DNA content as a predictor of response to chemotherapy in infants with unresectable neuroblastoma. N Engl J Med 311: 231–235.
16. Taylor SR, Blatt J, Costantino JP, Roederer M, Murphy RF (1988) Flow cytometric DNA analysis of neuroblastoma and ganglioneuroblastoma: a 10 year retrospective study. Cancer 62: 749–754.
17. Kusafuka T, Fukuzawa M, Oue T, Yoneda A, Okada A, Satani M (1994) DNA flow cytometric analysis of neuroblastoma:

distinction of tetraploidy subset. J Pediatr Surg 29: 543–547.
18. Tanaka T, Slamon DJ, Shimada H et al. (1991) A significant association of Ha-*ras p21* in neuroblastoma cells with patient prognosis. Cancer 68: 1296–1302.
19. Shimada H, Chatten J, Newton WA et al. (1984) Histopathologic prognostic factors in neuroblastic tumors: definition of subtypes of ganglioneuroblastoma and an age-linked classification of neuroblastomas. J Natl Cancer Inst 73: 405–416.
20. Nakagawara A, Arima-Nakagawara M, Scavarda J, Azar CG, Cantor AB, Brodeur GM (1993) Association between high levels of expression of the TRK gene and favorable outcome in human neuroblastoma. N Engl J Med 328: 847–854.
21. Nakagawara A, Zaizen Y, Ikeda K et al. (1991) Different genomic and metabolic patterns between mass screening-positive and mass screening-negative later-presenting neuroblastomas. Cancer 68: 2037–2044.
22. Hachitanda Y, Ishimoto K, Hata J, Shimada H (1994) One hundred neuroblastomas detected through a mass screening system in Japan. Cancer 74: 3223–3226.
23. Kusafuka T, Nagahara N, Oue T et al. (1995) Unfavourable DNA ploidy and Ha-*ras p21* findings in neuroblastomas detected through mass screening. Cancer 76: 695–699.
24. Bessho F, Hashizume K, Nakajo T, Kamoshita S (1991) Mass screening in Japan increased the detection of infants with neuroblastoma without a decrease in cases in older children. J Pediatr 119: 237–241.
25. Nishi Mo, Miyake H, Takeda T et al. (1992) Mass screening of neuroblastoma in Sapporo City, Japan. Am J Pediatr Hematol Oncol 14: 327–331.
26. Sawada T, Shikata T, Kawakatsu H, Sugimoto T (1992) Changes in the age distribution and incidence of patients with neuroblastoma before and after mass screening for neuroblastoma in infants in Japan. Med Pediatr Oncol 20: 424.
27. Evans AE, Baum E, Chard R (1981) Do infants with stage IV-S neuroblastoma need treatment? Arch Dis Child 56: 271–274.
28. Beckwith JB, Perrin EV (1963) In situ neuroblastoma: a contribution to the natural history of neural crest tumors. Am J Pathol 43: 1089–1104.
29. Ishimoto K, Kiyokawa N, Fujita H et al. (1990) Problems of mass screening for neuroblastoma: analysis of false-negative cases. J Pediatr Surg 25: 398–401.
30. Matsumura M, Tsunoda A, Nishi T, Nishihara H, Sasaki Y (1991) Spontaneous regression of neuroblastoma detected by mass screening. Lancet 338: 447–448.
31. Seeger RC, Wada R, Brodeur GM et al. (1988) Expression of N-*myc* by neuroblastoma with one or multiple copies of the oncogene. In: Evans AE, ed. Advances in neuroblastoma research 2. Alan R. Liss, New York, pp. 41–49.
32. Brodeur GM, Hayes FA, Green AA et al. (1987) Consistent N-*myc* copy number in simultaneous or consecutive neuroblastoma samples from sixty individual patients. Cancer Res 47: 4248–4253.
33. Hiyama E, Yokoyama T, Ichikawa T, Ishii T, Hiyama K (1990) N-*myc* gene amplification and other prognosis-associated factors in neuroblastoma. J Pediatr Surg 25: 1095–1099.
34. Sawada T, Matsumura T, Kawakatsu H et al. (1991) Long-term effects of mass screening for neuroblastoma in infancy. Am J Pediatr Hematol Oncol 13: 3–7.
35. Nishi M, Miyake H, Takeda T et al. (1987) Effects of the mass screening of neuroblastoma in Sapporo city. Cancer 60: 433–436.
36. Tuchman M, Lemineux B, Auray-Blais C et al. (1990) Screening for neuroblastoma at 3 weeks of age: methods and preliminary results from the Quebec Neuroblastoma Screening Project. Pediatrics 86: 765–773.
37. Lemieux B, Tuchman M, Leclerc JM et al. (1994) The Quebec neuroblastoma screening program: an update. In: Sawada T, Matsumura T, Kizaki, eds. Proceedings of the 3rd International Symposium on Neuroblastoma Screening, Kyoto, 1993. Department of Pediatrics, Kyoto Prefectural University of Medicine, Kyoto, pp 75–84.
38. Bernstein ML, Leclerc JM, Bunin G et al. (1992) A population-based study of neuroblastoma incidence, survival and mortality in North America. J Clin Oncol 10: 323–329.

Neuroblastoma

Jay Grosfeld

4

Introduction

Neuroblastoma is an embryonal tumour that evolves from neural crest cells. This neoplasm may arise at any site in the sympathetic nervous system, including the brain, the cervical region, the posterior mediastinum, para-aortic sympathetic ganglia, the pelvis and the adrenal medulla[1–3]. The material in this chapter will be limited to consideration of neuroblastoma occurring from the neonatal period until 1 year of age.

Epidemiology

Neuroblastoma is the second most common solid tumour of infancy and childhood, being exceeded in number only by brain tumours[4]. It is the most common abdominal malignancy noted in the newborn. Reports concerning the frequency of benign or malignant tumours seen in infants under 1 month of age indicate that teratomas are probably the most common neoplasms, followed by neuroblastoma, soft-tissue sarcoma, renal tumours, brain tumours, leukaemia and others[5,6]. Some 25%–30% of all patients with neuroblastoma are diagnosed in the first year of life. This tumour comprises 7%–14% of all childhood cancers[4–6]. Mass screening programs initiated in Japan evaluating the urinary levels of vanillylmandelic acid (VMA) and homovanillic acid (HVA) in infants at 6 months of age have uncovered a large number of cases of neuroblastoma[7]. The survival rate in these cases has been exceptionally high compared with survival rates of patients with neuroblastoma who present with clinical disease and are diagnosed by conventional measures[8]. The Japanese screening effort has doubled the incidence of neuroblastoma in young infants compared with that noted prior to the onset of screening, but has not decreased the number of cases observed in older children[9].

Most cases detected by screening have triploid chromosomes and almost never have other adverse findings such as N-*myc* amplification[10]. These cases probably represent the type of neuroblastic tumour that spontaneously regresses[9,10], and suggest that the increased number of neuroblastic tumours detected by screening represent instances of neuroblastoma that would otherwise regress and not present clinically[9–11]. Indeed, spontaneous regression of neuroblastoma has been observed in a subset of very young patients, particularly those under 1 year of age[12,13]. Regression may occur as a result of cytolysis of the tumour cell, causing haemorrhagic necrosis followed by eventual fibrosis and/or dystrophic calcification, or of maturation and transformation to a benign ganglioneuroma. Neonates with neuroblastoma in situ and infants classified as having stage IV-S disease may represent a group of patients with a single prezygotic mutation who have a high frequency of spontaneous tumour regression[14,15]. In contrast, a more aggressive sporadic form of neuroblastoma may be caused by a second somatic mutation of the tumour[14,15].

Familial cases of neuroblastoma have been observed in siblings, identical twins, and a mother and child[16–20]. A recent population-based study from Denmark reported an increased occurrence of neuroblastoma in the offspring of mothers at either end of the childbearing years (the very young and the old)[21]. In a case-control study Neglia et al. found no association with maternal age, birth weight or gestational age, but did show an increased rate of congenital anomalies in babies with neuroblastoma and a lower occurrence of prior fetal loss in their mothers than in control mothers[22]. Evidence of the embryonal development of this tumour, with secretion of metabolites from the tumour causing maternal hypertension, sweating, pallor, headaches and palpitations, is well documented[2,23]. Further evidence of the embryonal nature of neuroblastoma includes cases associated with antenatal death and instances in which placental invasion by the tumour has occurred, characterized by numerous emboli with tumour cells located in the vessels of the chorionic villi[24–28]. A specific chromosomal character type has not been observed in patients with neuroblastoma, although some chromosomal abnormalities are noted in a majority of neuroblastoma cells. This involves rearrangement or deletions of chromosome 1p36 and a number of other abnormalities in other chromosomes (e.g. chromosome 17)[23,29,30]. Double minutes as well as long non-banding staining regions have been observed in some neuroblastoma cell lines and may represent amplified cellular genes. Unique oncogenes are observed in certain neuroblastic tumours such as the N-*myc* and *ras* oncogenes (both being highly amplified)[31,32], suggesting that further chromosomal studies of this highly unusual paediatric tumour is advisable. Amplification of the N-*myc* oncogene in patients with neuroblastoma represents an important adverse prognostic finding[32–34]. In contrast, high levels of the *trk*proto-oncogene is associated with an improved diagnosis.

Cytogenetic studies of infants with neuroblastoma have shown that the majority of cases found by mass screening techniques in Japan have a triploid chromosome mode without structural abnormalities[29]. Structural abnormalities are much more common in children over the age of 1 year. Neuroblastoma has been observed in patients with Beckwith–Weidemann syndrome or pancreatic islet cell dysplasia and in babies born to mothers with seizure disorders who are taking phenylhydantoin[34–39]. Of babies born to mothers taking hydantoin, 10% will develop manifestations of fetal hydantoin syndrome[36–38]. These include mental retardation, growth deficiency and ocular hypertelorism. There is also an increased incidence of neuroblastoma in infants with fetal alcohol syndrome[39,40]. Alcohol has been established as a teratogen. In addition to neuroblastoma, adrenal carcinoma has been observed after maternal gestational alcohol abuse[41]. These substances may be both oncogenic and teratogenic in regard to the development of neural crest abnormalities. Neuroblastoma has also been observed in babies with Hirschsprung's disease involving the rectosigmoid, as well as in infants with total colonic aganglionosis[42–44]. These cases are more commonly associated with a primary tumour occurring in the mediastinum. The association of neuroblastoma and adrenocortical defects (Cushing's syndrome) due to adrenal hyperplasia has also been observed[45].

Embryology

Neuroblastoma arises from neural crest cells that form at the junction of the neural tube and epidermal tissues in the embryo[23,46]. As the neural tube forms, the neural crest cells can be observed as columns of cells that extend down the length of the embryo in the corners of the dorsolateral portion of the neural tube and migrate to a number of different areas, giving rise to a variety of cells. Neural crest cells are therefore multipotential precursors for cells that may be found in the adrenal medulla and sympathetic spinal ganglia, and for Schwann cells, meningeal tissues, peripheral neurons, the medullary C cells of the thyroid gland, melanocytes in the skin, chromaffin tissues and cells of the autonomic ganglia of the gastrointestinal tract and perhaps certain portions of membranous bone. Different regions of the neural crest tissues give rise to specific ganglia. The fate of any neural crest cell or group of cells is probably related to its initial position in the neural crest, with maturation and differentiation occurring after migration to a final resting site[44]. The cervical and sacral regions probably give rise to the parasympathetic systems, with mesenteric and submucosal nerve plexuses arising from craniocaudal migration of cervical neural crest cells, which arrive in the distal gut at 12 weeks' gestation. Thoracic and lumbar neural crest cells migrate and differentiate into the sympathetic ganglia and the adrenal medulla. Once the neural crest cells arrive at a specific site, differentiation into ganglia or malignant proliferation into neuroblastoma occurs and is probably determined by the local influences of the genome of the cells.

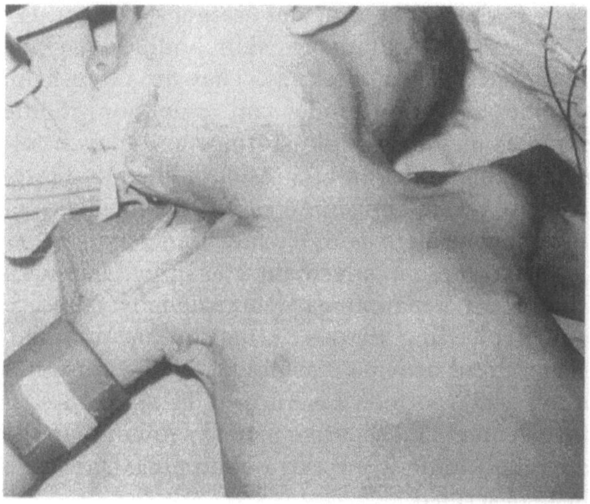

Figure 4.1 A mass in the left neck in a 4-month-old infant with cervical neuroblastoma. A biopsy was performed before the infant's transfer for definitive surgical excision. The patient is currently 17 years old and has no evidence of disease.

Ikeda et al. identified collections of neuroblasts in 7-week-old fetuses[47]. At 12 weeks nodules of neuroblasts are observed. The number and size of the neuroblastic nodules increase until the 15–17th fetal week. Guin et al. examined the adrenal glands from 92 fetuses aborted at 17–20 weeks' gestation and noted the presence of a neuroblastic adrenal nodule in each case[48]. Neuroblastoma in situ in the form of neuroblastic nodules in the adrenal glands (which may be larger than 3 mm in size and in some instances invade blood vessels) are seen in one in 180–260 newborn infants dying of congenital heart disease[49]. Other studies, in which careful sections of the adrenal gland in babies dying from other causes in the first 3 months of life were evaluated, showed that as many as one in 39 cases may have "neuroblastoma in situ". The incidence of neuroblastoma does not coincide with the high rate of appearance of these neuroblastic cells in young infants. These observations suggest that neuroblastoma in situ may undergo regression with differentiation and not present as a clinical case of neuroblastoma. Clinical tumour development may be related to defective regression or differentiation of microscopic neuroblastoma, which is found in the adrenal glands of 100% of fetuses studied at 10–20 weeks' gestation but is present in only one in 39 to one in 260 adrenal glands of newborns or infants less than 3 months old who die from other causes, and rarely thereafter[47–50].

Prenatal diagnosis

Neuroblastoma has rarely been detected as an unsuspected finding in the fetus on prenatal ultrasonography. However, when detected, these tumours generally follow a favourable course, with multiple favourable prognostic indicators such as low stage of disease, favourable biological markers including cellular DNA content and N-*myc* oncogene copy number, and favourable histology[51].

Clinical presentation

Although a handful of cases are observed in the neonate shortly after birth, the majority of patients with this neurogenic tumour present within the first 2–3 years of life[1–3,23,34,52]. The presence of a large nodular abdominal mass is the most common presenting finding, but many cases of neuroblastoma in the first year of life are nonadrenal in origin (neck, mediastinum, pelvis)[23] (Figure 4.1). Neuroblastoma may be associated with some unusual clinical manifestations, including "panda eyes" due to orbital metastases, opsoclonus/nystagmus (the "dancing-eye syndrome", which is probably related to an autoimmune phenomenon involving an antigen–antibody complex of IgG_3 and IgG_4), watery diarrhoea due to vasoactive intestinal polypeptide (VIP) secretion, Horner's syndrome in association with heterochromia as a result of a primary tumour arising in the cervical stellate ganglion, respiratory distress caused by a space-occupying mediastinal tumour (Figure 4.2) or severe abdominal distension (Figure 4.3), and hemiplegia related to tumour extension through the intervertebral foramina resulting in extradural compression and a pelvic mass which may result in either bladder or vascular compression[1–3,23,34].

Many of the cases that present in the newborn (as many as 30%) are associated with abdominal distension due to hepatomegaly and subcutaneous

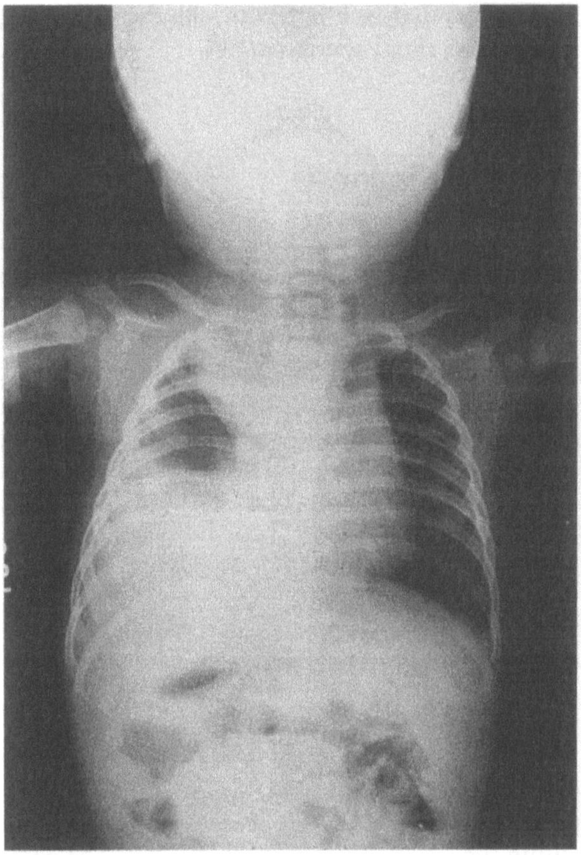

Figure 4.2 Chest radiograph (anteroposterior view) revealing the presence of a right upper mediastinal mass found to be a Stage II neuroblastoma. The patient achieved long-term survival following thoracotomy and resection.

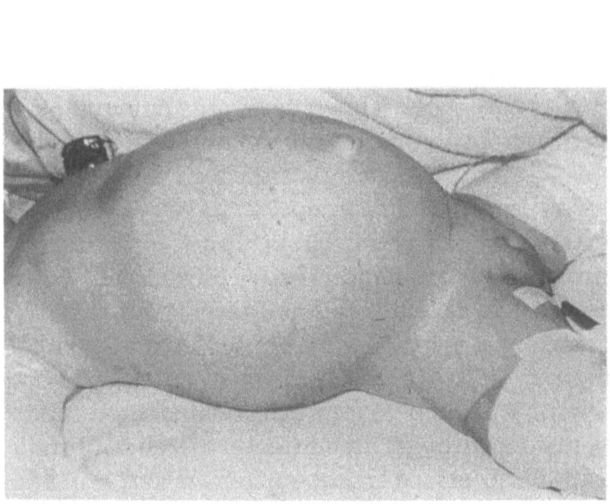

Figure 4.3 Photograph of a 6-week-old girl with significant abdominal distension, respiratory insufficiency and an enlarged nodular liver. The infant had stage IV-S neuroblastoma and died as a result of respiratory complications rather than tumour progression.

skin nodules (the unusual category of stage IV-S)[12,13,47–57]. Subcutaneous skin nodules may be scattered all over the body. They are often firm, mobile and non-tender on palpation. Some nodules may have a bluish tinge and blanch following manipulation as a result of liberating catecholamines. In congenital cases[2], the incidence of liver involvement is 65%, subcutaneous nodules 32% and bone involvement 3%. In patients with significant hepatomegaly, occasionally jaundice and a bleeding diathesis may be encountered. Generalized oedema resembling fetal hydrops has also been reported[2]. Instances of bilateral adrenal involvement and separate primary tumours in the abdomen and in an extra-abdominal site have been described[1,34,44].

Diagnostic tests

The radiological evaluation of infants with neuroblastoma includes chest radiograph, erect and recumbent abdominal radiographs, and computed tomography (CT) of the primary tumour site (neck, abdomen, pelvis, mediastinum) or magnetic resonance imaging, which has high accuracy and sensitivity[58]. Recently, three-dimensional reconstructions of spiral CT imaging has been reported to provide useful information that allows evaluation of the relationship to major blood vessels and resectability[59]. If the infant has a paraspinal tumour, magnetic resonance imaging is most rewarding in the evaluation of extradural tumour extension and may also document bone marrow involvement[34] and intraspinal extension. Bone marrow aspirate and biopsy may show rosettes of neuroblasts, and ^{99}mTc isotopic bone scan and ^{123}I metaiodobenzylguanidine (MIBG) scan will detect skeletal involvement[1,34]. The primary tumour often has areas of calcification on plain radiographs and may also pick up bone scanning isotopes[1,34]. Urine should be collected for catecholamines, VMA and HVA determination, and serum for neuron-specific enolase and serum ferritin levels. In patients with liver metastases, prothrombin time, partial thromboplastin time and platelet count should be obtained. A complete blood count is necessary for each patient to detect the presence of anaemia.

Table 4.1 Evans staging system

Stage	Description
I	Tumour confined to organ of origin
II	Tumour extends beyond organ of origin but does not cross the midline Unilateral lymph nodes may be involved
III	Tumour extends beyond midline Bilateral lymph nodes may be involved
IV	Distant metastases (skeletal, other organs, soft tissues, distant lymph nodes)
IVS	Would be stage I or II Remote disease confined to liver, subcutaneous tissues and bone marrow, but without evidence of bone cortex involvement

Table 4.2 St Jude staging system

Stage	Description
I	Localized tumour completely resected
IIA	Localized tumour resected with microscopic residual
IIB	Localized unresectable or partially resected tumour
IIIA	Disseminated metastases to liver, lymph node or skin, with no bone or bone marrow involvement
IIIB	Disseminated disease with one localized bone lesion but no bone marrow involvement
IIIC	Disseminated disease with bone marrow and/or generalized bone involvement

Table 4.3 Pediatric Oncology Group staging system

Stage	Description
A	Complete resection of primary tumour, with or without microscopic residual Intracavitary lymph nodes, not adherent to and removed with primary tumour, negative Liver negative
B	Grossly unresected primary tumour Nodes and liver as in stage A
C	Complete or incomplete resection of primary tumour Intracavitary nodes, not adherent to primary tumour, positive Liver as in stage A
D	Any dissemination of disease beyond intracavitary nodes, i.e. extracavitary nodes, liver, skin, bone marrow, bone
D (S)	Would be Evans stage I or II except for metastatic tumour in liver, bone marrow or skin

Staging

The staging criteria for neuroblastoma have undergone some changes over the years and vary somewhat according to the criteria used by any one cooperative tumour study group (Evans–CCG, St Jude–POG, IUCC, etc.)[1,23,34,60,61]. The Evans staging system is used by the Children's Cancer Group (CCG), of which our hospital is a member institution. All the staging schemes are in basic agreement regarding the categorization of a localized completely resectable lesion, instances of metastases to the bone cortex and infants with Evans stage IV-S, but some disagreement exists concerning other aspects of staging. The Evans system[60] (Table 4.1) places tumours with microscopic residual tumour and lymph node involvement in a stage II category, and tumours that are often large, cross the midline and are frequently not resectable in stage III. The St Jude classification[61] (Table 4.2) places unresectable tumours with gross residual disease in stage IIB, and subdivides stage III into:

A Lymph node, liver and skin metastases only
B Metastases to a single bone with normal bone marrow
C Generalized bone and bone marrow involvement

The Pediatric Oncology Group (POG) staging differs slightly from the St Jude system in that more emphasis is placed on whether lymph nodes are attached (localized) or unattached (remote) to the primary tumour in the same body cavity (Table 4.3). The European International Union Contra Cancer (IUCC) advocates both preoperative and postoperative staging using the TNM method, where T refers to tumour size, N to nodal status, and M to presence or absence of distal metastases[1,25] (Table 4.4). Recently, an international staging system (INSS) has been devised for neuroblastoma in hopes of developing a common set of criteria that can be evaluated worldwide[62,63] (Table 4.5). Recent reports by Haase et al.[64] highlight the ability of the INSS to differentiate patients with regional (stage 3) disease from those with a more favourable prognosis. Its implementation requires consistent standardized surgical involvement. The INSS may also provide a means of assessing a variety of biological characteristics that may then be incorporated into the overall prognosis. There is a general agreement that stage

Table 4.4 TNM clinical staging

Stage	Primary tumour	Lymph node involvement	Metastases
I	T1	N0	M0
II	T2	N0	M0
III	T1,T2 T3	N1 Any N	M0 M0
IV	T1,T2,T3	Any N	M1
V	T4	Any N	Any M

T1, tumour <5 cm; T2, tumour 5–10 cm; T3, tumour > 10 cm; T4, multicentric tumour; N0, nodes not involved; N1, nodes involved; M0, no metastases; M1, metastases present.

Table 4.5 International neuroblastoma staging system

Stage	Description
1	Localized tumour confined to area of origin Complete excision, with or without microscopic residual Ipsilateral and contralateral lymph nodes negative
2A	Unilateral tumour with incomplete excision Ipsilateral and contralateral lymph nodes negative
2B	Unilateral tumour with complete or incomplete excision Positive ipsilateral regional lymph nodes Contralateral lymph nodes negative
3	Tumour infiltrating across the midline with or without lymph node involvement Or unilateral tumour with contralateral lymph node involvement Or midline tumour with bilateral lymph node involvement
4	Dissemination of tumour to distant lymph nodes, bone, bone marrow, liver and/or other organs
4-S	Localized primary tumour as defined for stage 1 or 2 with dissemination limited to liver, skin and/or bone marrow

IV-S refers to infants under 1 year of age who would otherwise be characterized as having a stage I or II tumour but who also have unusual sites of remote disease, including multiple subcutaneous nodules, hepatic metastases and bone marrow involvement[60]. None of these cases have bone cortex metastases.

Pathology

Neuroblastoma commonly exhibits a haemorrhagic nesting of tumour cells, which are separated by fibrovascular bundles, with some necrosis and calcification[1,7]. Formation of densely speckled hyperchromatic nuclei with central fibrosis will result in rosette formation. In some instances, within the same patient, neuroblastoma is noted, with varying stages of maturation and differentiation to ganglioneuroblastoma and ganglioneuroma[1]. At times, undifferentiated neuroblasts appear as small round blue cells that may be difficult to differentiate from other tumour cell populations, including undifferentiated lymphoma, Ewing's tumour and certain instances of rhabdomyosarcoma[7]. Accurate diagnosis can usually be achieved by ultrastructural evaluation of the neuroblastoma cell, which demonstrates the presence of neurosecretory granules, neurotubules and neurofilaments[1,3,7]. Diagnosis can also be made by histological evaluation of bone marrow aspirates, which often demonstrate rosettes of neuroblastic tumour cells. More recently, immunocytological detection of bone marrow metastases using immunoperoxidase staining with monoclonal antibodies was more effective in detecting neuroblasts in the bone marrow than conventional histological evaluation[65,66]. In addition, neuroblasts can be detected in circulating blood using immunocytological techniques[67,68]. Immunodiagnostic evaluation also shows that neuron-specific enolase and serotonin are present in neuroblastic cells[69].

Prognostic markers

Generally the prognosis is better in infants less than 1 year of age than in older children. The site of the tumour is also important, and generally abdominal neuroblastoma has poorer prognosis than extra-abdominal tumours. The overall survival rate is also dependent on the clinical staging. Pathological classification of neuroblastoma has been revised in recent years in an effort to establish histological features that have prognostic value. Tumour grading and degrees of histological maturation have been modified and replaced by the Shimada classification system[70–72], which divides tumours into stroma-rich and stroma-poor categories (Table 4.6). The former are characterized by extensive Schwann-like spindle cell stroma with the appearance of a ganglioneuroblastoma. This favourable pattern may be diffuse, with immature cells uniformly distributed in an

Table 4.6 Shimada pathologic classification

	Favourable histology	Unfavourable histology
Stroma rich	Well differentiated Intermixed	Nodular
Stroma poor		
Age < 18 months	MKI < 200/5000	MKI < 100/5000
Age 18–60 months	MKI > 100/5000 Differentiating	MKI < 100/5000 Undifferentiated
Age > 5 years	None	All

MKI, mitosis–karyorrhexis index.

isolated well differentiated fashion, or intermixed throughout the tumour in microscopic clusters. The unfavourable stroma-rich tumours appear nodular. The three variables used to distinguish stroma-poor tumours into favourable or unfavourable categories include age at diagnosis, mitosis–karyorrhexis index (MKI) and neuroblast differentiation. The degree of differentiation is related to whether the neuroblast has developed nuclear and cytoplasmic features of ganglion cells: if 5% of the cells have a distinct rim of cytoplasm and a vesicular nucleus, the tumour is considered to be differentiating[71]. The MKI refers to the total number of necrotic tumour cells, cells with mitosis and cells with malformed, lobulated or pyknotic nuclei per 5000 cells examined[72]. The term "karyorrhexis" therefore refers to a variety of nuclear abnormalities that may indicate disturbed mitotic activity or borderline viability that may otherwise be difficult to detect histologically. The MKI varies with age so that a high MKI value in infants less than 18 months of age is >200/5000 cells, whereas >100/ 5000 cells is high for patients older than 18 months. Neuron-specific enolase is not a useful prognostic indicator in older children; however, elevated NSE levels (>100 ng/ml) in infants has been associated with a poor outlook. Neuroblastic cells secrete catecholamines and their by-products, including VMA, HVA, metanephrines and dopamine. Other biochemical tumour markers associated with neuroblastoma include cystathionine and elevated lactate dehydrogenase levels. These observations are non-specific, as cystathionine levels may also be elevated in patients with liver tumour and elevation of lactate dehydrogenase levels has been observed in some patients with lymphoma. Infants with an elevated serum ferritin level (>142 ng) have a guarded prognosis[73,74]. The excess ferritin is apparently produced by the tumour, and elevated serum ferritin levels are observed in patients with more advanced disease and in infants with hepatoblastoma. Although the majority of cases demonstrate catecholamine secretion (or its degradation by-products), an occasional neuroblastoma may be of parasympathetic origin and secrete acetylcholine rather than the catecholamines[1,3]. Like most other neural crest derived tumours, neuroblastoma has hormonal capacity and in some instances may secrete VIP, resulting in the hypokalaemic watery diarrhoea syndrome[75]. We therefore believe that neuroblastoma should probably be classified in the family of APUD tumours[3,25]. When tumour tissue is available for study, evaluation of DNA content of the neuroblasts by flow cytometry may be a useful prognostic guide. Unlike in most other malignant tumours, aneuploidy in neuroblastoma is associated with a better outlook than diploid[25]. In a study of the cellular DNA content of tumour cells in infants with neuroblastoma (by flow cytometry), Look et al. suggested that hyperdiploidy was associated with a more favourable diagnosis in infants less than 1 year of age but not in older patients[76].

Nakagawara et al. reported that amplification of N-*myc* oncogene in patients with neuroblastoma correlated inversely with age and tumour resectability and directly with prognosis[33]. More than 10 copies of the N-*myc* oncogene were observed in 66% of patients with neuroblastoma older than 1 year of age, compared with 13% at less than 1 year. N-*myc* amplification was associated with a lower resectability rate and increased mortality rate and was rarely seen in patients with stage I or II disease, but was more common in stage III and frequent (66%) in stage IV. Of interest was the fact that two of six patients with stage IV–S disease in this report had N-*myc* amplification[33]. In each instance this was associated with disease progression. The N-*myc* gene copy number is consistent for a given tumour at different times[77]. Seeger et al. confirmed these observations in an independent study indicating that amplification of more than 10 copies of N-*myc* oncogene was associated with advanced disease and a poor prognosis[32]. Stage IV–S tumours occur in infants of less than 1 year and have a high frequency of spontaneous tumour regression[48,49]. In contrast, more aggressive sporadic forms of neuroblastoma occur and may be caused by a second somatic mutation of the tumour[14,15].

Screening

The Japanese screening effort has doubled the incidence of neuroblastoma noted in young infants, but has not decreased the number of cases observed in older children[9]. Sawada described 170 cases of neuroblastoma in infants detected by screening. The study[11] included 49 infants (29%) with stage I tumours, 61 (36%) with stage II, 23 (14%) with stage III, 16 (9%) with stage IV and 21 (12%) with stage IV–S; 165 (97%) survived. Most cases detected by screening have triploid chromosomes and almost never have other adverse findings such as N-*myc* amplification[29]. These cases probably represent the type of neuroblastic tumour that spontaneously regresses[21,44], which suggests that the increased number of neuroblastic tumours detected by screening probably represents neuroblastoma that would otherwise regress and not present clinically[9,11,29]. Indeed, spontaneous regression of neuroblastoma has been observed in a subset of very young patients, particularly those under 1 year of age[12,13].

Neuroblastoma in infancy

Most newborn infants with neuroblastoma and 30% of infants with neuroblastoma less than 1 year of age have stage IV-S disease: more than 80% will have a long-term survival often without any specific therapy[12,13]. Age is a very important independent prognostic factor in patients with neuroblastoma[74]. Infants less than 1 year of age have a significantly improved outlook[1–3,31,34]. At the J.W. Riley Hospital for Children in Indianapolis[34], 76% of children younger than 1 year of age have survived, compared with 32% of children older than 1 year of age (Figure 4.4). This compares very well with studies from the Children's Cancer Study Group[52], where the survival for infants less than 1 year of age was 72%. This favoured outlook in the first year of life extends across all stages, including infants with stage IV metastatic disease, of whom almost half survive despite having bone cortex metastases[54]. This is in contrast to a survival rate of less than 10% for children over 1 year of age with stage IV tumours. For most infants with stage I neuroblastoma, complete surgical excision of the primary tumour is the only therapy required[1,31,34]. There is no evidence to suggest that chemotherapy improves the outlook for infants with completely excised stage I tumours. In patients with stage II disease, complete excision may not always be possible and microscopic tumour residual may be left behind, particularly in thoracic primary tumours with extension into intervertebral foramina, or abdominal or pelvic paraspinal tumours. If the patient has normal tumour markers, fewer than three copies of the N-*myc* oncogene, increased *trk* levels and aneuploid tumour chromosomal mode, no other therapy is necessary. However, if the tumour has more than 10 copies of N-*myc* oncogene, diploid DNA flow cytometry, and/or elevated serum ferritin levels (>142 ng), even in the infant age group, the residual disease should be treated with an intensive chemotherapy regimen using cis platin, Adriamycin, Cytoxan and etoposide (VP-16)[34]. This may be of particular importance if the regional lymph nodes are also involved[31]. Although resection of the primary tumour in association with intensive chemotherapy results in improved survival in patients with stage III tumours, the efficacy of surgical resection of the primary tumour in patients with stage IV disease remains a somewhat clouded issue[78,82]. In our experience at J.W. Riley Hospital for Children, the only survivors of stage IV disease have had excision of the primary tumour[78,81]. Matsumura et al.[79] in an evaluation of the role of surgery for metastatic neuroblastoma reported that seven of 11

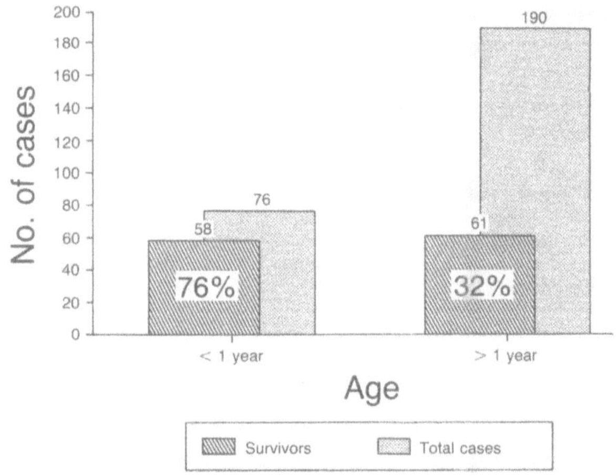

Figure 4.4 Bar chart showing a significantly improved survival rate for infants less than 1 year of age with neuroblastoma. Of 76 infants with neuroblastoma younger than 1 year, 58 (76%) survived , compared with only 61 of 190 (32%) cases older than 1 year. (From Grosfeld[34])

infants less than 1 year of age with stage IV disease who underwent complete but delayed primary resection of the tumour remained disease free for more than 5 years. In addition, infants less than 1 year of age had a better initial response to chemotherapy than older children. Of patients with stage IV disease who were younger than 1 year, 50% had no evidence of residual tumour at the time of delayed primary or second-look surgery compared with only 22% of cases older than 1 year. These observations suggest that resolution of metastases may have more impact on length of survival than surgical excision of the primary tumour. Aggressive surgical resection of the tumour should be attempted when disseminated disease is controlled by chemotherapy. These authors concluded that delayed primary tumour resection was of significant benefit in babies younger than 1 year and those with unfavourable Shimada histology[80]. Paul et al. reported a 5 year survival rate of 75% among stage IV patients less than 1 year of age, compared with a 10.5% survival rate in infants older than 1 year following multimodal treatment with MADDOC therapy (nitrogen mustard, vincristine, dacarbazine, doxorubicin, Cytoxan and cisplatin) and etoposide (VP-26) and cisplatin for relapse[83] (Figure 4.5). Of 78 babies less than 1 year of age, 24 (31%) had stage IV disease, which is a lower incidence than that observed in older children (Figure 4.6): 18 (75%) of them survived. All six patients without bone metastases and 12 of 16 with bone cortex involvement are alive. Five infants were less than 3 months of age at the time of diagnosis. However, the survival rate was similar in babies diagnosed and treated less than 6 months and more than 6 months of age at biopsy. Because of a significantly improved prognosis in these infants with stage IV disease using this treatment regimen, Paul et al.[83] do not advocate the use of bone marrow transplantation in babies less than 1 year of age. Reports by Kretschmar et al.[84] and Nickerson et al.[54] also note an improved survival rate in babies with stage IV neuroblastoma who were less than 1 year of age at diagnosis. Jereb et al.[85] in a retrospective study of 112 patients with neuroblastoma who were less than 2 years of age noted that infants with tumours at non-adrenal primary sites (neck, pelvis) had better prognosis. This correlates well with our own experience, in which babies with primary tumours arising in the neck, pelvis and mediastinum have a better survival rate than infants with primary abdominal tumours[1,34]. Survival rates in Jereb's review were 100% (10/10) for infants with stage I disease, 78% (21/27) for stage II, 87% (13/15) for stage III, and 88% (7/8) for stage IV-S without therapy. Although only 18% of infants less than 2 years old with stage IV tumours survived, this was significantly better than the 2% survival rate noted in children older than 2 years with metastatic disease (Figure 4.5). Survival rate of infants between 0 and 5 months was similar to that of patients diagnosed and treated between 6 months and 1 year. A recent report by Haase et al.[86] in

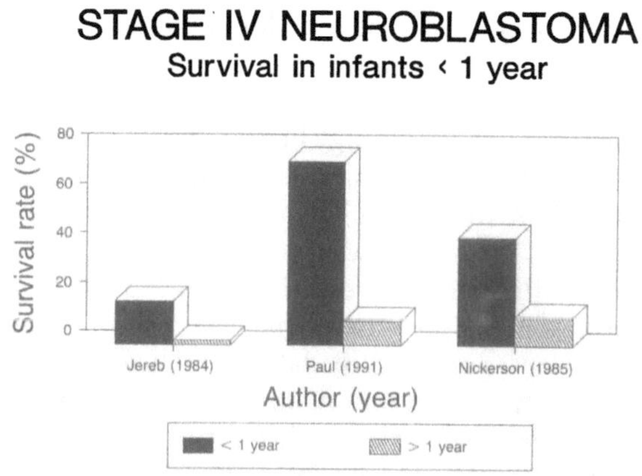

Figure 4.5 Bar chart showing improved survival rate in infants less than 1 year of age with stage IV neuroblastoma in three separate reports[54,83,85]. Recent aggressive multidrug treatment has resulted in significantly improved results (75% survival rate). (From Paul et al.[83])

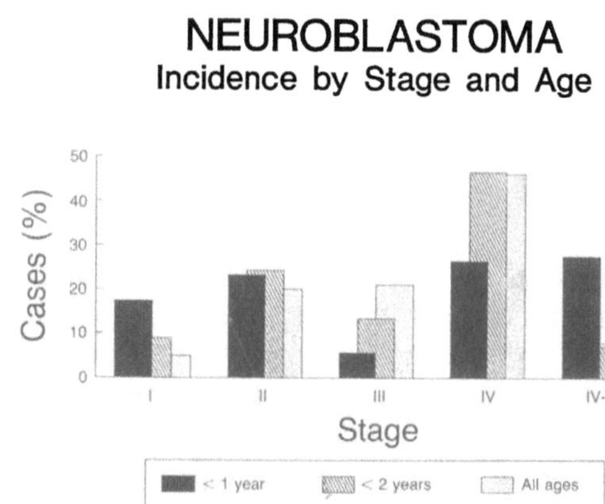

Figure 4.6 Bar chart showing the incidence of neuroblastoma by stage and age. Stages I and IV-S are more common in the first year of life. Almost 50% of the cases seen after 1 year of age have distant metastases (stage IV). There is a gradual reduction of stage I and increase of stage III cases with advancing age. (Data from Paul et al.[83] (< 1 year), Jereb et al.[85] (< 2 years) and Grosfeld[34] (all ages))

children over 1 year of age documented a clear survival advantage if the primary tumour was resected in patients with stage IV disease receiving an intensive four-drug chemotherapy regimen (cisplatin, etoposide, doxorubicin and cyclophosphamide). A median survival rate of 20 months (range 8–47 months) was achieved in 23 of 39 patients with complete resection (59%), compared with six of 23 (26%) with partial excision: 14 of the 39 children required an ipsilateral nephrectomy to achieve complete resection, and 12 of these 14 are disease-free survivors. No difference in survival rate was related to the timing of the surgical procedure or the site of the primary stage IV tumour[86]. Shamberger et al. confirmed this observation in a study of 18 children with stage III and 42 with stage IV neuroblastoma[87]. Although there was no difference in survival based on timing of operation, resection was safer if carried out after initial chemotherapy. The operative complication rate was higher in patients undergoing primary tumour resection at the time of diagnosis[87]. The Children's Cancer Study Group has observed that infants under 1 year of age with stage IV disease and more than 10 copies of the N-*myc* oncogene have rapidly progressive disease and often succumb despite chemotherapy. Therefore, in selected cases with poor prognostic factors, more intense chemotherapy regimens, complete resection of the primary tumour and perhaps bone marrow transplantation may be necessary to attain a cure in infants with stage IV disease who are younger than 1 year of age.

Stage IV-S

In contrast to cases of stage IV neuroblastoma with bone metastasis, the survival rate of infants with stage IV-S disease with remote metastases to the liver and subcutaneous tissue is greater than 80%[1–3,31,34] (Table 4.7). Many cases of neuroblastoma that occur in neonates are stage IV-S. These cases may represent as many as 30% of all cases that present in the first year of life (Figure 4.6). Significant tumour in the liver in neonates with stage IV-S disease may be present because the liver is a preferential site for tumour metastases in the fetus, where 93% of blood flow bypasses the uninflated lungs in utero, with a high flow occurring through the sinus venosus. The hepatic reticuloendothelial system may act as a trap for circulating tumour cells that bypass the pulmonary circulation. Although most patients with stage IV-S disease do well, infants that fail to survive often die from complications of the disease rather than from tumour progression. Complications of severe hepatomegaly include respiratory insufficiency as a result of significant elevation of the diaphragm by a large liver filled with tumour, renal compromise due to compression by the mass, and vomiting leading to protein–calorie malnutrition and aspiration pneumonia[34,54,55,78]. Infants less than 3 months of age have more symptoms related to hepatomegaly and tolerate therapy less well than older infants. Most cases of stage IV-S neuroblastoma complicated by respiratory insufficiency as a result of significant diaphragmatic elevation from hepatomegaly and tumour infiltration benefit from treatment with low-dose irradiation to the liver. Radiotherapy in the range of 600 R is well tolerated[54,55,78] with initial doses of 100–150 cGy/day. Initial doses are followed by a delay in therapy for 2 weeks and then, if no subjective regression in liver size is seen, the remaining dose can be administered. Although higher doses of irradiation have been used (3300 R) this practice has resulted in considerable morbidity, including development of multiple rib chondromas, chest and pelvic hypoplasia, radiation nephritis and hepatic fibrosis, and has been abandoned[55]. Although some early reduction in the size of the bulky tumour-filled liver is seen and peripheral oedema may resolve in a few weeks, complete resolution may take 6–15 months[31,34,54,78]. Resolution of liver mass is probably more related to the natural course of the disease than to radiotherapy. Although insertion of a Dacron reinforced silastic sheet to create a ventral abdominal wall hernia to make room for the enlarged liver has been advo-

Table 4.7 Survival in stage IV-S neuroblastoma

Author	Year	No. of cases	No. of survivors	%
D'Angio et al.[57]	1971	16	14	88
Breslow and McCann[52]	1971	19	18	95
Nitschke et al.[56]	1983	11	11	100
Jereb et al.[85]	1984	8	7	88
Nickerson et al.[54]	1985	35	31	89
Blatt et al.[55]	1987	11	8	73
Grosfeld[34]	1991	21	17	81

cated by some investigators, we have not found this technique to be very effective[89]. Mortality due to septic complications following insertion of silastic has been observed[57,78]. Total parenteral nutrition (TPN) is a useful therapeutic adjunct in infants with stage IV-S disease, as the enlarged liver elevates the diaphragm and changes the oesophagogastric angle, resulting in symptomatic gastro-oesophageal reflux. This may result in significant vomiting, and may increase the risk of aspiration and decrease caloric intake, leading to malnutrition[1,34]. TPN allows for adequate caloric intake, reduces the risk of infection from immunosuppression due to malnutrition, and may permit completion of chemotherapy courses if the patient requires it. Low-dose irradiation to the liver is useful in many cases, but the administration of cyclophosphamide at 5 mg/kg body weight may serve the same purpose[34]. Symptom resolution may take several weeks to occur following administration of chemotherapy. Regression of the tumour follows the same slow process (6–15 months) seen after treatment with radiotherapy. Treatment of stage IV-S neuroblastoma remains controversial. Survival of these unusual infants with hepatic metastases, subcutaneous nodules and in some instance bone marrow involvement without evidence of bone cortex is greater than 80%, often without specific treatment[12,13]. Patients with multiple subcutaneous nodules seem to have the most favourable outlook. This may be due to an increased immunological stimulus as a response to tumour being present in multiple sites. Increased uptake of major histocompatibility complex (MHC) class I antigen by neuroblastoma cells in vitro and in vivo appears to influence outcome favourably. Although most infants with stages I-IV neuroblastoma show a low level of class I MHC surface antigen expression, infants with stage IV-S disease show normal levels that are similar to those of control tissues[90]. MHC class I antigens may play a role in tumour immunosurveillance, and this may be why stage IV-S patients do so well. This suggests that class I MHC surface antigen expression reflects a more benign tumour behaviour. Sugio et al. reported that down-modulation of MHC class I antigen expression was associated with high levels of expression and amplification of N-*myc* oncogene in patients with advanced disease (stage III and IV)[91]. Although a significant number of babies with stage IV-S disease have tumour cells detected in the bone marrow, this occurrence has not adversely affected survival rate. A number of paediatric cancer centres avoid the use of either chemotherapy or irradiation in these cases. However, if tumour cells are recovered from the marrow aspirate and elevated serum ferritin and/or other adverse tumour markers (>10 copies of N-*myc*) are noted, an aggressive chemotherapy regimen is probably in order. Interventional therapy is indicated in stage IV-S disease with complications, whereas more aggressive chemotherapy is required in the usual case in which the tumour demonstrates more than 10 copies of N-*myc* oncogene and/or an elevated serum ferritin level (>142 ng/ml). Hann et al., evaluating biological differences between patients with stage IV and stage IV-S disease, indicated that elevated serum ferritin levels and E-rosette inhibition was higher in the former group[73]. Amplification of N-*myc* may occur in as many as one in 12 patients with a stage IV-S tumour who, despite having a good prognostic stage, develop progressive disease and die. This indicates that highly selected cases should be treated more aggressively, using multidrug chemotherapy as if they had a stage IV tumour. Some patients with stage IV-S neuroblastoma have survived without resection of the primary tumour and the site of primary tumour may not be identified in others , but given the information now available regarding the improved outlook for patients with stage IV tumours following complete resection of the primary tumour, resection of the primary neoplasm should also be performed in high-risk stage IV-S cases with poor prognostic markers when feasible.

A better understanding of the development and biological behaviour of the neural crest cell, improved insight regarding of the immune aspects of neuroblastoma, clarification of the role of screening programmes (e.g. at 12–18 months of age), refinements in combined therapy (particularly in the very young infant) and a more careful selection of certain patients for more aggressive treatment based on advanced stage, unfavourable Shimada tumour histology, elevated serum tumour markers, diploid DNA flow cytometry and more than 10 copies of N-*myc* oncogene may prove useful in further reducing the mortality rate of this highly unusual and potentially lethal paediatric malignancy in the first year of life.

References

1. Grosfeld JL (1986) Neuroblastoma. In: Ravitch MM, Welch K, Randolph JG, Rowe MI, O'Neill JA, eds. Pediatric surgery, 4th edn. Year Book Medical, Chicago, pp 283–293.
2. Pochedly C (1976) Neuroblastoma in infancy. In: Pochedly C, ed. Neuroblastoma. Publishing Sciences Group, Acton MA, pp 22–23.
3. Grosfeld JL (1986) Neuroblastoma in infancy and childhood. In: Hays DM, ed. Pediatric Surgical Oncology. Grune and Stratton, Orlando, pp 63–85.
4. Stiller CA, Parkin DM (1992) International variation in the incidence of neuroblastoma. Int J Cancer 52: 538–543.
5. Young JL, Ries LG, Silverberg E (1986) Cancer incidence, survival and mortality for children under 15 years of age. Cancer 58: 598–602.
6. Bader JL, Miller RW (1979) US cancer incidence and mortality in the first year of life. Am J Dis Child 133: 157–159.
7. Sawada T, Kidowaki T, Sakamoto I (1984) Neuroblastoma: mass screening for early detection and its prognosis. Cancer 53: 2731–2735.
8. Sawada T (1986) Outcome of 25 neuroblastomas revealed by screening in Japan. Lancet i: 377.
9. Bessho F, Hashizume K, Nakajo T, Kamoshita S (1991) Mass screening in Japan increased the detection of infants with neuroblastoma without a decrease in cases in older children. J Pediatr 119: 237–241.
10. Ishimoto K, Kiyokawa N, Fujita H et al. (1990) Problems of mass screening for neuroblastoma: analysis of false negative cases. J Pediatr Surg 25: 398–401.
11. Sawada T (1989) Present status of mass screening for neuroblastoma. Pediatr Rev 22: 336–356.
12. Haas D, Ablin AR, Miller C, Zoger S, Matthay KK (1988) Complete pathologic maturation and regression of stage IV-S neuroblastoma without treatment. Cancer 62: 818–825.
13. Evans AE, Baum E, Chard R (1981) Do infants with stage IV-S neuroblastoma need treatment? Arch Dis Child 56: 271–274.
14. Knudson AG Jr, Strong LC (1972) Mutation and cancer: a model for Wilms' tumour of the kidney. J Natl Cancer Inst 48: 313–324.
15. Knudson AG Jr, Meadows AT (1980) Regression of neuroblastoma IV-S: a genetic hypothesis. N Engl J Med 302: 1254–1256.
16. Chatten J, Voorhees ML (1967) Familial neuroblastoma. Report of a kindred with multiple disorders including neuroblastomas in four siblings. N Engl J Med 277: 1230–1236.
17. Hardy P, Nesbit M (1972) Familial neuroblastoma: report of a kindred with a high incidence of infantile tumors. J Pediatr Surg 80: 74–77.
18. Wagget J, Aherne G, Aherne W (1973) Familial neuroblastoma. Report of two sib pairs. Arch Dis Child 48: 63–75.
19. Gerson JM, Chatten J, Eisman S (1974) Familial neuroblastoma: a follow-up. N Engl J Med 290: 1487.
20. Pegelow CH, Ebbin AJ, Powars D, Towner JW (1975) Familial neuroblastoma. 87: 763–765.
21. Carlsen NLT (1986) Epidemiological investigation on neuroblastoma in Denmark 1943–1980. Br J Cancer 54: 977–988.
22. Neglia JP, Smithson WA, Gunderson P, King FL, Singher LJ, Robison LL (1988) Prenatal and postnatal risk factors for neuroblastoma. A case control study. Cancer 61: 2202–2206.
23. Voute P, Wadman S, Von Patten W (1970) Congenital neuroblastoma; symptoms in the mother during pregnancy. Clin Pediatr 9: 206–207.
24. Potter E, Parish JM (1942) Neuroblastoma in a still born fetus. Am J Pathol 18: 141–151.
25. Birner W (1966) Neuroblastoma as a cause of antenatal death. Am J Obstet Gynecol 82: 1388–1391.
26. Anders D, Kinderman G, Pfeiffer U (1973) Metastasizing fetal neuroblastoma with involvement of the placenta simulating erythroblastosis: report of two cases. J Pediatr 82: 50–53.
27. Strauss L, Driscoll SG (1964) Congenital neuroblastoma involving the placenta: report of two cases. Pediatrics 34: 23–31.
28. Weinberg T, Radman HM (1943) Fetal dystocia due to neuroblastoma of adrenals with metastases to liver. Am J Obstet Gynecol 46: 440–445.
29. Ishimoto K, Kiyokawa N, Fujita H et al. (1990) Problems of mass screening for neuroblastoma: analysis of false negative cases. J Pediatr Surg 25: 398–401.
30. Gilbert F, Feder M, Balaban G et al. (1984) Human neuroblastoma and abnormalities of chromosomes 1 and 17. Cancer Res 44: 5444–5449.
31. Pizzo PA, Miser JS, Cassady JR, Filler RM (1989) Solid tumors of childhood. In: Devita VT, Helman S, Rosenberg SA, eds. Cancer, Principles and Practice, 3rd edn. JP Lippincott, Philadelphia, pp 1525–1536.
32. Seeger RC, Brodeur GM, Sather H et al. (1985) Association of multiple copies of the N-*myc* oncogene with rapid tumor progression in neuroblastoma. N Engl J Med 313: 1111–1116.
33. Nakagawara A, Ikeda K, Tsuda T, Higashi H (1987) N-*myc* oncogene amplification and prognostic factors of neuroblastoma in children. J Pediatr Surg 22: 895–898.
34. Grosfeld JL (1991) Neuroblastoma: a 1990 overview. Pediatr Surg Int 6: 9–13.
35. Emery LG, Shields M, Shah NR, Garbes A (1983) Neuroblastoma associated with Beckwith-Wiedemann syndrome. Cancer 52: 176–179.
36. Grotting JC, Kassel C, Demner L (1979) Nesidioblastosis and congenital neuroblastoma. Arch Pathol Lab Med 103: 642–646.
37. Pendergass TW, Hanson JW (1976) Fetal hydantoin syndrome and neuroblastoma. Lancet ii: 150.
38. Sherman S, Roizen N (1976) Fetal hydantoin syndrome and neuroblastoma. Lancet ii: 517.
39. Seeler RA, Israel JN, Royal JE, Kaye CI, Rao S, Abulaban M (1979) Ganglioneuroblastoma and fetal hydantoin-alcohol syndromes. Pediatric 63: 524–527.
40. Kinney H, Faix R, Brazy J (1980) The fetal alcohol syndrome and neuroblastoma. Pediatrics 66: 130–132.
41. Hornstein L, Crowe C, Gruppo R (1977) Adrenal carcinoma in a child with a history of fetal alcohol syndrome. Lancet ii: 1292.
42. Carachi R, Auldist AW, Chow CW (1982) Neuroblastoma and Hirschsprung's disease. Z Kinderchir 35: 24–25.
43. Gaisie G, Kook SO, Young IW (1979) Coexistent neuroblastoma and Hirschsprung's disease: another manifestation of neurocristopathy. Pediatr Radiol 8: 161–163.
44. Michna BA, McWilliams NB, Kurmmel TM, Hartenberg MA, Salzberg AM (1988) Multifocal ganglioneuroblastoma coexistent with total colonic aganglionosis. J Pediatr Surg 23: 57–59.
45. Blatt J, Lee A, Taylor SR (1988) Neuroblastoma associated with adrenocortical defects. Pediatrics 82: 790–792.
46. Crowder RE (1957) The development of the adrenal gland in man with special reference to the origin and ultimate location of cell types and evidence in favour of the "cell migration" theory. Contrib Embryol 36: 195–210.
47. Ikeda Y, Lister J, Buyukpamukcu M (1981) Congenital neuroblastoma, neuroblastoma in-situ and the normal fetal development of the adrenal. J Pediatr Surg 16: 636–644.
48. Guin GH, Gilbert EF, Jones B (1968) Incidental neuroblastoma in infants. Am J Clin Pathol 51: 126–136.

49. Beckwith JB, Perrin EV (1963) In-situ neuroblastoma: a contribution to the natural history of neural crest tumours. Am J Pathol 43: 1089–1104.
50. Turkel SB, Itabashi HH (1974) The natural history of neuroblastic cells in the fetal adrenal gland. Am J Pathol 76: 225–244.
51. Ho PT, Estroff JA, Kozakewich H et al. (1993) Prenatal detection of neuroblastoma: a ten year experience from the Dana-Farber Cancer Institute and Children's Hospital. Pediatrics 92: 358–364.
52. Breslow B, McCann B (1971) Statistical estimation of prognosis for children with neuroblastoma. Cancer Res 31: 2098–2103.
53. Stokes SH, Thomas PRM, Perez CA, Vietti TJ (1984) Stage IV-S neuroblastoma – results with definitive therapy. Cancer 53: 2083–2086.
54. Nickerson HJ, Nesbit ME, Grosfeld JL, Baehner R, Sather H, Hammond D (1985) Comparison of stage IV and IV-S neuroblastoma in the first year of life. Med Pediatr Oncol 13: 261–268.
55. Blatt JB, Deutsch M, Wollman MR (1987) Results of therapy in stage IV-S neuroblastoma with massive hepatomegaly. Int J Radiat Oncol Biol Phys 13: 1467–1471.
56. Nitschke R, Humphry GB, Sexauer CL, Smith EI (1983) Neuroblastoma: therapy for infants with good prognosis. Med Pediatr Oncol 11: 154–158.
57. D'Angio GJ, Evans AE, Koop CE (1971) Special pattern of widespread neuroblastoma with a favourable prognosis. Lancet i: 1046–1049.
58. Tanabe M, Yoshida H, Ohnuma N, Iwai J, Takatani H (1993) Imaging of neuroblastoma in patients detected by mass screening using urinary catecholamine metabolites. J Pediatr Surg 25: 610–624.
59. Plumley DA, Grosfeld JL, Kopecky KK, Buckwalter KA, Chazevaughan W (1994) The role of spiral (helical) computerized tomography with three dimensional reconstruction in pediatric solid tumours. J Pediatr Surg 30: 317–321.
60. Evans AE, D'Angio GJ, Randolph JG (1971) A proposed staging for children with neuroblastoma. Cancer 27: 374–378.
61. Hayes FA, Green AA, Hutsu HO, Kumar M (1983) Surgicopathologic staging of neuroblastoma: prognostic significance of regional lymph node metastases. J Pediatr 102: 59–62.
62. Brodeur GM, Seeger RC, Barrett A et al. (1988) International criteria for diagnosis, staging and response to treatment in patients with neuroblastoma. J Clin Oncol 6: 1874–1881.
63. Haase GM (1991) Staging systems for neuroblastoma: a look at the old and the new. Pediatr Surg Int 6: 14–18.
64. Haase GM, Atkinson JB, Stram DO, Lukens JN, Matthay KK (1995) Surgical management and outcome of locoregional neuroblastoma: comparison of the children's cancer group and the international staging systems. J Pediatr Surg 30: 289–295.
65. Moss T, Reynolds P, Sather HN, Romansky SG, Hammond GD, Seeger RC (1991) Prognostic value of immunocytologic detection of bone marrow metastases in neuroblastoma. N Engl J Med 324: 219–226.
66. Nageu J, Kigasawa H, Zomioka K, Kogu N, Nishihira H, Nagao T (1994) Immunocytochemical detection of bone marrow-invasive neuroblastoma cells. Eur J Haematol 53: 74–77.
67. Sanders DG, Wiley FM, Moss TJ (1991) Serial immunocytologic analysis of blood for tumor cells in two patients with neuroblastoma. Cancer 67: 1423–1427.
68. Moss TJ, Sanders DG (1990) Detection of neuroblastoma cells in blood. J Clin Oncol 8: 736–740.
69. Makinen J (1972) Microscopic patterns as a guide to prognosis of neuroblastoma of childhood. Cancer 29: 1637–1646.
70. Seltzer PM, Marangos PJ, Parka AM et al. (1983) Raised neuron specific enolase in serum of children with metastatic neuroblastoma: a report from the Children's Cancer Study Group. Lancet ii: 361–363.
71. Shimada H, Chatten J, Newton WH Jr et al. (1984) Histopathological prognostic factors in neuroblastoma: definition of subtypes of ganglioneuroblastoma and an age-linked classification of neuroblastoma. J Natl Cancer Inst 73: 405–416.
72. Chatten J, Shimada H, Sather HN, Wong KY, Siegel SE, Hammond D (1988) Prognostic value of histopathology in advanced neuroblastoma: a report from the Children's Cancer Study Group. Hum Pathol 19: 1187–1198.
73. Hann HW, Evans AE, Cohen IJ, Leitmeyer JE (1981) Biologic differences between neuroblastoma stages IV-S and IV: measurement of serum ferritin and E-rosette inhibition in 30 children. N Engl J Med 305: 425–429.
74. Evans AE, D'Angio GJ, Propert K, Anderson J, Hann HL (1987) Prognostic factors in neuroblastoma. Cancer 59: 1853–1859.
75. Bloom SR, Polak JM, Pearse AGE (1973) Vasoactive intestinal polypeptide and watery diarrhoae syndrome. Lancet ii: 14–16.
76. Look AT, Hayes FA, Nitschke R, McWilliams NB, Green AA (1984) Cellular DNA content as a predictor of response to chemotherapy in infants with unresectable neuroblastoma. N Engl J Med 311: 231–235.
77. Brodeur GM, Hayes FA, Green AA et al. (1987) Consistent N-*myc* copy number in simultaneous or consecutive neuroblastoma samples from sixty individual patients. Cancer Res 47: 4248–4253.
78. Grosfeld JL, Schatzlein M, Ballantine TVN, Weetman RM, Baehner RL (1978) Metastatic neuroblastoma: factors influencing survival. J Pediatr Surg 13: 59–65.
79. Matsumura M, Atkinson JB, Hays DM et al. (1988) An evaluation of the role of surgery in metastatic neuroblastoma. J Pediatr Surg 23: 448–453.
80. Smith EI, Krous HF, Tunell WP, Hitch DC (1980) The impact of chemotherapy and radiation on secondary operations for neuroblastoma. Ann Surg 191: 561–569.
81. Grosfeld JL, Ballantine TVN, Baehner RL (1978) Experience with "second-look" operations in pediatric solid tumours. J Pediatr Surg 13: 375–380.
82. Starz A, Finkelstien J, Grosfeld JL et al. (1983) An evaluation of the role of surgery in disseminated neuroblastoma: a report from the Children's Cancer Study Group. J Pediatr Surg 18: 147–151.
83. Paul SR, Tarbell NJ, Kory B, Kretschmar CS, Lavally B, Grier HE (1991) Stage IV neuroblastoma in infants: longterm survival. Cancer 67: 1493–1497.
84. Kretschmar CS, Frantz CN, Rosen EM, Cassady JR, Levey R, Sallan SE (1984) Improved prognosis for infants with stage IV neuroblastoma. J Clin Oncol 2: 799–803.
85. Jereb B, Bretsky SS, Vogel R, Helson L (1984) Age and prognosis in neuroblastoma: review of 112 patients younger than two years. Am J Pediatr Hematol Oncol 6: 233–243.
86. Haase GM, O'Leary MC, Ramsay NKC et al. (1991) Aggressive surgery combined with intensive chemotherapy improves survival in poor risk neuroblastoma. J Pediatr Surg 26: 1119–1124.
87. Shamberger RC, Allarde-Segundo M, Kozakewich HPW, Grier HE (1991) Surgical management of stage III and IV neuroblastoma: resection before or after chemotherapy? J Pediatr Surg 26: 1113–1118.
88. Suita S, Zaizen Y, Kaneko M et al. (1994) What is the benefit of aggressive chemotherapy for advanced neuroblastoma with N-*myc* amplification? A report from the Japanese study group for the treatment of advanced neuroblastoma. J Pediatr Surg 29: 746–750.
89. Schnaufer L, Koop CE (1975) Silastic abdominal patch for

temporary hepatomegaly in stage IV-S neuroblastoma. J Pediatr Surg 10: 73–75.
90. Squire R, Fowler CL, Brooks SP, Rich GA, Cooney DR (1990) The relationship of class I MHC antigen expression to stage IV-S disease and survival in neuroblastoma. J Pediatr Surg 25: 381–386.
91. Sugio K, Nakagawara A, Sasazuki T (1991) Association of expression between N-*myc* gene and major histocompatibility complex class I gene in surgically resected human neuroblastoma. Cancer: 1384–1388.

Mesoblastic Nephroma and Wilms' Tumour

Prem Puri and V. Kalidasan

5

Introduction

The most common renal tumour encountered in the first month of life is congenital mesoblastic nephroma, which was described by Bolande et al.[1] in 1967. Congenital mesoblastic nephroma was diagnosed in 2.8% of patients enrolled in the National Wilms' Tumor Study (NWTS)[2]. A review of the NWTS also reveals that of 3340 patients registered in the study 27 with renal neoplasms were not more than 30 days old[3]. Of these 27 patients, 18 had mesoblastic nephroma, one had malignant rhabdoid tumour of the kidney, four had Wilms' tumour and four had non-neoplastic lesions. Neonatal Wilms' tumour is extremely rare, and has been reported to account for 0.1%–1.5% in most series[4–6].

Pathology

Bolande recognized congenital mesoblastic nephroma as a unique lesion that was benign in nature with a tendency to local infiltration. It could be distinguished clinically and pathologically from true congenital Wilms' tumour by its usually benign behaviour, a preponderance of mesenchymal derivatives and lack of the malignant epithelial components typical of Wilms' tumour. However, the tumour does have a locally infiltrative tendency, which distinguishes it from hamartomas with more limited growth potential. Beckwith[7] believes that the fetal kidney in congenital mesoblastic nephroma becomes stimulated to a fibromatous or leiomyomatous development as distinct from a true nephroblastoma and therefore behaves differently. He predicted that this tumour would have a pathological spectrum with classic benign congenital mesoblastic nephroma at one extreme and unequivocally malignant spindle cell sarcomas at the other, with intermediate lesions of indeterminate biological significance.

Congenital mesoblastic nephroma is usually solid and unilateral, and can attain a very large size. Typical mesoblastic nephroma tends to be firm to hard in consistency, whorled and pale yellow to whitish-grey in colour, with a bulging surface when cut. There is no evidence of necrosis or haemorrhage. Microscopically, typical mesoblastic nephroma is composed of uniform spindle-shaped cells, which are arranged in bundles and surround nephrons. Atypical and more aggressive mesoblastic nephromas (cellular variants) tend to be soft fleshy tumours with areas of gross haemorrhage and necrosis without well recognizable normal glomeruli or tubules[8]. Cystic degeneration may be noted. The cells are larger and exhibit atypia and mitotic activity. Perinephric extension may be seen in the atypical tumours. Congenital mesoblastic nephroma may occasionally be confused with rhabdoid variants of Wilms' tumour. Careful light microscopy is usually sufficient to establish the exact nature of the tumour; rarely, electron microscopy or immunocytochemical studies are needed[9].

Molecular characterization of congenital mesoblastic nephromas has been attempted, to compare it with Wilms' tumour. Mesoblastic nephroma did not express N-*myc* oncogene or the suppressor gene *WT1* seen in Wilms' tumour, and no loss of heterozygosity was found[10]. Gaillard et al.[11] have reported their findings on the nucleolar organizing regions in mesoblastic nephroma. Silver staining of nucleolar organizing region (Ag-NOR) proteins was used in an attempt to determine cellular proliferative activity. The cellular variants of congenital mesoblastic nephroma showed significantly greater number of Ag-NOR dots, compared with the typical and less cellular variants. These authors have suggested that Ag-NOR dots may be used in conjunction with other criteria to predict tumour behaviour and modify therapy. DNA ploidy and flow cytometric measurement of DNA have been attempted in mesoblastic nephroma, and DNA content may be another useful guide to management[12]. Chromosomal aberrations have been found in congenital mesoblastic nephroma[13,14]. Similarities between the karyotypes of congenital mesoblastic nephroma and leiomyoma have been shown[14]. Additional copies of chromosome 11 have been frequently found, as well as other less common abnormalities; there is some evidence that trisomy 11 may be found in association with the cellular variant of the tumour[15].

Renin production and hypertension have been reported as common features of congenital mesoblastic nephroma[16,17]. Several investigators have reported distinctive patterns of immunoreactive renin staining, suggesting that mesoblastic nephromas are a source of increased renin production. The most intense staining for renin was observed within areas of recognizable cortex trapped within the tumour. Renin was localized in cells of the walls of vessels running up to the glomeruli. Hypercalcaemia (and nephrocalcinosis) has been reported as a paraneoplastic phenomenon, which seems to disappear after nephrectomy[18,19].

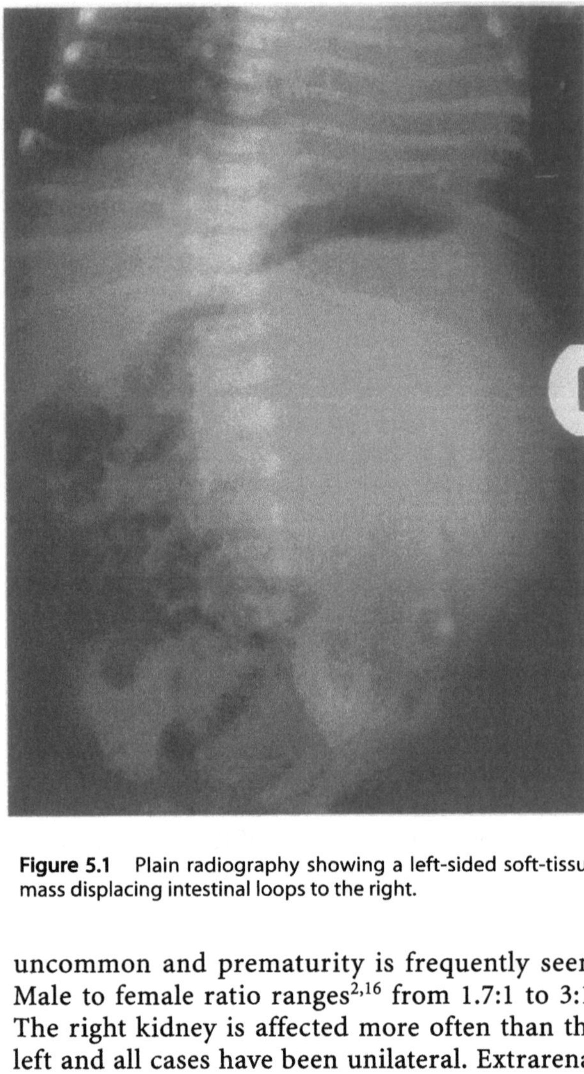

Figure 5.1 Plain radiography showing a left-sided soft-tissue mass displacing intestinal loops to the right.

Clinical features

Congenital mesoblastic nephroma presents in the neonatal period as a large non-tender abdominal mass. About 25% of these tumours are diagnosed in the first 3 days of life. More tumours are now being diagnosed by antenatal ultrasonography, but as yet there is no evidence to alter the management of the pregnancy or the treatment of the tumour[20]. Maternal polyhydramnios is not uncommon and prematurity is frequently seen. Male to female ratio ranges[2,16] from 1.7:1 to 3:1. The right kidney is affected more often than the left and all cases have been unilateral. Extrarenal extension of the tumour has been found at surgery in 15%–20% of cases. Some patients present with hypertension and congestive cardiac failure. Haematuria is a rare presentation. Haemorrhagic shock and disseminated intravascular coagulation have been noted in a few cases[21]. Bleeding may be associated with tumour rupture and haemoperitoneum[22]. Associated congenital anomalies were seen in 14% of patients in an NWTS survey[2].

Diagnosis

Plain radiography of the abdomen shows a large soft-tissue abdominal mass that may rarely show calcification (Figure 5.1). Sonography demon-

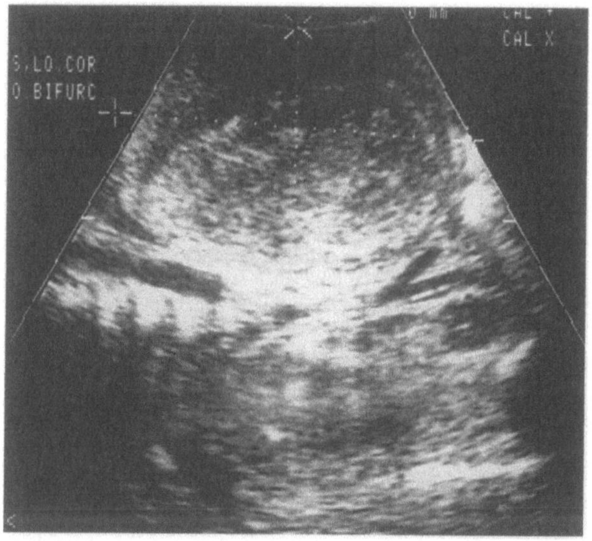

Figure 5.2 Ultrasonography demonstrates a mixed echogenic mass.

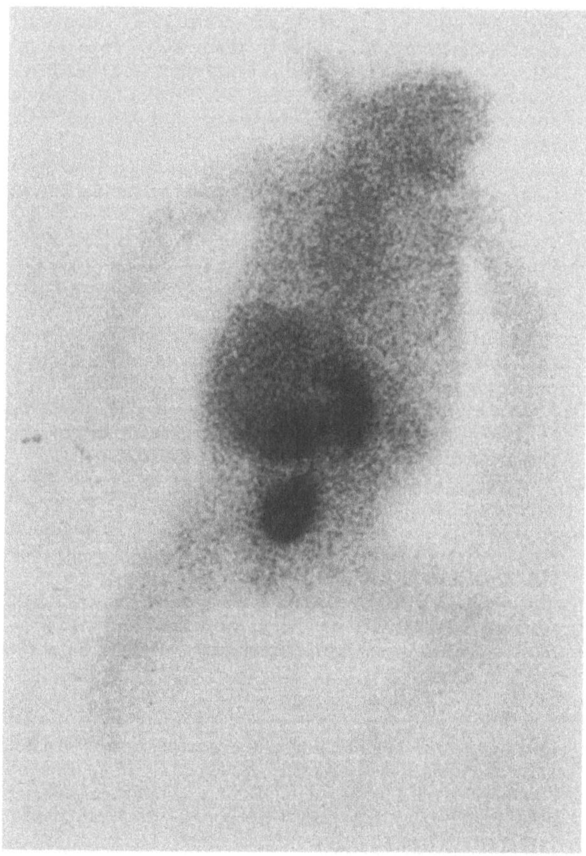

Figure 5.3 Renal scintigraphy (dimercaptosuccinate) shows function in the renal mass.

strates the solid nature of the tumour and its renal origin; most commonly a mixed echogenic mass is seen (Figure 5.2). Congenital mesoblastic nephroma should be easily distinguishable from hydronephrosis and renal cystic disorders. Congenital mesoblastic nephroma is the only primary renal tumour with function demonstrable by renal scintigraphy: excretion of radionuclide is due to functioning nephrons trapped in the tumour (Figure 5.3)[23]. Computed tomography may be needed to delineate the anatomy, especially in exophytic tumours that involve one pole of the kidney, which may be amenable to treatment by partial nephrectomy. Tumour biopsy is not needed. Congenital mesoblastic nephroma has been reported in a solitary kidney, but true mesoblastic nephroma does not seem to present in a bilateral manner[24].

Treatment

The treatment of congenital mesoblastic nephroma is excision. Radiotherapy has never been advocated, but some children have been treated with chemotherapy for the cellular variants of the tumour. However, adjuvant chemotherapy seems to be unnecessary even where there has been tumour rupture: local recurrence is rare. Distant metastases have been reported but are extremely uncommon[25]. A review of 38 patients with the cellular variant of mesoblastic nephroma by Gormley et al.[26] showed that seven children had recurrence and three died. They found pathologically positive surgical margins to be the only statistically significant predictor of recurrent disease. Frozen section may help in obtaining tumour-free margins during surgery. However, recent studies in molecular biology may shed further light on tumour behaviour and add criteria for further therapy after surgery. Partial nephrectomy may be performed in selected cases, and in this event obtaining a tumour-free margin is very important[27]. Currently, surgery is the only therapy needed, and chemotherapy should be reserved for the rare recurrence. However, if the tumour is discovered to be a Wilms' tumour on pathological examination further management will be dictated by the nature of the tumour and its stage as outlined in the NWTS protocol for Wilms' tumour.

Complications

The main complication relating to surgery appears to be operative rupture, which has a reported incidence as high as 10% in some series[2]. The nature of congenital mesoblastic nephroma is to infiltrate the capsule of the kidney and go beyond it locally, and therefore perioperative rupture is the commonest complication encountered during the mobilization and removal of the tumour. It would seem that nephrectomy alone is a treatment of choice for congenital mesoblastic nephroma even when there has been intraoperative rupture. Hypotension from blood loss is another complication, which can be avoided with meticulous surgical technique during the process of ligating and dividing the renal pedicle. In the past, complications related to chemotherapy and radiotherapy were unacceptably high in this age group. These modalities should be used only if a nephroblastoma or a congenital mesoblastic nephroma with a cystic appearance and a lot of haemorrhage in it is suspected. Local recurrence is unusual, and adequate margins should be allowed when resecting the tumour in order to remove it whole. If unusual cellularity of the tumour is reported by the pathologist in an infant over 3 months of age or the tumour is unusually cystic with haemorrhage at the time of surgery, local recurrence of the tumour should be looked for, and a second operation may be necessary 3–6 months later.

Prognosis

Survival rate in these patients is very good. Several studies have shown follow-up for several years with no recurrence of disease.

References

1. Bolande RP, Brough AJ, Izant RJ (1967) Congenital mesoblastic nephroma of infancy. A report of 8 cases and the relationship to Wilms' tumour. Pediatrics 40: 272–278.
2. Howell CG, Othersen HB, Kiviat NE, Norkool P, Beckwith JB, D'Angio GJ (1982) Therapy and outcome in 51 children with mesoblastic nephroma: a report of the National Wilms' Tumor Study. J Pediatr Surg 17: 826–831.
3. Hrabovsky EE, Otherson HB, de Lorimer A, Kelalis P, Beckwith JB, Takashima J (1986) Wilms' tumour in the neonate: a report from the National Wilms' Tumor Study. J Pediatr Surg 21: 385–387.
4. Crom DB, Wilimas JA, Green AA, Pratt CB, Jenkins JJ, Behm FG (1989) Malignancy in the neonate. Med Pediatr Oncol 17: 101–104.
5. Campbell AN, Chan HSL, O'Brien A, Smith CR, Becker LE (1987) Malignant tumors in the neonate. Arch Dis Child 62: 19–23.
6. Ritchey ML, Azizkhan RG, Beckwith JB, Hrabovsky EE, Haase GM (1995) Neonatal Wilms' Tumor. J Pediatr Surg 30: 856–859.
7. Beckwith JB (1974) Mesenchymal renal neoplasms of infancy revisited. J Pediatr Surg 9: 803–805.
8. Chan HSL, Mancer K, Weitzman SS (1987) Congenital mesoblastic nephroma: a clinicoradiologic study of 17 cases representing the pathologic spectrum of the disease. J Pediatr 111:65.
9. Weeks DA, Beckwith JB, Mierau GW, Zuppan CW (1991) Renal neoplasms mimicking rhabdoid tumour of kidney. A report from the National Wilms' Tumor Study Pathology Center. Am J Surg Pathol 15: 1042–1054.
10. Tomlinson GE, Argyle JC, Velasco S, Nisen PD (1992) Molecular characterization of congenital mesoblastic nephroma and its distinction from Wilms' tumour. Cancer 70: 2358–2361.
11. Gaillard D, Bouvier R, Sonsino E et al. (1992) Nucleolar organizer regions in congenital mesoblastic nephroma. Pediatr Pathol 12: 811–821.
12. Barrantes JC, Toyn C, Muir KR et al. (1991) Congenital mesoblastic nephroma: possible prognostic and management value of assessing DNA content. J Clin Pathol 44: 317–320.
13. Schofield DE, Yunis EJ, Fletcher JA (1993) Chromosome aberrations in mesoblastic nephroma. Am J Pathol 143: 714–724.
14. Carpenter PM, Mascarello JT, Krous HF, Kaplan JW (1993) Congenital mesoblastic nephroma: cytogenic comparison to leiomyoma. Pediatr Pathol 13: 435–441.
15. Mescarello JT, Cajulis TR, Krous HF, Carpenter PM (1994) Presence or absence of trisomy 11 is correlated with histologic subtype in congenital mesoblastic nephroma. Cancer Genet Cytogenet 77: 50–54.
16. Yokomori K, Hori T, Takemura T, Tsuchida Y (1988) Demonstration of both primary and secondary reninism in renal tumours in children. J Pediatr Surg 23: 403–409.
17. Malone PS, Duffy PG, Ransley PG, Risdon RA, Cook T, Taylor M (1989) Congenital mesoblastic nephroma, renin production and hypertension. J Pediatr Surg 24: 599–600.
18. Woolfield NF, Abbott GD, McRae CU (1988) A mesoblastic nephroma with hypercalcaemia. Aust Pediatr J 24: 309–310.
19. Angulo JC, Lobez JT, Ereno C, Flores N (1991) Congenital mesoblastic nephrom, nephrocalcinosis and hypertrophic pyloric stenosis. J Surg Oncol 48: 142–144.
20. Matsumura M, Nishi T, Sasaki Y, Yamada R, Yamamoto H, Ohhama Y (1993) Prenatal diagnosis and treatment strategy for congenital mesoblastic nephroma. J Pediatr Surg 28: 1607–1609.
21. Zach TL, Cifuentes RF, Strom RL (1991) Congenital mesoblastic nephroma, hemorrhagic shock and disseminated intravascular coagulation in a newborn infant. Am J Perinatol 8: 203–205.
22. Goldberg J, Liu P, Smith C (1994) Congenital mesoblastic nephroma presenting with hemoperitoneum and shock. Pediatr Radiol 24: 54–55.
23. Kirks DR, Kaufman RA (1989) Function with mesoblastic nephroma: imaging-pathologic correlation. Pediatr Radiol 19: 136–139.

24. Nicholson DA, Gupta SC (1990) Case report: congenital mesoblastic nephroma occurring in a solitary kidney. Clin Radiol 41: 211–213.
25. Heidelberger KP, Ritchey ML, Dauser RC, McKeever PE, Beckwith JB (1993) Congenital mesoblastic nephroma metastatic to the brain. Cancer 72: 2499–2502.
26. Gormley TS, Skoog SJ, Jones RB, Maybee D (1989) Cellular congenital mesoblastic nephroma: what are the options? J Urol 142: 479–483.
27. Kalidasan V, Mammen A, Hutson JM, Kelly JH, Auldist AW (1994) Congenital mesoblastic nephroma: treatment options. Pediatr Surg Int 9: 524–525.

Liver Tumours

Yechiel Sweed and Jehuda A. Bar-Maor

6

Introduction

Neonatal primary hepatic tumours are rare, and few cases are reported in both small and large series[1–4]. Benign tumours, including haemangioendothelioma and mesenchymal hamartoma, account for the majority of hepatic lesions; hepatic malignancies are extremely rare[5–7]. This low incidence of malignancy in the neonatal period is different from that of infancy and childhood in which two-thirds of patients present with hepatoblastoma and hepatocarcinoma[1]. Liver tumours of the newborn pose a challenge to all disciplines of paediatric practice. The benign vascular lesions can reach a large size before discovery, and may present with a life-threatening complication such as congestive heart failure, whereas the malignant tumours are unresectable in half the patients at the time of diagnosis[8,9]. A combined management plan by surgeons, neonatologists, oncologists and anaesthetists have minimized morbidity and mortality rates in both patient groups, although the prognosis for patients with malignant disease is still poor[1,9]. As a rule, complete hepatic resection is necessary for cure in malignant tumours, and surgical removal is the treatment of choice for many benign lesions that can be safely resected[1,3]. However, vascular lesions of the liver can now be successfully treated without surgical resection in most patients, whereas in patients with malignant tumours chemotherapy has a significant effect on survival rate as it is potentially life-saving in initially unresectable cases and is the only effective method to eliminate diffuse metastases before surgery[8,10–12]. The survival rate of patients with disease unresectable by standard methods has improved with total hepatectomy and liver transplantation[13].

Prenatal diagnosis

The increasing utilization of high-resolution ultrasonography has resulted in the ability to diagnose congenital anomalies and tumours at an earlier embryonal age. The more common diseases associated with embryonal hepatomegaly include infectious diseases (e.g. cytomegalovirus and toxoplasmosis), congenital haemolytic anaemia (e.g. spherocytosis), congestive heart failure and metabolic diseases (e.g. galactosaemia and tyrosinaemia).

Liver tumours in the fetus can cause hepatic enlargement or simply a change in the sonographic appearance of this organ[14,15]. Fetal benign or malignant liver tumours have typical echogenic findings. Among the tumours are benign hepatic haemangioma, with hypoechogenic sonographic appearance[16]; hepatoblastoma, which is the most frequent hepatic malignancy in fetal life, with its predominant echogenic sonographic appearance[17]; and mesenchymal hamartoma, which generally appears as an irregular mass with solid and cystic components[18]. Another benign hepatic fetal lesion is the solitary hepatic cyst, which can be diagnosed antenatally[19] but is often diagnosed as an incidental finding at surgery in the elderly[20]. Hepatic calcifications can occur with both hamartomas and hepatoblastomas[14,21], but

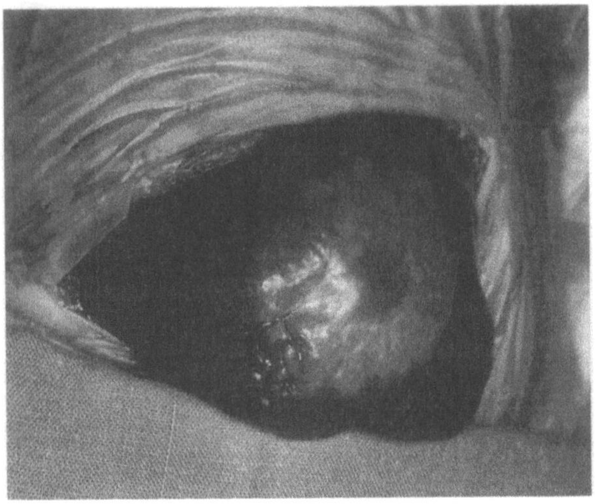

Figure 6.1 Macroscopic appearance of haemangioendothelioma of the liver showing a bull's-eye feature.

are more frequently associated with intrauterine infections and thrombosis of the portal and hepatic venous systems[22,23].

In evaluation of a fetus with a right abdominal solitary or multicystic mass, other fetal conditions which are more frequent and are not associated with the liver must be considered, including multicystic renal malformations (e.g. hydronephrosis, renal cysts and cystic dysplasia), congenital gastrointestinal atresias and stenosis, and bowel obstructions caused by other mechanical or neuronal abnormalities (e.g. meconium ileus or Hirschsprung's disease). Choledochal cyst can also be diagnosed prenatally and should be included in the differential diagnosis[24]. The recognition of any abdominal mass should alert the physician to the need for early neonatal intervention after appropriate evaluation.

Benign tumours

Infantile haemangioendothelioma

Hepatic haemangioendotheliomas are the commonest benign liver tumours of the neonatal period and infancy[25], the majority being diagnosed before 6 months of age with 85% of patients symptomatic by 2 months of age[26]. Females are affected twice as commonly as males[8]. Haemangiomas involving the liver can pose life-threatening complications in the first year of life[27,28]. The most lethal is high-output congestive heart failure, due to large intrahepatic arteriovenous communications, which can be refractory to conservative therapy with up to 90% mortality rate[2,26]. Aggressive medical management with hepatic artery ligation or embolization has improved survival rates significantly[29].

Pathology

Haemangiomatous hepatic lesions range from 1 to 15 cm in diameter, are non-encapsulated and can be either solitary or multicentric[2,25] (Figure 6.1). The solitary hepatic haemangioendothelioma is a less common lesion with a better prognosis because it is usually not associated with congestive heart failure[8]. Weinberg and Finegold[30] reviewed 1256 paediatric patients with primary hepatic tumours, and found that 13% had vascular tumours of the liver. Two histological patterns of hepatic haemangioendothelioma were described by Dehner and Ishak[2]. Type I haemangioendothelioma, the most common vascular lesion, is usually characterized by channels of varying size, lined by a single layer of endothelial cells in a myxomatous stroma that also includes small bile ducts. Regression of this histological type is frequent. Type II haemangioendothelioma appears more aggressive, with budding structures lined by endothelial cells that are larger, and more pleomorphic and hyperchromatic, than those of type I and can be confused with angiosarcoma of the adult. Unlike angiosarcoma, however, type II haemangioendotheliomas have frequently demonstrated cavernous differentiation, fibrosis and calcification – features associated with regression[30]. Many tumours show features of both types of histological lesion[2] (Figure 6.2). Although the majority of infants with haemangioendothelioma have benign lesions, a few cases of angiosarcoma have been reported in early childhood[31]. Thus it is not possible to predict with full confidence the ultimate course of a hepatic haemangioendothelioma from the histology of the lesion[30,32].

The natural evolution of hepatic lesions is difficult to discern because of the frequent need for intervention. Typically the evolution of the haemangioendotheliomas of the liver parallels that of skin lesions. They proliferate and undergo rapid enlargement during the first 6 months of life,

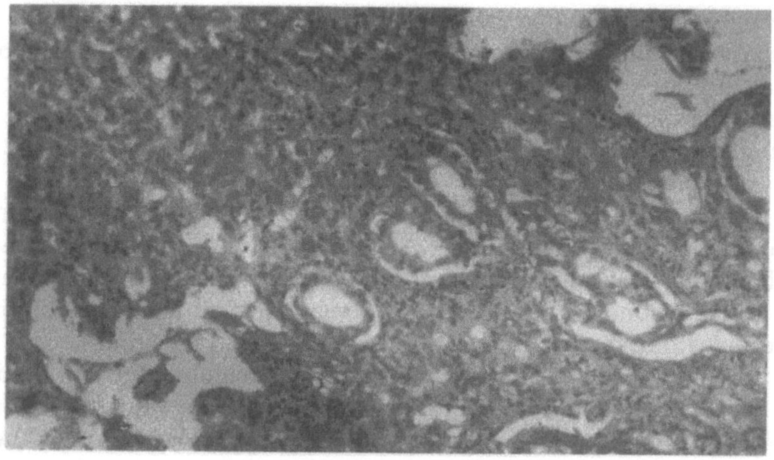

Figure 6.2 Histological appearance of haemangioendothelioma from the patient in Figure 6.1, showing intercommunicating vascular channels lined by endothelial cells with ill-defined margins protruding into the liver parenchyma, and focal bile duct proliferation.

followed by slow growth and stabilization at 1 year of age and later spontaneous regression[8,26,33,34]. The time course for involution is variable: most lesions have started to regress by 2–3 years of age, and over 75% of lesions resolve by the age of 5–7 years[26,33,35]. Although this evolution and spontaneous involution appears in some patients, respiratory distress occurs in about half by 6 weeks of age, and some fatalities occur as a result of congestive heart failure despite medical treatment[34].

Clinical presentation

Hepatomegaly is the usual presentation of haemangioendothelioma in the neonate and is commonly associated with congestive heart failure in the absence of congenital heart disease[29]. A typical presentation consists of a triad of hepatomegaly, congestive heart failure and cutaneous haemangiomas[2,8,36,37]. The hepatomegaly is usually in excess of that expected from the congestive heart failure, and medical treatment of cardiac failure has little effect on liver size[27]. Often a bruit is heard over the liver. Haematological abnormalities associated with the tumour include thrombocytopenia[38–40], anaemia[27,34,41] and coagulopathy[28,36]. Primary hepatic symptoms and signs such as jaundice[42] or hepatic and portal hypertension[26,43] are uncommon.

Congestive heart failure occurs in two-thirds of patients and is a high-output heart failure[8]. It is caused mainly by the arteriovenous shunting of blood from the hepatic artery to hepatic veins through the abnormal lesions, but may be exacerbated by expansion of the plasma volume or accompanying anaemia[44]. The haemodynamic changes of this large left-to-right shunt include decreased peripheral resistance, decreased diastolic blood pressure, increased cardiac output and widened pulse pressure[27]. A rare presentation of hepatic haemangioma is fatal intraperitoneal haemorrhage as a result of spontaneous rupture of the lesion, which usually occurs within the first 2 weeks of life[45,46].

Diagnosis

The diagnosis of hepatic haemangioendothelioma can usually be made by typical physical and laboratory findings in an infant less than 6 months old. The triad of hepatomegaly, high-output cardiac failure and cutaneous haemangiomas is strongly suggestive of hepatic haemangioma. The laboratory findings usually reveal normal liver function tests except for a raised level of serum bilirubin in one-third of patients[8], and coagulopathy secondary to platelet sequestration (Kasabach–Merritt syndrome) in about half of these infants[29]. Confirmation of diagnosis can be obtained by abdominal ultrasonography, ^{99m}Tc radionuclide scan, computed tomography of the liver (CT) or selective hepatic arteriography[25,36,40,47]. Initial radiological investigations should include plain radiography of the abdomen and chest, which usually show cardiomegaly with or without increased pulmonary vascular markings and an enlarged liver that may contain calcifications, respectively[27].

Abdominal ultrasonography may show multiple areas of non-homogeneity throughout the liver, which represent multiple masses within the parenchyma[48]. On the real-time view, the areas are shown to be rounded nodular densities[41]. A dilated proximal abdominal aorta and large draining hepatic veins on ultrasonography indicates arteriovenous shunting within the hepatic mass[48]. Technetium-99m scan of a multicentric haemangioendothelioma will reveal multiple diffuse lesions in both lobes of the liver, with less activity compared with the normal liver during the first flow of the study, whereas in delayed static studies the reverse is seen[49].

CT with a rapid-sequence technique is considered to be pathognomonic for haemangioendothelioma of liver and is as specific as angiography for the diagnosis of this lesion[25,41]. CT before injection of contrast medium reveals round or oval homogeneous masses, with CT Housefield units lower than those of the surrounding liver. After intravenous bolus injection of contrast medium the lesions are enhanced to a greater degree than the normal liver, and on delayed scans the lesions become isodense with the normal liver[36].

Selective angiography is valuable in diagnosis and can also be useful in treatment; however, it is invasive. It can be performed through the umbilical artery in the newborn, or through puncture of the femoral artery in the infant. It may reveal the vascular character of the lesion, its early venous drainage and the tortuosity of the vessels, and may give an indication of whether the lesion is resectable[40].

Magnetic resonance imaging (MRI) has been used to evaluate disseminated haemangiomatosis and the extent of visceral involvement, including the liver[50]. It has been found to be accurate in the assessment of vascular liver tumours in adults[51], and has an advantage over CT because it does not use ionization radiation.

The differential diagnosis of hepatic haemangioendothelioma should include neuroblastoma with diffuse metastases to the liver and hepatoblastoma. MRI is helpful for liver imaging and especially in differentiating haemangiomas and malignant tumours[52,53]. The absence of a primary tumour, with normal vanillylmandelic acid levels and negative bone marrow and bone scans, helps to differentiate this tumour from neuroblastoma. Normal α-fetoprotein levels distinguish these patients from those with hepatoblastoma.

Treatment

In the absence of symptoms no treatment is necessary, but the patient must be carefully observed for cardiac failure, respiratory distress and massive hepatomegaly. The initial management of a symptomatic patient includes diuretics and digitalis for congestive heart failure, with corticosteroids to control coagulopathy and reduce tumour size. Steroid therapy in the form of prednisone, 2–5 mg/kg per day, has been the most widely used therapeutic measure since the first report[35,54] in 1969–70. However, some patients do not respond to steroid therapy[55,56]. Recently, the use of Interferon Alfa-2a[39], or cyclophosphamide[57], have been reported to improve the condition of patients refractory to the first mode of medical treatment. The daily subcutaneous injections of Interferon Alfa-2a (up to 3 million units per square metre of body surface) for 9–14 months[39], or the cyclophosphamide therapy at a dose of 10 mg/kg per day for 3 consecutive days, 5 weeks apart[41,57], have both produced dramatic response and early regression of life-threatening hemangiomas of infancy[39,57].

Failure to respond to medical management necessitates hepatic artery occlusion, either surgically[34,56] or by angiographic embolization[58,59]. It is important to emphasize that the length of life between onset of symptoms and death for those who die without surgical intervention is only 1 month, which gives a short time for the trial of any regimen that is not as definitive as ligation or embolization of the hepatic artery[8]. The success rates of non-invasive surgical treatment by ligation[60] or embolization[8] of the hepatic artery are 72%–75% and 62%, respectively.

Radiotherapy in doses from 200 to 2000 mCi has been widely used[25,27], although this should be reserved as a last resort in the sequence of therapeutic trials because of the potential long-term side-effects, including a low risk (1%) of induced malignant conditions[40,61].

Surgical resection is rarely feasible because of the huge size and diffuse nature of these lesions, and is recommended mainly for localized angiomas (solitary haemangioendotheliomas), especially if they are complicated by intraperitoneal haemorrhage[62]. Other indications for hepatic lobectomy or local resection of localized haemangioma are congestive heart failure that is unresponsive to medical therapy, and lesions undifferentiable from a malignant growth[8,28]. Essentially, hepatic haemangiomas can be divided into resectable and non-resectable groups only on the basis of angiographic findings. Large localized lesions can be successfully treated with ligation or embolization of the appropriate left or right hepatic artery[58,63]. Liver transplantation may be required in infants with haemangioendotheliomas supplied mainly by the portal vein[25].

Prognosis

The survival rate of infants with haemangioendothelioma has improved dramatically, from 30% in 1972[27] to 80% in 1988[25]. This improvement has been attributed mainly to the early treatment of infants by ligation or embolization of the hepatic artery[56,58], as well as to medical treatment with Interferon Alfa-2a or cyclophosphamide[25,41,57]. Patients with localized hepatic haemangioma have a far better prognosis than those with multicentric haemangioendothelioma, with an overall survival rate of 94% in the former group compared with 40% in the latter.

Mesenchymal hamartoma

Mesenchymal hamartoma is an uncommon benign developmental anomaly of the liver that affects newborns, infants and young children, and usually presents in the first year of life[29,64]. It is the second most common benign liver tumour (following haemangioma) seen in infancy[65]. Mesenchymal hamartoma has an excellent long-term prognosis[65–68]. However, neonates still compose a high-risk group of patients, especially those with a prominent angiomatous tissue compound inside their tumour[3,64,69,70].

Pathology

The lesion appears grossly as a large solitary rounded or irregular mass and mostly arises in the right lobe of the liver[29]. This is often large[64], measuring more than 8 cm in diameter, with an average weight of 1300 g. It can be deeply embedded within the parenchyma, but often protrudes from the liver to become pedunculated on a broad base[71]. Although the tumour is sharply demarcated from the adjacent liver parenchyma, it has no definite capsule. On section, the tumour is composed of multiple cysts filled with a yellowish fluid or mucoid material. Microscopic examination reveals large cystic spaces with non-epithelial lining, although in some cases there is a bile-duct-type lining composed of flattened or cuboidal epithelium. The cysts are surrounded by dense fibrous connective tissue septa, and interspersed in a loose myxoid stroma containing prominent ground substance, mesenchymal cells, blood vessels and proliferation of bile ducts. Within the interstitium and between the cysts there are usually islands of compressed liver tissue[65]. This tumour-like lesion is usually benign, and no cases with progressive cellular proliferation, or cellular atypism to suggest neoplasia, have been reported[30]. In a few cases, the hamartomas are highly vascularized and behave clinically and radiologically like a haemangioendothelioma[69,70].

The exact pathogenesis of mesenchymal hamartoma is not clear, but the prevalent theory is that it represents an aberrant development of primitive mesenchyme in the portal tracts, probably from the bile ducts[71].

Clinical presentation and diagnosis

The commonest presenting symptom is a progressive abdominal distension of 1–2 months duration[65]. Other symptoms include poor appetite and respiratory distress as a result of congestive heart failure and/or impaired diaphragmatic excursion from the underlying hepatic mass[29,70,72]. Some patients are asymptomatic and the tumour is discovered incidentally at autopsy or on routine physical examination[65]. Examination reveals a right upper quadrant mass or hepatomegaly in all patients, associated with dilated superficial abdominal veins or cachexia in a few cases[73,74].

Laboratory evaluation is not helpful in making the diagnosis, and results of liver function tests are usually within normal limits. High serum levels of α-fetoprotein were measured in five of seven patients reported in Japan[75] and in one case reported in the USA[76]. In all these patients the high levels rapidly decreased to normal – after resection of the tumour in the first group and after medical treatment in the patient reported from the USA.

The diagnosis is usually suggested by CT and by ultrasonography[65]. Ultrasonography typically reveals a collection of fluid-filled spaces with septa and some echogenic foci[77]; CT usually shows an intrahepatic cyst mass with smooth margins and a septate central cystic area. It supports the results of ultrasonography by showing the extent of the hepatic mass and its relationship to adjacent structures[47,78]. Angiography may be useful, showing in most cases a hypovascular cystic mass, but is not necessary[65,68]. Technetium-99m radionuclide scan may be helpful in showing an intrahepatic mass with decreased uptake.

The differential diagnosis of mesenchymal hamartoma is limited and includes malignant mesenchymoma with a cystic component, and a rare lesion of cystic hepatoblastoma[79]. Malignant mesenchymoma of the liver, which is also called undifferentiated sarcoma of the liver, is mainly seen in the older age group, and most patients present with abdominal pain in contradistinction to mesenchymal hamartoma of the liver[80,81]. Teratomas and simple cysts of the liver must also be differentiated, and these lesions will usually show calcifications on plain radiography or ultrasonography[77].

Treatment and prognosis

Once the diagnosis is made, removal of the lesion is recommended because these lesions grow to a large size and compress adjacent organs[68]. Extirpation by enucleation of the lesion can be accomplished if the tumour can easily be dissected from the surrounding liver tissue[29,75]. This surgical approach decreases blood loss, and normal liver tissue is saved. However, in most cases, simple excision of the mass with surrounding rim of normal liver tissue, or a formal hepatic lobectomy, is necessary[3,65,68]. With a huge lesion deeply situated close to the vena cava or the hepatic veins, or when the lesion is bulging across to the opposite lobe, marsupialization of the cysts into the peritoneal cavity may be employed[3,82]. This tumour has been reported to respond to cyclophosphamide therapy, but this should be considered only in life-threatening angiomatous tumours[76].

The long-term prognosis of these patients is excellent, with no evidence of recurrence[75]. Surgical morbidity and mortality rates are low, mostly associated with operative complications[64]. Excessive blood loss is the most common complication during and immediately after operation. Other postoperative complications include profound hypoglycaemia, ascites and biliary fistula[83].

Malignant liver tumours: hepatoblastoma and hepatocarcinoma

Primary hepatic tumours in newborns, infants and children are the third most common intra-abdominal neoplasm, next only to neuroblastoma and Wilms' tumour[84]. Two-thirds of these tumours are malignant, and account for 0.2%–2.8% of all primary malignancies in infancy and childhood from European and North American series[1,30,85]. Hepatoblastoma and hepatocellular carcinoma are the commonest hepatic malignancies, with the former being predominantly encountered before 3 years of age, and the latter in older children with a second peak before 2 years of age[1,9,86,87]. In the neonatal period, most of the patients with hepatic malignancy have hepatoblastoma; and only a few cases have hepatocarcinoma[1,4,88–90]. Males are affected twice as frequently as females. A few familial cases have been reported[91,92], and an epidemiological relationship to geographical location has been described[93]. Although the incidence of hepatoblastoma appears to be relatively constant throughout the world, with rates between 0.5 and 1.5 per million population per year, the incidence of hepatocellular carcinoma shows more geographical variation: it is more frequent than hepatoblastoma in some populations of Eastern Asia and Latin America[94].

Congenital malignant liver tumours are very rare. Four newborns with liver tumours (three hepatoblastomas and one hepatocellular carcinoma) among 375 children with hepatic neoplasia have been reported by Exelby et al.[1] in a national survey of American Academy of Pediatrics, Surgical Section, in 1974. Campbell et al.[5] reported one case of neonatal hepatoblastoma among 56 cases of liver tumours over a 60 year period in Toronto, and Gauthier et al. cited two cases with liver tumour that were diagnosed at birth in a review of 29 cases over a 13 year period[85].

Various congenital defects and acquired disorders are associated with liver tumours, with an incidence of 10%–20%[5,9,84,87,95–99] (Table 6.1). This association is similar to the increased incidence of congenital defects in other embryonal tumours, including Wilms' tumour, rhabdomyosarcoma and germ-cell tumours.

Although the causes of liver tumours have not yet been clearly identified, there is a suggestion

Table 6.1 Anomalies and defects associated with childhood hepatic tumours

Anomalies and syndromes	Associated disorders	Congenital liver disorders
Hemihypertrophy	Polyposis coli	Biliary atresia
Haemangioma	—	Neonatal hepatitis
Beckwith–Weidemann syndrome	—	Hereditary tyrosinaemia
Adenomatoid renal dysplasia	Osteoporosis	—
Congenital absence of kidney	Androgen therapy	Glycogen storage disease
		Von Gierke disease
Fetal alcoholic syndrome	Fanconi's anaemia	Lipid storage disease

that hepatoblastoma is a malignant tumour related to maldevelopment, which may be associated with 11p to 5q mutations, whereas hepatocellular carcinoma is more usually a complication of metabolic, inflammatory or other disorders, which damage the liver and lead to cirrhosis[95].

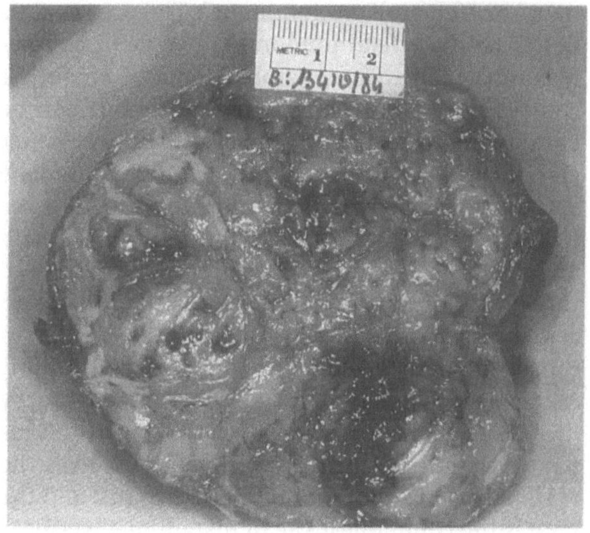

Figure 6.3 Cross-section through a hepatoblastoma showing grey fleshy tumour tissue with necrotic and haemorrhagic areas.

Pathology

Hepatoblastoma

Hepatoblastoma involves the right lobe of the liver in 75% of cases and is more often unifocal than hepatocarcinoma. In one-third of patients it involves both lobes[1]. The gross appearance of hepatoblastoma consists of a lobulated, usually solitary, mass surrounded by a fibrous pseudocapsule and separated from the normal parenchyma of the liver. Tortuous prominent vessels may course over the tumour surface. On cross-section, some necrotic or haemorrhagic areas may be seen; however, cystic areas are uncommon[85] (Figure 6.3). Microscopic studies often show extension of the tumour outside the gross margins together with intravascular invasion[30] (Figure 6.4). The lesions are classified by most workers, according to the Ishak and Glunz classification, as pure epithelial hepatoblastoma or mixed hepatoblastoma. The latter contains both epithelial and mesenchymal tissue. The pure epithelial lesions are further divided into "embryonal cell predomi-

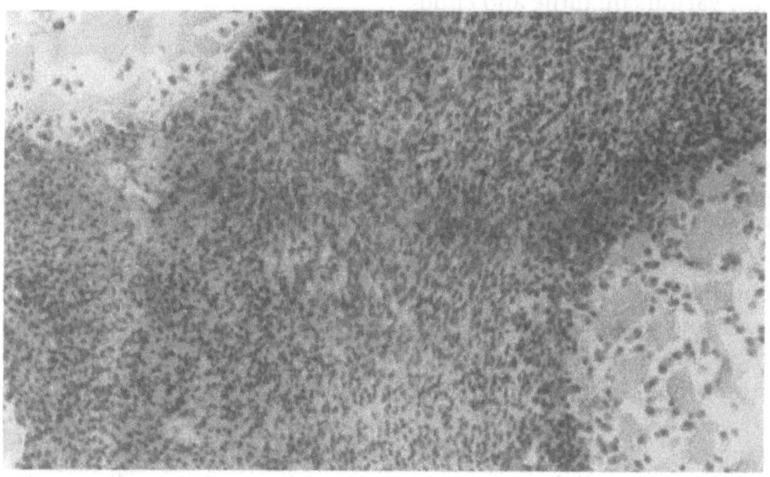

Figure 6.4 Histological findings of hepatoblastoma showing sheets of primitive small cells and two areas of osteoid formation.

nant" or "fetal cell predominant". The prognosis is better with the fetal-predominant type of hepatoblastoma than with hepatoblastoma of any other cell type. This is true only if the tumour can be completely resected[30,99]. There are two other classifications. The Kasai and Watanabe classification divides hepatoblastoma into three histological subtypes: fetal, embryonal and anaplastic[100]. Gonzalez-Crussi et al.[101] described three histological subtypes: fetal, embryonal, and a macrotrabecular type with features similar to those of hepatocellular carcinoma of adults. Metastasis to other parts of the liver occurs by direct extension, via intrahepatic vascular or lymphatic channels. Extrahepatic spread involves the regional lymph nodes in the porta hepatis, and the lung is the commonest site of distant metastasis.

Hepatocellular carcinoma

This tumour involves the right lobe of the liver in most patients; however, it is often extensively invasive and multicentric at the time of diagnosis, and so resection is possible in less than 30% of patients[1,9]. On cross-section, haemorrhage and necrosis within the tumour is found more often than in hepatoblastoma, and pseudoencapsulation is less noticeable. The tumour is often bile stained[30]. Hepatocarcinoma shows histological features identical to those of liver cell carcinoma in adults; thus, it is usually called the "adult" type of primary epithelial liver tumour of children. A distinctive variant of hepatocellular carcinoma is known to occur in the non-cirrhotic liver of older children and young adults and is called "fibrolamellar" carcinoma[87]. Various infantile and childhood diseases, including giant cell hepatitis and biliary atresia, predispose to cirrhosis, but these diseases do not appear to place the child at risk for hepatocellular carcinoma, and reports of associated hepatoma are rare[30]. An exception is the chronic form of hereditary tyrosinaemia, in which it is estimated that 30% of children will develop hepatoma[96]. In most reports, the prognosis of hepatocellular carcinoma has been as grave in children as in adults, owing to the advanced stage of disease at diagnosis. The distinctive variant of fibrolamellar carcinoma has a more favourable prognosis[102].

The vital importance of pathology review by expert paediatric pathologist is well demonstrated in the study by Mann et al.[95], in which 14% of the cases originally registered as malignant liver tumours were excluded later on histological ground: they were found to be metastatic malignant tumours arising in extrahepatic sites or nonmalignant hepatic disorders. Moreover, specialist pathology reviews have changed or refined the initial diagnosis in 50% of cases, and in 40% the initial opinion of a panel of paediatric pathologists on the subtype of tumour was not unanimous[95]. Difficulties in diagnosis can result in delay, and poor diagnosis in maltreatment.

Clinical presentation

Most infants with hepatoblastoma or hepatocellular carcinoma will present with an asymptomatic abdominal mass, progressive abdominal distension or hepatomegaly[95]. However, a few patients at an older age may present with advanced signs of malignant disease, including nausea, vomiting, abdominal pains, pallor, weight loss, anorexia and weakness[1,29,86]. Abdominal pain may be caused by ischaemic infarction, or by haemorrhage within the tumour, resulting in capsular pain[103]. Jaundice is an infrequent symptom, being extremely rare in hepatoblastoma[1]. Other rare clinical manifestations include shock resulting from rupture of the tumour with internal bleeding[85,94] and precocious puberty in young males, which is usually associated with hepatoblastoma[104–106]. The latter is the result of abnormal production of human chorionic gonadotrophin and high serum levels of testosterone, produced either by the testicular Leydig cells or by the tumour itself[107].

Diagnosis

Most infants with liver tumours are diagnosed after birth. Diagnosis is made on physical examination and certain biochemical and radiological investigations. An abdominal mass is palpable in more than 90% of cases, and a quarter of these patients are diagnosed on routine physical examination[29,85].

Laboratory studies often reveal anaemia, thrombocytosis, and normal or slightly increased levels of liver enzymes[84,97,108]. The serum bilirubin level is rarely elevated and appears only in cases with advanced liver disease. The most significant laboratory advance in recent years is the measure-

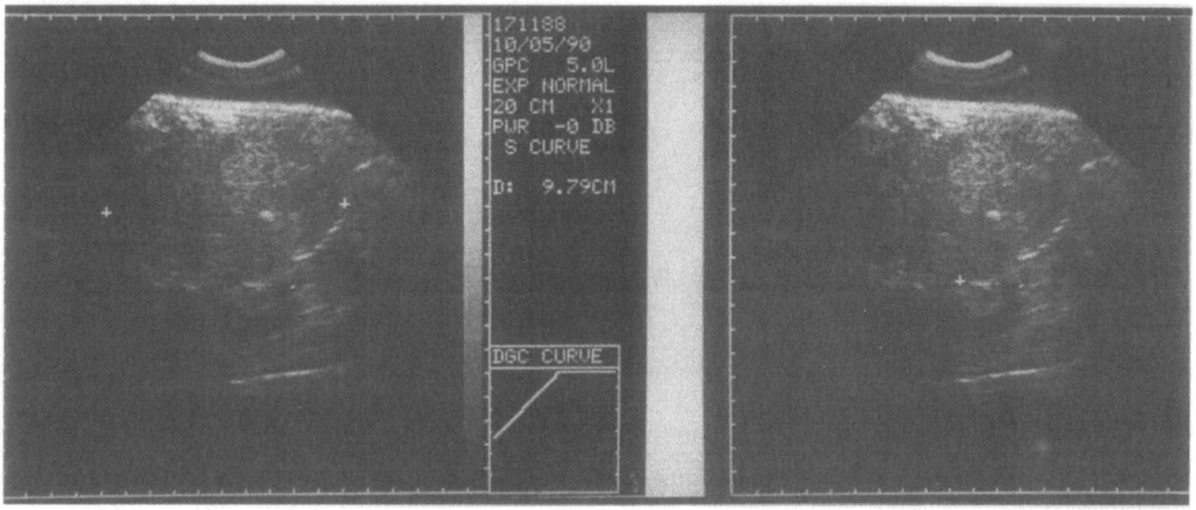

Figure 6.5 Ultrasonographic findings of hepatoblastoma showing a large hypoechoic mass with small round hyperechoic areas and focal calcification.

ment of serum α-fetoprotein level, which is found to be elevated in more than 80% of patients with hepatoblastoma and hepatocarcinoma[85,94]. This is an α-globulin produced by embryonic hepatocytes and normally present in the serum of fetuses and normal infants in the first few days of life[109]. It is a very useful tumour marker for diagnosis, and when positive can be used to follow the patient by serial determinations, either following chemotherapy treatment before surgery or after resection of the liver tumour[110,111]. This protein is a sensitive indicator for local residual tumour, recurrence or distant metastases, although there is no correlation between initial α-fetoprotein levels and tumour size, weight, differentiation, stage of disease or survival time[112,113]. Other malignant tumours of infancy associated with high serum levels of α-fetoprotein include yolk sac tumours, teratomas and embryonal carcinomas.

The most useful radiological investigations for assessing tumour localization and resectability are ultrasonography, CT, MRI and angiography[114–117]. However, the initial evaluation must include plain radiographs of abdomen and chest. Abdominal radiographs usually demonstrate hepatomegaly and may show calcifications; chest radiographs may reveal lung metastases, although CT is far more sensitive in this respect[118]. Ultrasonography has emerged as the major diagnostic tool, and correctly predicts the extent and resectability of liver tumours in most patients[114] (Figure 6.5). Although both hepatoblastoma and cystic hepatoblastoma have a characteristic ultrasonographic appearance[114,119], there are reports of similarities in echo patterns between malignant and benign tumours[120]. Intraoperative ultrasonography during hepatic resection has been reported in five patients, including a newborn with hepatoblastoma[4]. In this group, the operative strategy had to be changed in all cases despite extensive preoperative evaluation, including preoperative ultrasonography.

CT can give superior information in these infants concerning origin, extent, resectability and type of hepatic tumour[116,117]. It also provides accurate information on vascularity and spread of tumour outside the liver. Angiography, preferably performed via an umbilical artery, is essential if resection is being considered, but only if the other imaging studies have not excluded the possibility of resection. It provides a vascular map to assist in the planning of resection: there is a high percentage of vascular anomalies. CT combined with angiography can also provide valuable information on the blood supply to the hepatic mass (Figure 6.6). The introduction of digital subtraction angiography has reduced the examination time and the dosage of contrast medium and gives improved visualization of the portal venous anatomy[121] (Figure 6.7).

Patency of the interior vena cava can be assessed either by ultrasonography or by venacavograph, although the latter may be misleading as it is difficult to distinguish between

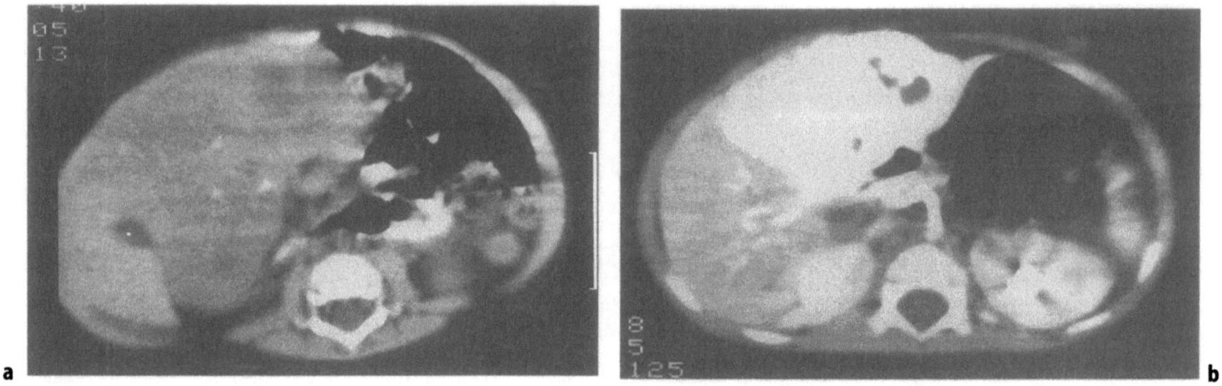

Figure 6.6 **a** Computed tomography of the liver at the level of the gall bladder showing a huge low-density mass with calcifications within it in the left liver lobe. The mass is expanding beyond the liver border. **b** Computed tomography combined with angiography of the liver obtained during injection of contrast media into the superior mesenteric artery. The left liver lobe mass is intensely enhanced, showing small cystic areas within it.

extrinsic compression and invasion of the tumour. However, venacavography should be applied routinely before surgery to the rare patient whose tumour occupies the caudate lobe, because of the common direct involvement of adjacent major vessels[122]. Isotope liver scan is limited in value as it lacks specificity and often fails to illustrate the full extent of the disease. MRI provides sophisticated and detailed information about the internal architecture of the liver mass and the liver haemodynamic status[123].

Ultrasonography, CT, MRI and angiography provide accurate imaging information on the origin of tumour, extension, type and vascular map, but are not definitive in determining resectability; infants should have the benefit of

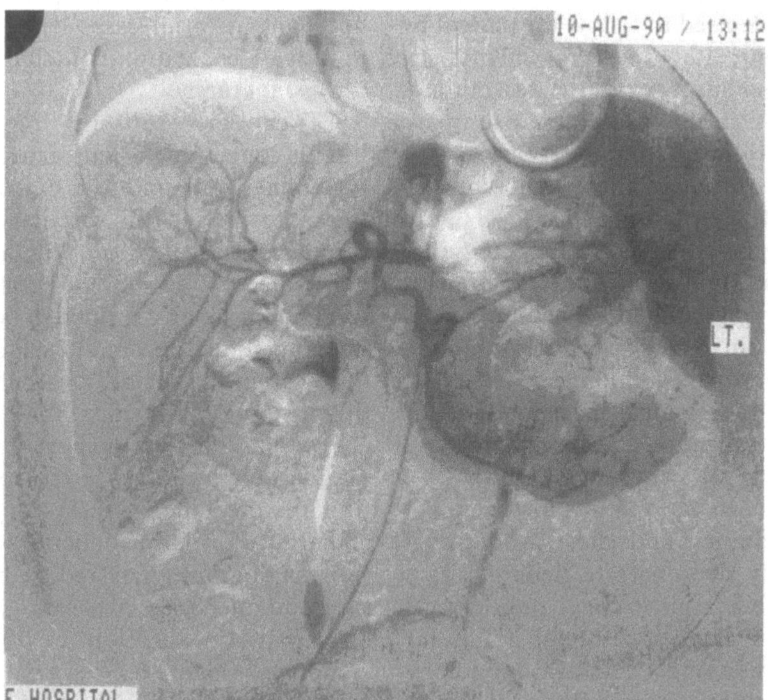

Figure 6.7 Digital subtraction angiography of the coeliac trunk showing a large mass of the left liver lobe supplied by the gastroduodenal artery.

laparotomy, because some tumours will be found to be resectable despite appearing otherwise on imaging[4,103,114]. Three-dimensional reconstruction of spiral CT has been reported to provide useful information that allows evaluation of the relationship to major blood vessels and of resectibility[115].

Staging

Clinical staging in malignant liver tumours is helpful for prognosis and interpreting results from various studies. Table 6.2 illustrates one of the clinical staging schemes[10].

Table 6.2 Clinicopathological staging system

Stage	Description
I	Complete resection
II	Microscopic residual tumour • Intrahepatic • Extrahepatic
III	Gross residual tumour • Primary completely resected, nodes positive and/or tumour spill • Primary not completely resected, and/or nodes positive and/or tumour spill
IV	Metastatic disease • Primary completely resected • Primary not completely resected

Treatment

Complete resection of the hepatic malignant tumour at the time of initial laparotomy should be the primary surgical goal, as it offers the best opportunity for cure[10,97,124]. However, nearly half of all cases with hepatic cancer are unresectable at the time of diagnosis as a result of bilobar involvement of the tumour, large size and the presence of distal metastases[1]. For this group of patients, preoperative chemotherapy has been used by many investigators in an attempt to increase the percentage of patients amenable to complete resection[11,125–127]. Assessment of resectability of hepatic tumours is still being debated in the medical literature. Most surgeons adhere to the concept that resectability should be determined only on the basis of complete and formal exploration of the abdomen; others believe that this information can be accurately obtained from the preoperative diagnostic imaging studies, including ultrasonography, CT, MRI, angiography and needle biopsy for histological confirmation[10,127–129].

In a prospective study of patients with stage II–IV hepatic cancer (using the staging system shown in Table 6.2), King et al.[10] have reported that patients who underwent incomplete primary resection at initial operation had a better prognosis than those who were only biopsied on first exploration and underwent resection at second-look operation. Survival rates were 58% and 41% respectively, although with no statistically significant difference. They have also found that patients with delayed hepatic resections have an increased risk of postoperative complications[10]. Others prefer to administer preoperative chemotherapy to all patients with unresectable tumour[85,127,129]. Black et al.[11] no longer advocate immediate resection of hepatoblastoma, whether the tumour is resectable or unresectable at presentation, and recommend chemotherapy before surgery in all cases.

Chemotherapeutic protocols for hepatoblastoma and hepatocarcinoma involve several agents given both systemically and intra-arterially[1,85,125,126,130]. The most frequently used agents are vincristine, Adriamycin, actinomycin D, cyclophosphamide, 5-fluorouracil and cisplatin (C-DDP). Of these agents, Adriamycin and cisplatin, used either alone or in combination, are considered the most effective drugs for hepatoblastoma. However, therapeutic response in patients with hepatocarcinoma remains poor[10,126,127,131]. As a result of the high toxicity of these agents, which mainly include bone marrow suppression and cardiac toxicity, and because the population is extremely young, including newborns and infants, it is important to develop a regimen with the highest therapeutic index and minimal toxicity.

Langevin et al.[127] have reported the use of cisplatin and Adriamycin by continuous infusion in a group of six patients including a newborn. A dramatic clinical response was obtained in all cases, including shrinkage of the tumour, decrease in α-fetoprotein levels, disappearance of lung metastases on CT, and histological evidence of substantial tumour necrosis in the surgically resected lobes. This response appeared with only minimal toxicity. These toxic medications for newborns and infants with a body weight of less than 10 kg should be given according to their body weight[127]. Infants with a body weight of more than

10 kg should receive this treatment according to their body surface area[10,11], using the conversion factor 30 kg = 1 m^2. M-mode echocardiograms, creatinine clearance and audiogram should be obtained in each patient to assist in treating and preventing cardiotoxicity, nephrotoxicity and audiotoxicity[127]. Appropriate hydration at the time of treatment is mandatory to prevent renal complications.

There are different clinical and laboratory criteria for the appropriate time of surgical intervention following chemotherapy[10,11,127,129]. These criteria include:

1. α-Fetoprotein level decreased to less than 1% of the initial value, or beginning to increase before reaching 1%[11]
2. Greater than 50% reduction in tumour size on follow-up CT[10,127]
3. Absence of metastatic disease[129]

In most patients, these changes appear within 10–12 weeks of treatment[11,127].

Operative technique

Present techniques of hepatic resection are based on the true segmental and lobar anatomy of the liver, as was first accurately described by Goldsmith and Woodburne[132]. A good knowledge of the liver anatomy is a prerequisite for anatomical surgery of this organ[133,134].

Following induction of general anaesthesia with endotracheal intubation, peripheral arterial and central venous pressure catheters are inserted by percutaneous puncture, in addition to one or two other intravenous cannulas, which should be placed in the upper extremities. Other monitoring devices should include pulse oximeter and end-tidal capnograph to identify air emboli during the liver resection, nasopharyngeal and rectal temperature probes, and urinary catheters[135]. Constant communication and close cooperation with the paediatric anaesthesiologist is very important to recognize and respond to any complication, including large volume shifts, bleeding or air emboli, which can mean disaster to these small patients.

The standard incision is a right subcostal incision extended across the midline to form an inverted chevron. Newborns and infants rarely require a thoracic extension, but if necessary it should be done through the right eighth intercostal space[136]. At laparotomy, the tumour is biopsied and frozen section carried out to confirm the malignancy. Once resectability has been determined, the porta hepatis is dissected and individual branches of the portal vein, hepatic artery and hepatic duct to the lobe of liver to be excised are isolated, ligated and divided. The entire liver is then mobilized and freed from all its attachments to permit proper identification of the many draining hepatic veins that empty into the inferior vena cava along its retrohepatic course. Following the vascular and biliary isolation of the specimen, at the porta hepatis, the liver is divided along the intersegmental plane, developing bundles of vessels and bile ducts, which are ligated or clipped. This part of the dissection may proceed either by the finger-fracture technique[85,103] or by ultrasonic dissection[137]. The hepatic veins can be dissected and divided as the last stage of the hepatic resection, either extrahepatically[138] or intrahepatically[134]. Dissection of the hepatic veins is dangerous in that there is a major risk of tearing or penetrating either the large hepatic veins or the vena cava, causing massive bleeding which can be difficult to control. Therefore, it was suggested that the dissection of hepatic veins should be preceded by total clamping of the hepatic vessels and of the suprahepatic and infrahepatic vena cava, described by Huguet et al. as "normothermic hepatic total vascular exclusion"[139]. Another major complication that can occur at the initial stage of hepatic vein dissection is air embolism. This can usually be prevented by appropriate positive end-expiratory pressure (PEEP) ventilation. Clamping of the porta hepatis may be necessary during the liver resection (Pringle manoeuvre), especially if bleeding is excessive. This temporary inflow occlusion of structures in the free edge of the lesser sac can be well tolerated[140] for a period of longer than 30 min.

Several technical innovations have been suggested to diminish blood loss and to allow more complete tumour resection. These include hepatic vascular exclusion with hypothermic perfusion of the liver with lactated Ringer's solution[139,141], the use of marked normovolaemic haemodilution anaesthesia with relative hypotension and moderate hypothermia[142], and the use of profound hypothermia with circulation arrest[143,144]. However, there is considerable morbidity with the last technique[143]. Hypothermia during hepatic resection has a beneficial effect as it causes a decrease in metabolic rate and provides cerebral protection in the event of major blood loss[141,144,145]. It also increases the safe ischaemic time for the liver when isolated, and thus minimizes postoperative liver dysfunction[110].

Drainage of the upper abdomen by sump drains is more effective at removing accumulations of blood and bile. Biliary tract decompression is recommended only in selected cases, as a result of increased incidence of sepsis[136].

Postoperative complications and management

Excessive blood loss is the most common complication during and immediately after major liver surgery and has a significant effect on the perioperative morbidity and mortality rates[1,70,85]. Other common metabolic and haematological disturbances include hypoglycaemia, hypoproteinaemia and jaundice. These complications must be anticipated and prevented by standard intravenous administration of dextrose, albumin and fresh frozen plasma to all patients in the initial postoperative management[103]. In addition, careful monitoring of the prothrombin time and serum albumin and blood glucose levels will prevent coagulopathy and neurological complications[146].

A minor degree of jaundice can be expected following large hepatic resection because of decrease in functioning liver tissue. However, increasing bilirubin levels may indicate severe liver damage and/or septicaemia. Markedly elevated bilirubin levels after surgery are considered a poor prognostic sign[147]. Jaundice may also be caused by obstruction to the extrahepatic biliary system. In the early postoperative period this may be due to a blood clot, but a late onset suggests stricture of the bile duct[110]. Hypoglycaemia coagulopathy and hypoproteinaemia reflect both loss of functioning liver tissue and increased fibrinolysis with a loss of plasma proteins at the resection site of the liver[136]. Septicaemia remains a significant complication: the raw liver surface is a good medium for bacterial growth, and disruption of the biliary tree provides a potential source of bacteria. Thus, prophylactic antibiotic cover should be routine and should include broad-spectrum cover for gram-negative and anaerobic organisms. In addition, septicaemia can reflect an underlying process such as pneumonia or a subphrenic abscess. Other relatively frequent postoperative complications include biliary fistula, wound infection and small bowel obstruction[138,148]. These complications can be managed non-operatively in most patients, and surgical intervention is rarely needed.

Long-term assessment after hepatic surgery include ^{99m}Tc radionuclide liver scan to assess regeneration, serial measurements of α-fetoprotein, chest radiography and abdominal ultrasonography to detect recurrence[9,10]. α-Fetoprotein levels should be routinely determined, weekly until the level is normal, monthly for 1 year, 2-monthly for a further year and then 6-monthly[111]. Failure of α-fetoprotein level to return to normal after resection of the lesion is a very sensitive indicator of residual tumour at either a local or a metastatic site[113,149]. King et al.[10] have reported that measurements of serum α-fetoprotein level were more accurate than second-look laparotomy in predicting the presence of residual disease[10].

A rise of α-fetoprotein level after its return to normal, or any suggestion of intra-abdominal recurrence by ultrasonography, merits investigation including CT of the abdomen and chest for local recurrence or lung metastases. Subsequently it warrants second-look laparotomy for further tumour resection, and in some cases chest exploration for excision of pulmonary metastases[113]. Some surgeons prefer second-look laparotomy for all patients with liver malignancy[10].

Radiotherapy has been used as an adjunctive therapy in the tumour bed of a few patients with liver tumours[126]. However, it appears to have greater adverse effects on the young child's liver than on adult livers[150], and is therefore an inappropriate treatment for the newborn patient[62].

Orthotopic liver transplantation for hepatoblastoma and hepatocellular carcinoma can now be considered for children, if the tumour involves vessels and other vital structures which preclude partial hepatic resection[151]. However, if extensive evaluation for metastases demonstrates spread beyond the liver, the patient should be considered untreatable by transplantation. Initial poor results due to tumour recurrence have been improved by modification of immunosuppression regimens with cyclosporine. Iwatsuki et al.[152] have reported that the 5 year survival rate of adult patients with hepatocellular carcinoma treated by orthotopic liver transplantation was the same as the survival rate of patients who underwent hepatic resection.

There are several reports on successful liver transplantation in children with hepatic tumours[153,154], but the clinical follow-up of these patients is of short duration.

Prognosis

The prognosis of hepatic malignancy improved in the past 10 years both for children who underwent complete extirpation of liver cancer and for patients with primarily incomplete resection of hepatoblastoma or hepatocellular carcinoma. There is an over 50% cure rate for children in the first group[9,85,155], and improved survival rate, from 12% to 48% in the second group[10,156]. The long-term survival rate for newborns and neonates is difficult to determine because of the small number of cases in most series[1,4,85,127].

References

1. Exelby PR, Filler RM, Grosfeld JL (1975) Liver tumors in children in the particular reference for hepatoblastoma and hepatocellular carcinoma: American Academy of Pediatrics, Surgical Section Survey – 1974. J Pediatr Surg 10: 329–337.
2. Dehner LP, Ishak KG (1971) Vascular tumours of the liver in infants and children. A study of 30 cases and review of the literature. Arch Pathol 92: 101–111.
3. Ehren H, Mahour GH, Isaacs H (1983) Benign liver tumors in infancy and childhood: report of 48 cases. Am J Surg 145: 325–329.
4. Thomas BL, Krummel TM, Parker GA et al. (1989) Use of intraoperative ultrasound during hepatic resection in pediatric patients. J Pediatr Surg 24: 690–693.
5. Campbell AN, Chan HSL, O'Brien A et al. (1987) Malignant tumours in the neonate. Arch Dis Child 62: 19–23.
6. Isaacs H (1987) Congenital neonatal malignant tumours. A 28 year experience at Children's Hospital of Los Angeles. Am J Pediatr Hematol Oncol 9: 121–129.
7. Hartman GE, Shochat SJ (1989) Abdominal mass lesions in the newborn's diagnosis and treatment. Clin Perinatol 16: 123–135.
8. Becker JM, Heitler MS (1989) Hepatic hemangioendotheliomas in infancy – collective review. Surg Gynecol Obstet 168: 189–200.
9. Giacomantonio M, Ein SH, Mancer K et al. (1984) Thirty years of experience with pediatric primary malignant liver tumors. J Pediatr Surg 19: 523–526.
10. King DR, Ortega J, Campbell J et al. (1991) The surgical management of children with incompletely resected hepatic cancer is facilitated by intensive chemotherapy. J Pediatr Surg 26: 1074–1081.
11. Black CT, Cangir A, Choroszy M, Andrassy RJ (1991) Marked response to preoperative high dose cis-platinum in children with unresectable hepatoblastoma. J Pediatr Surg 26: 1070–1073.
12. Pazder R, Bready B, Langir A (1993) Pediatric hepatic tumours: clinical trials conducted in the United States. J Surg Oncol 3: 127–130.
13. Tugge EP, Tugge DU, Reyes J et al. (1992) Resection including transplantation for hepatoblastoma and hepatocellular carcinoma: impact on survival. J Pediatr Surg 27: 292–296.
14. Romero R (1988) Hepatomegaly. In: Romero R, Pilu G, Jeahthy P, Ghidiri A, Hobbins JC, eds. Prenatal diagnosis of congenital anomalies. Appleton and Lange, East Norwalk, Connecticut, pp 249–251.
15. Petrikovsky BM, Cohen HL, Scimeca P, Belluci E (1994) Prenatal diagnosis of focal nodular hyperplasia of the liver. Prenat Diagn 14: 406–409.
16. Berdon WE, Baker DH (1969) Giant hepatic hemangioma with cardiac failure in the newborn infant. Radiology 62: 1523–1528.
17. Cremin BJ, Nuss D (1974) Calcified hepatoblastoma in a newborn. J Pediatr Surg 9: 913–915.
18. Hirata GI, Matsunaga ML, Medeari AL et al. (1990) Ultrasonographic diagnosis of a fetal abdominal mass: a case of a mesenchymal liver hamartoma and a review of the literature. Prenat Diagn 10: 507–512.
19. Alcalay M, Dan U, Kessler A et al. (1991) Prenatal ultrasonic diagnosis of hepatic cyst. Pediatr Surg Int 6: 146–147.
20. Flagg RS, Robinson DW (1967) Solitary nonparasitic hepatic cysts. Arch Surg 95: 964–973.
21. Abramson SJ, Lack EF, Teele RL (1982) Benign vascular tumors of the liver in infants: sonographic appearance. AJR Am J Roentgenol 138: 629–632.
22. Shackelford GD, Kirks DR (1977) Neonatal hepatic calcification secondary to transplacental infection. Radiology 122: 753–757.
23. Hawass ND, El Badawi MG, Fatani JA et al. (1990) Fetal hepatic calcification. Pediatr Radiol 20: 528–535.
24. Howell CG, Templeton JM, Weiner S et al. (1983) Antenatal diagnosis and early surgery for choledochal cyst. J Pediatr Surg 18: 387–393.
25. Holcomb GW, O'Neill JA, Mahboubi S (1988) Experience with hepatic hemangioendothelioma in infancy and childhood. J Pediatr Surg 23: 661–666.
26. Jackson C, Greene HL, O'Neill JA et al. (1977) Hepatic hemangioendothelioma. Am J Dis Child 131: 74–77.
27. McLean RH, Moller JH, Warwick WJ et al. (1972) Multinodular hemangiomatosis of the liver in infancy. Pediatrics 49: 563–573.
28. Pereyra R, Andrassy CRJ, Mahour GH (1982) Management of massive hepatic hemangiomas in infants and children: a review of 13 cases. Pediatrics 70: 254–258.
29. Guzzetta PC, Randolph JG (1989) Pediatric hepatic surgery. Surg Clin North Am 69: 251–257.
30. Weinberg AG, Finegold MJ (1986) Primary hepatic tumours in childhood. In: Finegold MJ, ed. Pathology of neoplasia in childhood and adolescence. WB Saunders, Philadelphia, pp 333–372.
31. Falk H, Herbert JT, Edmonds L et al. (1981) Review of four cases of childhood hepatic angiosarcoma – elevated environmental arsenic exposure in one case. Cancer 47: 382–391.
32. Strate SM, Rutledge JC, Weinberg AC (1984) Delayed development of angiosarcoma in multinodular infantile hepatic hemangioendothelioma. Arch Pathol Lab Med 108: 943–944.
33. Lampe I, Latourette HB (1959) Management of hemangiomas in infants. Pediatr Clin North Am 6: 511–521.
34. DeLorimier AA, Simpson EB, Baum RS et al. (1967) Hepatic artery ligation for hepatic hemangiomatosis. N Engl J Med 277: 333–337.
35. Touloukian RJ (1970) Hepatic hemangioendothelioma during infancy: pathology diagnosis and therapy with prednisone. Pediatrics 45: 71–76.

36. Dachman DH, Lichtenstein JE, Friedman AC et al. (1983) Infantile hemangioendothelioma of the liver: a radiologic–pathologic–clinical correlation. Am J Radiol 140: 1091–1096.
37. Leonidas JC, Staus L, Beck AR (1973) Vascular tumours of the liver in newborns. Am J Dis Child 125: 507–510.
38. Shim WKT (1968) Hemangiomas of infancy complicated by thrombocytopenia. Am J Surg 116: 869–906.
39. Ezekowitz RAB, Phil D, Mulliken JB et al. (1992) Interferon Alfa-2a therapy for life-threatening hemangiomas of infancy. N Engl J Med 326: 1456–1463.
40. Cohen RC, Myers NA (1986) Diagnosis and management of massive hemangiomas in childhood. J Pediatr Surg 21: 6–9.
41. Cornelius AS, Womer RB, Jakacki R (1989) Multiple hemangioendotheliomas of the liver. Med Pediatr Oncol 17: 501–504.
42. Yohannan MD, Abdulla AMA, Patel PJ (1990) Neonatal hepatic hemangioendothelioma: presentation with jaundice and microangiopathic haemolytic anaemia. Eur J Pediatr 149: 804–805.
43. Linderkamp O, Hopner F, Klose H et al. (1976) Solitary hepatic hemangioma in a newborn infant complicated by cardiac failure, consumptive coagulopathy, microangiopathic hemolytic anemia and obstructive jaundice. Eur J Pediatr 124: 23–29.
44. Margileth AM, Muceles M (1965) Cutaneous hemangiomas in children: diagnosis and conservation management. JAMA 194: 523–526.
45. Chitayat D, Schwartz KO, Daniels-Phillips E (1979) Fatal bleeding due to spontaneous rupture of a cavernous hepatic hemangioma. Harefuah 97: 75–76.
46. Sewell JH, Weiss K (1961) Spontaneous rupture of hemangioma of the liver: a review of the literature and presentation of illustrative case. Arch Surg 83: 729–733.
47. Moss AA, Clark RF, Palubinskas AJ et al. (1971) Angiographic appearance of benign and malignant hepatic tumours in infants and children. AJR Am J Roentgenol 113: 61–69.
48. Abramson SJ, Lack EE, Teele RL (1982) Benign vascular tumours of the liver in infants: sonographic appearance. AJR Am J Roentgenol 138: 629–632.
49. Front D, Royal HD, Israel O et al. (1981) Scintigraphy of hepatic hemangiomas: the value of Tc-99m labelled red blood cells. J Nucl Med 22: 684–687.
50. Montgomery SP, Guillot AP, Barth RA (1990) MRI of disseminated neonatal hemangiomatosis: case report. Pediatr Radiol 20: 204–205.
51. Rummeny E, Weissleder R, Stark DD et al. (1989) Primary liver tumors: diagnosis by MR imaging. AJR Am J Roentgenol 152: 63–72.
52. McFarland EG, Mayo-Smith WW, Saini S, Hahn PF, Goldberg MA, Lee MJ (1994) Hepatic hemangiomas and malignant tumours: improved differentiation with heavily T-2 weighted conventional spin-ECHO MR imaging. Radiology 193: 43–47.
53. Stewart B, Mulker MF, Foley M, Weilopolski PA, Finn JP (1994) Fast MR imaging of the liver: quantitative comparison of techniques. Radiology 193: 37–42.
54. Goldberg SJ, Fonkalsrud E (1969) Successful treatment of hepatic hemangioma with corticosteroids. JAMA 208: 2473–2474.
55. Nguyen B, Shandling B, Ein S et al. (1982) Hepatic hemangioma in childhood: medical management or surgical management. J Pediatr Surg 17: 576–579.
56. Davenport M, Hansen L, Heaton ND et al. (1995) Hemangioendothelioma of the liver in infants. J Pediatr Surg 30: 44–48.
57. Hurvitz CH, Alkally AL, Sloninsky L et al. (1985) Cyclophosphamide therapy in life-threatening vascular tumors. J Pediatr 109: 360–363.
58. Johnson DH, Vinson AM, Wirth FH et al. (1984) Management of hepatic hemangioendothelioma of infancy by transarterial embolization: a report of two cases. Pediatrics 73: 546–549.
59. Burrows PE, Rosenberg HC, Chuang HS (1985) Diffuse hepatic hemangiomas: percutaneous transcatheter embolization with detachable silicone balloons. Radiology 156: 85–88.
60. Davenport M, Hansen L, Heaton ND, Howard ER (1995) Hemangioendothelioma of the liver in infants. J Pediatr Surg 30: 44–48.
61. Haselow RE, Nesbit M, Dehner LP et al. (1978) Second neoplasms following megavoltage radiation in a pediatric population. Cancer 42: 1185–1191.
62. Irving IM (1990) Abdominal tumors. In: Lister J, Irving IM, eds. Neonatal surgery. Butterworths, London, pp 122–141.
63. Stanley P, Grinell VS, Staunton RE et al. (1983) Therapeutic embolization of infantile hepatic hemangioma with polyvinyl alcohol. AJR Am J Roentgenol 141: 1047–1051.
64. Stocker JT, Ishak KG (1983) Mesenchymal hamartoma of the liver: report of 30 cases and a review of the literature. Pediatr Pathol 1: 245–267.
65. DeMaioribus CA, Lally KP, Sim K et al. (1990) Mesenchymal hamartoma of the liver. A 35 year review. Arch Surg 125: 598–600.
66. Maresh R (1903) Uber ein Lymphangiom der Leber. Z Heilk 24: 39–50.
67. Edmondson HA (1956) Differential diagnosis of tumors and tumor-like lesions of liver in infancy and childhood. Am J Dis Child 91: 168–186.
68. Raffensperger JG, Gonzalez-Crussi F, Skeehan T (1983) Mesenchymal hamartoma of the liver. J Pediatr Surg 18: 585–587.
69. Lanuza A, Perez-Candela V, Ceres L et al. (1980) Hepatic hamartoma in a newborn. Pediatr Radiol 9: 111–112.
70. Smith WL, Ballantine TVN, Gonzalez-Crussi F (1978) Hepatic mesenchymal hamartoma causing heart failure in the neonate. J Pediatr Surg 13: 183–185.
71. Dehner LP, Ewing SL, Saumer HW (1975) Infantile mesenchymal hamartoma of the liver. Arch Pathol 99: 379–382.
72. Srouji MN, Chatten J, Schulman WM et al. (1978) Mesenchymal hamartoma of the liver in infants. Cancer 42: 2483–2489.
73. Ishida M, Tsuchida Y, Saito S et al. (1966) Mesenchymal hamartoma of the liver. Case report and literature review. Ann Surg 164: 175–182.
74. Silber DL, Soper RT, Kent T (1970) Life threatening mesenchymal hamartoma of the liver. J Pediatr Surg 5: 471–472.
75. Ito H, Kishikawa T, Toda T et al. (1984) Hepatic mesenchymal hamartoma of an infant. J Pediatr Surg 19: 315–317.
76. Alkalay AL, Puri AR, Pomerance JJ et al. (1985) Mesenchymal hamartoma of the liver responsive to cyclophosphamide therapy: therapeutic approach. J Pediatr Surg 20: 125–128.
77. Rosenbaum DM, Mindell HJ (1980) Ultrasonographic findings in mesenchymal hamartoma of the liver. Radiology 138: 425–427.
78. Ros PR, Goodman ZD, Ishak KG et al. (1986) Mesenchymal hamartoma of the liver: radiologic–pathologic correlation. Radiology 158: 619–623.
79. Stanley RJ, Dehner LP, Hesker AE (1973) Primary malignant mesenchymal tumors (mesenchymoma) of the liver in childhood: an angiographic–pathologic study of three cases. Cancer 32: 973–984.
80. Stocker JT, Ishak KG (1978) Undifferentiated (embryonal) sarcoma of the liver. Cancer 42: 336–348.
81. Newman KD, Schisgall R, Reaman G, Guzzetta PC (1989) Malignant mesenchymoma of the liver in children. J Pediatr Surg 24: 781–783.
82. Randolph JG, Altman RP, Arensman RM et al. (1978) Liver

resection in children with hepatic neoplasms. Ann Surg 187: 599–605.
83. Yandza T, Valayer J (1986) Benign tumors of the liver in children: analysis of a series of 20 cases. J Pediatr Surg 21: 419–423.
84. Clatworthy HW, Schiller M, Grosfeld JL (1974) Primary liver tumours in infancy and childhood. Arch Surg 109: 143–147.
85. Valayer J, Lemerle J (1986) Tumeurs du foie. In: Alagille D, Odieure M, eds. Maladies du foie et des voies biliaries chez l'enfant. Flammarion, Paris, pp 239–259. Cited by Gauthier F, Valayer J, LeThai B et al. (1986) Hepatoblastoma and hepatocarcinoma in children: analysis of a series of 29 cases. J Pediatr Surg 21: 424–429.
86. Ishak K, Glunz PR (1967) Hepatoblastoma and hepatocarcinoma in infancy and childhood: report of 47 cases. Cancer 20: 396–422.
87. Lack EE, Neave C, Vawter GF (1983) Hepatocellular carcinoma. Cancer 52: 1510–1515.
88. Alpert ME, Seeler RA (1970) Alpha-fetoprotein in embryonal hepatoblastoma. J Pediatr 77: 1058.
89. Foster JH, Berman MM (1977) Solid liver tumors. WB Saunders, Philadelphia.
90. Misugi K, Okajima H, Misugi N et al. (1967) Classification of primary malignant tumors of the liver in infancy and childhood. Cancer 20: 1760–1771.
91. Surendran N, Radhakrishna K, Chellam VG (1989) Hepatoblastoma in siblings. J Pediatr Surg 24: 1169–1171.
92. Napoli VM, Campbell WG Jr (1977) Hepatoblastoma in infant sister and brother. Cancer 39: 2647–2650.
93. Parkin DM, Stiller CA, Drager GJ et al. (1988) The international incidence of childhood cancer. Int J Cancer 42: 511–520.
94. Chen WJC, Lee JC, Hung WT (1988) Primary malignant tumor of liver in infants and children in Taiwan. J Pediatr Surg 23: 457–461.
95. Mann JR, Kasthuri N, Raafat F et al. (1990) Malignant hepatic tumours in children: incidence, clinical features and aetiology. Paediatr Perinat Epidemiol 4: 276–289.
96. Weinberg AG, Mize CE, Worthen HG (1976) The occurrence of hepatoma in the chronic form of hereditary tyrosinaemia. J Pediatr Surg 88: 434–438.
97. Filler RM, Hagen J (1981) Liver tumors. Surg Clin North Am 61: 1209–1217.
98. Altman RP, Schwartz AD (1983) Malignant disease of infancy, childhood and adolescence, 2nd edn. WB Saunders, Philadelphia, p 524.
99. Green DM (1985) Diagnosis and management of malignant solid tumors in infants and children. Martinus Nijhoff, Boston, pp 410–438.
100. Kasai M, Watanabe I (1970) Histologic classification of liver cell carcinoma in infancy and childhood and its clinical evaluation. A study of 70 cases collected in Japan. Cancer 25: 551–553.
101. Gonzalez-Crussi F, Upton MP, Maurer HS (1982) Hepatoblastoma. Attempt at characterization of histologic subtypes. Am J Surg Pathol 6: 599–612.
102. Craig JR, Peters RL, Edmondson HA et al. (1980) Fibrolamellar carcinoma of the liver. A tumor of adolescents and young adults with distinctive clinicopathologic features. Cancer 46: 372–379.
103. Joyce AD, Howard ER (1989) Hepatobiliary tumours of childhood: investigation and management. In: Spitz L, Wurnig P, Angerpointner TA, eds. Progress in pediatric surgery 22. Springer-Verlag, Berlin, pp 69–93.
104. Nakagawara A, Ikeda K, Hayashida Y et al. (1982) Immunocytochemical identification of human chorionic gonadotropin and α-fetoprotein producing cells of hepatoblastoma associated with precocious puberty. Virchows Arch A Pathol Anat 398: 45–51.
105. Behrle FC, Mantz FA, Olsen RL (1963) Virilization accompanying hepatoblastoma. Pediatrics 32: 265–271.
106. Hirota M, Iwafuchi M, Oshawa Y et al. (1982) Gonadotropin producing hepatoblastoma. J Jpn Soc Pediatr Surg 18: 1147–1152.
107. Galifer RB, Sultan C, Margueritte G et al. (1985) Testosterone-producing hepatoblastoma in a 3 year old boy with precocious puberty. J Pediatr Surg 20: 713–714.
108. Nickerson HJ, Silberman TL, McDonald TP (1980) Hepatoblastoma, thrombocytosis and increased thrombopoietin. Cancer 45: 315–317.
109. Tsuchida Y, Endo Y, Saito S et al. (1978) Evaluation of α-fetoprotein in early infancy. J Pediatr Surg 13: 155–156.
110. Davidson PM, Waters KD, Brown TCK, Auldist AW (1988) Liver tumors in children. Pediatr Surg Int 3: 377–381.
111. McIntyre KR, Vogel CL, Primack A et al. (1976) Effect of surgical and chemotherapeutic treatment on α-fetoprotein levels in patients with hepatocellular carcinoma. Cancer 37: 677–683.
112. Purves LR (1976) Alpha fetoprotein and the diagnosis of liver cell cancer. In: Cameron HM, Linsell DA, Warwick GP, eds. Liver cell cancer. Elsevier, Amsterdam, pp 61–79.
113. Black CT, Luck SR, Musemeche CA, Andrassy RJ (1991) Aggressive excision of pulmonary metastases is warranted in the management of childhood hepatic tumors. J Pediatr Surg 26: 1082–1086.
114. DeCampo M, DeCampo JF (1988) Ultrasound of primary hepatic tumours in childhood. Pediatr Radiol 19: 19–24.
115. Plumky DA, Grosfeld JL, Kopecky KK, Buckwalter KA, Glaze Vaughan W (1994) The role of spiral (helical) computerized tomography with three dimensional reconstruction in pediatric solid tumours. J Pediatr Surg 30: 317–321.
116. Korobkin M, Kirks DR, Sullivan DC et al. (1981) Computed tomography of primary liver tumours in children. Radiology 139: 431–435.
117. LeBerge JM, Laing FC, Federle MP et al. (1984) Hepatocellular carcinoma: assessment of resectability by computed tomography and ultrasound. Radiology 152: 485–490.
118. Miller JH, Gates GF, Stanley P (1977) The radiologic investigation of hepatic tumors in childhood. Radiology 124: 451–458.
119. Miller JH (1981) The ultrasonographic appearance of cystic hepatoblastoma. Radiology 138: 141–143.
120. Brunelle F, Chaumont P (1984) Hepatic tumors in children: ultrasonic differentiation of malignant from benign lesions. Radiology 150: 695–699.
121. Foley DW, Stewart ET, Milbrath JA et al. (1983) Digital subtraction angiography of the portal venous system. AJR Am J Roentgenol 140: 497–499.
122. Takayama T, Makuuchi M, Kosuge T et al. (1991) A hepatoblastoma originating in the caudate lobe radically resected with the inferior vena cava. Surgery 109: 208–213.
123. Ohtomo K, Itai Y, Yoshirawa K et al. (1987) Hepatic tumours: dynamic MR imaging. Radiology 163: 27–31.
124. Randolph JG, Altman RP, Arensman RM et al. (1978) Liver resection in children with hepatic neoplasms. Ann Surg 187: 599–605.
125. Weinblatt ME, Siegal SE, Siegal MM et al. (1982) Preoperative chemotherapy for unresectable primary hepatic malignancies in children Cancer 50: 1061–1064.
126. Quinn JJ, Altman AJ, Robinson HT et al. (1985) Adriamycin and cisplatin for hepatoblastoma. Cancer 56: 1926–1929.
127. Langevin AM, Pierro A, Liu P et al. (1990) Adriamycin and cis-platinum administered by continuous infusion preoperatively in hepatoblastoma unresectable at presentation. Med Pediatr Oncol 18: 181–184.
128. Tsuchida Y, Bastos JC, Honna T et al. (1990) Treatment of disseminated hepatoblastoma involving bilateral lobes.

J Pediatr Surg 25: 1253–1255.
129. Filler RM, Ehrlich PF, Greenberg ML et al. (1991) Preoperative chemotherapy in hepatoblastoma. Surgery 110: 591–597.
130. Ogita S, Tokiwa K, Taniguchi H, Takahashi T (1987) Intraarterial injection of antitumor drugs dispersed in lipid contrast medium: a choice for initially unresectable hepatoblastoma in infants. J Pediatr Surg 22: 412–414.
131. Perilongo G, Uni A (1989) Hepatoblastoma. Med Pediatr Oncol 17: 144–148.
132. Goldsmith NA, Woodburne RT (1957) The surgical anatomy pertaining to liver resection. Surg Gynecol Obstet 105: 310–318.
133. Tsuchida Y, Hashimoto H, Iwanaka T et al. (1989) Left hepatic trisegmentectomy for intralobar hepatoblastoma located close to the hepatic hilum. J Pediatr Surg 24: 1167–1168.
134. Bismuth H (1982) Surgical anatomy and anatomical surgery of the liver. World J Surg 6: 3–9.
135. Estrin JA, Belani KG, Karnavas AG et al. (1986) A new approach to massive blood transfusions during pediatric liver resection. Surgery 99: 664–670.
136. Stone HH (1975) Major hepatic resections in children. J Pediatr Surg 10: 127–135.
137. Putnam CW (1989) Techniques of ultrasonic dissection in resection of the liver. Surg Gynecol Obstet 157: 474–478.
138. Price JB, Schullinger JN, Sontulli NV (1982) Major hepatic resections for neoplasia in children. Arch Surg 117: 1139–1141.
139. Huguet CH, Nordliner B, Galopin JJ et al. (1978) Normothermic hepatic vascular exclusion for extensive hepatectomy. Surg Gynecol Obstet 147: 689–693.
140. Nordlinger B, Douvin D, Javardin L et al. (1980) An experimental study of survival after two hours of normothermic hepatic ischemia. Surg Gynecol Obstet 150: 859–864.
141. Fortner JG, Shiy MH, Kinne DW et al. (1974) Major hepatic resection using vascular isolation and hypothermic perfusion. Ann Surg 180: 644–652.
142. Schaller RT, Schaller JJ, Furman EB (1984) The advantages of hemodilution anesthesia for major liver resection in children. J Pediatr Surg 19: 705–710.
143. Ein SH, Shandling B, Williams WG et al. (1981) Major hepatic tumour resection using profound hypothermia and circulation arrest. J Pediatr Surg 16: 339–342.
144. Chang JHT, Janik JS, Burrington JD et al. (1988) Extensive tumor resection under deep hypothermia and circulatory arrest. J Pediatr Surg 23: 254–258.
145. Brown KB, Auldist AW, Davidson PM (1988) Anaesthetic considerations in liver tumor resection in children. Pediatr Surg Int 4: 11–15.
146. McDermott WV Jr (1967) Major hepatic resection in diagnostic techniques and metabolic problems. Surgery 54: 56–66.
147. Balasegaram M (1979) Hepatic resection for malignant tumours. Surg Rounds 2: 14–44.
148. Bar-Maor JA, Kam I, Sweed Y, Shashony G (1988) Resection of primary liver tumours in children. Harefuah 114: 594–598.
149. Pitchard J, Da Curha A, Cornbleet MA, Carter CJ (1982) Alpha-fetoprotein monitoring of response to adriamycin in hepatoblastoma. J Pediatr Surg 17: 429–430.
150. Kasai M, Watanabe I (1986) Liver tumurs. In: Voute PA, Barrett A, Bloom HL et al., eds. Cancer in children. Springer-Verlag, Berlin.
151. Whitington PF (1990) Advances in pediatric liver transplantation. Adv Pediatr 37: 357–379.
152. Iwatsuki S, Starzl TE, Sheahan DG et al. (1991) Hepatic resection versus transplantation for hepatocellular carcinoma. Ann Surg 214: 221–229.
153. Iwatsuki S, Gordon RD, Shaw BW et al. (1985) Role of liver transplantation in cancer therapy. Ann Surg 202: 401–407.
154. Colonna JO II, Ray RA, Goldstein Li et al. (1986) Orthotopic liver transplantation for hepatobiliary malignancy. Transplantation 42: 561–562.
155. Evans AE, Land VS, Newton WA et al. (1982) Combination chemotherapy (vincristine, adriamycin, cyclophosphamide, and 5-fluorouracil) in the treatment of children with malignant hepatoma. Cancer 50: 821–826.
156. Haas J, Maczynski A, Krailo M et al. (1984) Histopathology and prognosis in childhood hepatoblastoma and hepatocarcinoma. Cancer 64: 1082–1095.

Soft-Tissue Sarcoma

Peter Frey

7

Introduction

Soft-tissue sarcomas are malignant mesenchymal or soft-tissue tumours that not only behave aggressively with infiltrative growth at the site of the tumour – as most soft-tissue tumours do – but also metastasize and show a definite malignant histological pattern, which is often difficult to determine with certainty. Soft-tissue sarcomas are thought to originate from undifferentiated mesenchymal cells, being the initial cells for the development of connective tissue, muscle, fat, tendon and nerve tissue, as well as vascular and lymphatic structures. The undifferentiated initial mesenchymal cells can either develop into differentiated cells of the above-mentioned soft tissues, becoming malignant secondarily, or become malignant in the undifferentiated state or in a state that does not allow recognition of the cell line they belong to. These tumours are classified as undifferentiated sarcoma. A simplified adaptation to the neonatal age group of the classification of benign and malignant soft-tissue tumours by Stout and Lattes[1] and Krementz and Munchmore[2] is shown in Table 7.1.

Table 7.1 Simplified classification of soft-tissue tumours relevant to the neonatal age group

Tissue of origin	Benign form	Malignant form
Fibrous tissue	Fibroma Congenital fibromatosis[a] Congenital myofibromatosis[a]	Fibrosarcoma
Muscular tissue		
Striated	Rhabdomyoma	Rhabdomyosarcoma
Smooth	Leiomyoma	Leiomyosarcoma[b]
Vascular structures	Haemangioma Lymphangioma Benign haemangiopericytoma	Malignant haemangiopericytoma
Unknown origin		Undifferentiated sarcoma

[a] With locally infiltrative growth.
[b] Very rare in neonates.

Epidemiology

The aetiology of soft-tissue sarcoma is still unknown. Chromosomal aberration[3,4], viruses[2,5], irradiation[6] and lack of immune response[7] have been discussed as aetiological agents. In the adult population, soft-tissue sarcomas are relatively uncommon malignancies, forming approximately 0.5%–1% of all malignancies and having an incidence of 0.8% per 100 000 population[2]. In the neonatal population, however, the situation differs, with a reported incidence[8] of 36.5 per million live births or approximately one in 27 000. Barson[9] estimates a prevalence of neonatal neoplasia of one in 12 500 to one in 17 300 total births. Half of these neoplasms are diagnosed within 24 h of birth, and two-thirds during the first week[10]. Malignancies in the neonatal period are believed to represent 1%–1.9% of all paediatric malignancies[11,12] and account for one death per 6.24 million live births[13]. Soft-tissue sarcoma is estimated to represent 11.1%–15.7% of all neonatal malignancies[10,12,14]. Approximately 17% appear in childhood and 2% of these in the neonatal period[15]. The site of origin differs widely. As the tissue of origin is derived from the mesenchyme, which is present in all regions of the body, no real preference in predilection of the site can be expected. In a com-

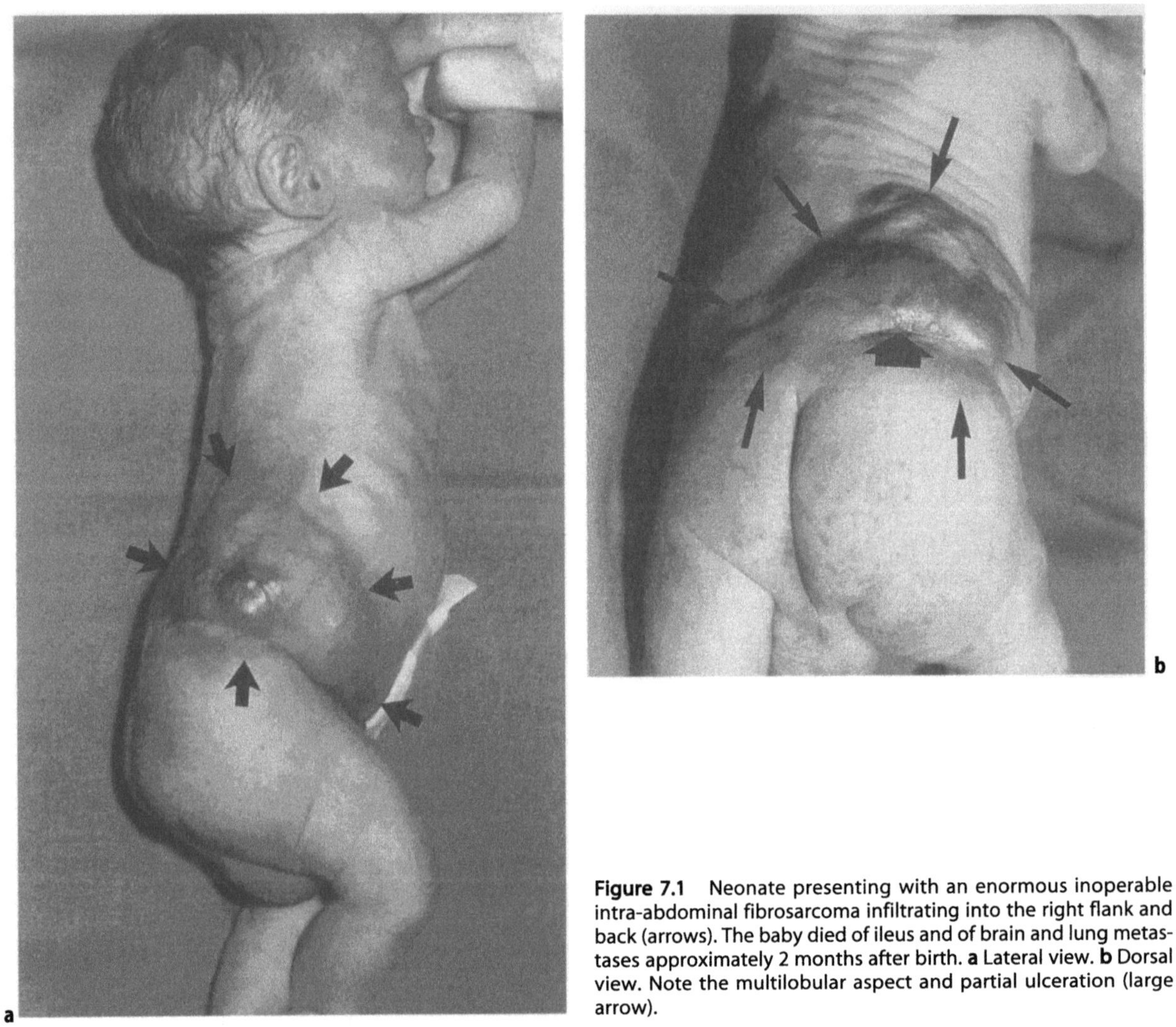

Figure 7.1 Neonate presenting with an enormous inoperable intra-abdominal fibrosarcoma infiltrating into the right flank and back (arrows). The baby died of ileus and of brain and lung metastases approximately 2 months after birth. **a** Lateral view. **b** Dorsal view. Note the multilobular aspect and partial ulceration (large arrow).

bined series of 48 neonates with the diagnosis of soft-tissue sarcoma[10–12,14,16], 25% occurred in the head and neck, 23% in the trunk, 19% in the lower limbs, 8% each in the urogenital system and upper limbs, and 6% in the abdomen. Commonest in children are rhabdomyosarcoma and undifferentiated sarcoma, which predominantly arise in the head and neck region and in the pelvis[2]. Generally, soft-tissue sarcomas (with the exception of rhabdomyosarcoma) grow relatively slowly, and commonly appear as painless small to medium-sized lesions. Neoplasms arising within muscular structures or in the abdominal or thoracic cavity are often recognized only when they have grown to a considerable mass and have become palpable or are interfering with the function of an organ by compression (Figure 7.1). Proper examination would reveal macroscopic lesions in the first 24 h of life in the majority of cases. Soft-tissue sarcomas have been diagnosed prenatally[17].

Once suspected, histopathological diagnosis and grading must follow without delay. In small lesions, excision biopsy is recommended; however, incisional biopsies should be undertaken in the larger lesions before complete surgical excision is attempted. The site of the incisional biopsy should be carefully chosen not to compromise further radical surgery. Needle biopsy may provide enough tissue for histological diagnosis, but there is a danger of tumour spread along the needle tract. Most soft-tissue sarcomas can be diagnosed by light microscopy using conventional staining techniques. Diagnosis may be difficult in up to 15% of cases[2], but electron microscopy[2], immunohistochemistry[18,19] and molecular biology[20] may help. With computed tomography and magnetic resonance imaging, it is possible to detect the exact anatomical position, extension of the tumour and metastases. Angiography can help to diagnose the tumour and to evaluate its relationship to major blood vessels before operation. Isotope scanning may detect metastatic spread. Accurate staging is essential because prognosis seems to be related to the anatomical localization, the size and the histopathological grading of the tumour[2,21]. However, it has to be stressed that neonatal soft-tissue sarcomas do not necessarily behave similarly to their adult counterparts. They are staged applying the TNM (tumour nodes metastasis) system, with additional tumour grading (G)[22]. Tumour size seems to be a good indicator for local recurrence and survival; however, prognosis is better predicted by anatomical location and histological grade[2]. The classification and staging of soft-tissue sarcomas is summarized in Table 7.2. The most frequently encountered forms in the neonatal period are fibrosarcoma followed by rhabdomyosarcoma and undifferentiated sarcoma. Malignant haemangiopericytomas are less often seen, and leiomyosarcoma is extremely rare in the neonatal period; therefore only fibromyosarcoma, rhabdomyosarcoma and undifferentiated sarcoma will be discussed in detail here.

Table 7.2 TNM classification and staging of soft tissue sarcoma

Stage	Histological grade of malignancy	Tumour size	Lymph node involvement	Distant metastases
Ia	G1	T1	N0	M0
Ib	T1	T2	N0	M0
IIa	G2	T1	N0	M0
IIb	G2	T2	N0	M0
IIIa	G3	T1	N0	M0
IIIb	G3	T2	N0	M0
IIIc	G1	T1	M1	
IVa	G1	T3	N0 or N1	M0
IVb	G1	T1	M1	

G1, low; G2, moderate; G3, high; T1, <5 cm; T2, >5 cm; T3, involving surrounding structures; N0, no lymph node involvement; N1, local or distant lymphatic metastases; M0, no distant metastases; M1, distant metastases. From Krementz and Munchmore[2].

Fibrosarcoma

Fibrosarcomas are malignant neoplasms arising from fibrous tissue. Over 80% of patients suffering from these neoplasms are over 20 years of age when diagnosis is established[23,24]. The histologically typical cell pattern of fibrosarcoma consists of spindle-shaped fibroblasts, aggressively infiltrating the surrounding tissues and forming pseudocapsules. In neonates, fibrosarcomas also represent the most common soft-tissue sarcomas and are histologically almost identical to the adult form, although their cells are more primitive looking, having a more rounded shape and being less pleomorphic – in other words being less mature[25–27]. Unlike in adults, a direct relationship between the histological appearance of the tumour and the final outcome is not evident in neonates[28]. Neonatal tumours are predominantly located in the distal parts of the upper and lower limbs, whereas in adults the common sites are the trunk, the thigh and the knee[25,27,29,30]. However, they have rarely been described in the abdomen, in the oral cavity[31] and in the lungs[32] in neonates. Contrary to findings in adults, metastasizing fibrosarcomas are very seldom seen in neonates, occurring in only about 8%–13% of cases diagnosed in early childhood[23,25,28,33]. Therefore, and owing to the lack of correlation between histology and prognosis, fibrosarcoma in neonates represents a separate entity differing from the adult form, not only because of its anatomical distribution, but also because it has a better prognosis even following less aggressive treatments[34]. Because these tumours rarely metastasize and have a tendency for only local recurrence, Dehner[35] prefers to use the term "congenital fibrosarcoma-like fibromatosis" (CFLF), rather than congenital fibrosarcoma. Others are reluctant to call fibrosarcoma "fibromatosis" because of its aggressive nature and its ability to metastasize, although it does so less frequent than when occurring in adults[36]. It has to be stressed that on occasion it is impossible or extremely difficult to distinguish histopathologically low-grade fibrosarcoma from the – by definition – benign infantile or congenital fibromatosis and myofibromatosis. The latter show very aggressive infiltrative growth locally, with occasional recurrence after surgery, but without metastatic tendency in neonates[13] (Figure 7.2). The generally suggested treatment of fibrosarcoma in neonates is radical surgery. An early wide local excision, well within healthy tissue, should be performed in the hope of preventing local recurrence, which is reported to occur in 16%–47% of cases[25,28,35]. However, in many patients the lesion

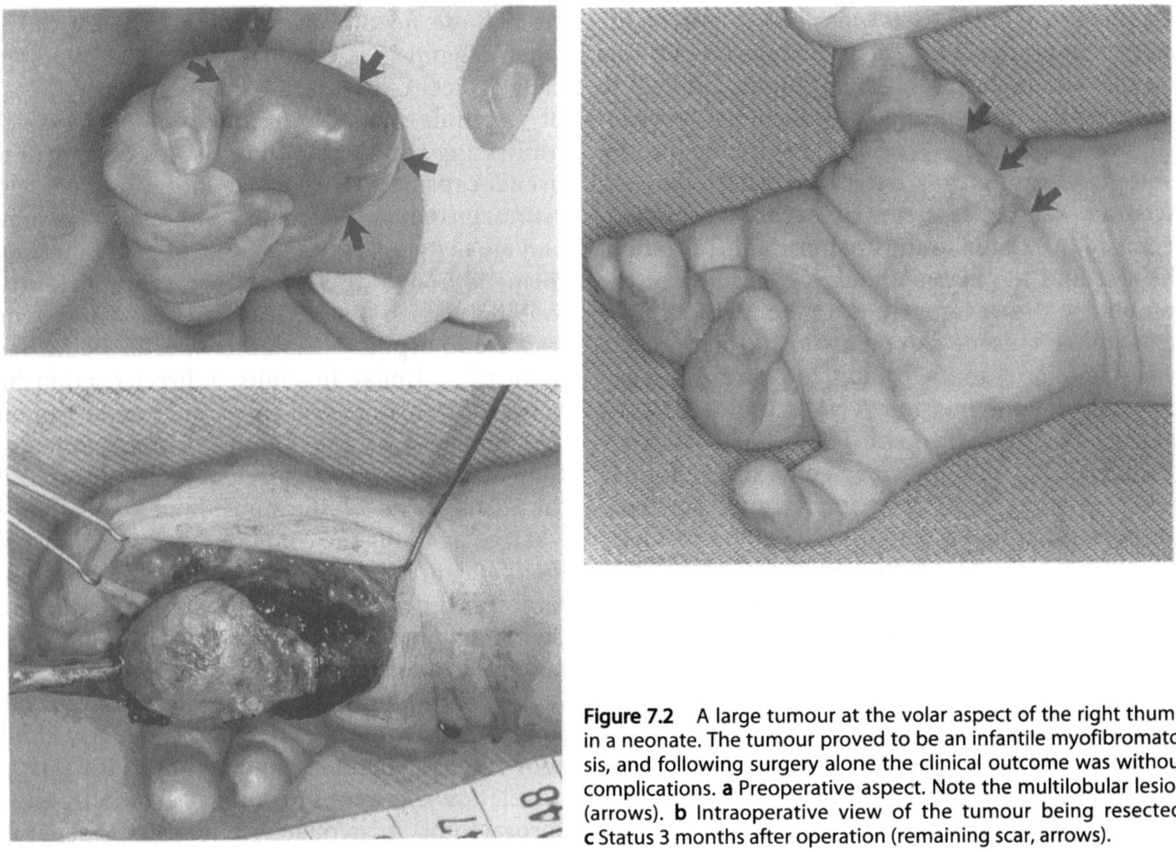

Figure 7.2 A large tumour at the volar aspect of the right thumb in a neonate. The tumour proved to be an infantile myofibromatosis, and following surgery alone the clinical outcome was without complications. **a** Preoperative aspect. Note the multilobular lesion (arrows). **b** Intraoperative view of the tumour being resected. **c** Status 3 months after operation (remaining scar, arrows).

can be adequately removed or recurrent tumour controlled only by amputation or disarticulation of a limb or part of it. In unresectable tumours, or if extensible mutilation or amputation is required for adequate resection, preoperative and postoperative chemotherapy may be used. Although there is not much evidence to indicate improved success rate with adjuvant chemotherapy or radiotherapy following surgery[23,25,27], Ninane et al.[34] reported excellent response to preoperative treatment of fibrosarcoma using a combination of vincristine, actinomycin D and cyclophosphamide (VAC)[37]. Salloum et al.[16] advocated the use of additional chemotherapy in particular cases (fibrosarcoma with the pathological features of malignant fibrous histiocytoma) to reduce existent risk, albeit small, of distant metastases. Preoperative chemotherapy, to make radical excision feasible, was suggested by Hays et al.[38] in the 1970s. Blocker et al.[28] reported a series of 52 neonatal patients with an overall mortality rate of 12%. Metastatic disease was also found in 12%. In 11 patients with fibrosarcoma of the upper extremity, there was no death or metastatic disease. Of 26 patients with the lesion situated at the lower extremity, two (8%) died and three (11%) had metastatic disease. In the 15 patients with axial lesions (head, neck, trunk, abdomen), four (27%) died and three (20%) had metastases.

In summary, fibrosarcoma in the newborn is a rare tumour. The treatment of choice is wide local excision, which can often be a mutilating procedure. Chemotherapy and radiotherapy may be of additional help in treating a tumour which shows a high tendency for local recurrence. Metastases and fatal outcome are relatively rare.

Rhabdomyosarcoma

Rhabdomyosarcoma is a soft-tissue tumour arising from striated muscle. Stout[39] first described it as a separate entity in 1946. Rhabdomyosarcoma is the most common soft-tissue tumour in children, accounting for approximately 8% of all solid tumours. They are generally diagnosed[40,41] before the age of 5–6 years, with a second peak between 15 and 19 years of age, probably due to the increased frequency of paratesticular tumours[41]. In the neonatal period, rhabdomyosarcomas are the second most common mesenchymal tumours after fibrosarcoma, accounting for approximately 3% of all rhabdomyosarcomas in childhood[42]. Neonatal rhabdomyosarcomas are seen in 17.9% of tumours described in the first year of life[41], with the head and neck region being the predominant primary site in neonates, followed by the urogenital tract[43]. Rhabdomyosarcomas are commonly hard or fleshy, white, well vascularized tumours, aggressively infiltrating the surrounding tissues. Cystic or myomatous and necrotic areas can be observed within the tumour, which is never surrounded by a true capsule, although occasionally a pseudocapsule may be observed. Rhabdomyosarcomas are diagnosed either at routine clinical examination of the newborn or when they manifest themselves by increasing mass effect on surrounding organs and vital structures. Prenatal diagnosis of rhabdomyosarcoma in the 36th gestational week has also been reported[7]. Tumours arising from the urogenital tract are often presented as botryoides lesion with a grape-like multinodular shape (Figure 7.3). Computed tomography and magnetic resonance imaging are excellent additional diagnostic means to detect and evaluate local infiltration and metastatic disease.

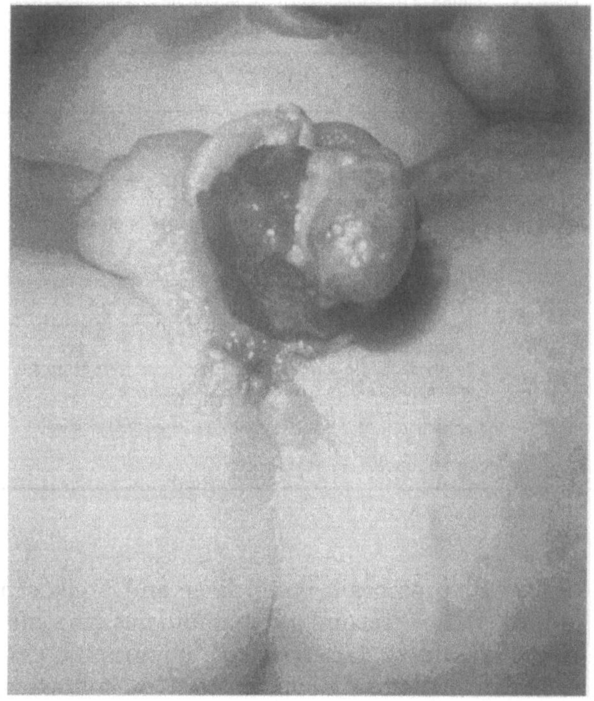

Figure 7.3 Sarcoma botryoides of the vagina. (Courtesy of Mr Prem Puri)

Histologically, neonatal rhabdomyosarcomas are commonly embryonal, of which the botryoid form is a variant. The morphology of the embryonal rhabdomyosarcoma corresponds to that of skeletal muscle between the 7th and 10th fetal week. The histological forms are at one extreme characterized by the undifferentiated "small blue or round cells" and at the other by well differentiated rhabdomyosarcoma cells[35]. The histologically alveolar type has morphology similar to that of striated muscle of the 8th to 12th fetal week and is rarely encountered in the neonatal period[11,41]. Palmer et al.[44] suggest a new histological classification, distinguishing monomorphous, anaplastic and mixed pathological types. The first group shows uniform size of tumour cell. The second group is characterized by enlarged and bizarre mitotic figures and has a very poor prognosis. These tumours have been divided[45] into subgroups I with only scattered anaplastic cells, and II with foci or large sheets of anaplastic cells and a poorer prognosis than subgroup I. The third mixed group, representing the majority of rhabdomyosarcomas (80%), has a relatively good prognosis.

Therapy for rhabdomyosarcoma consists of surgical excision, chemotherapy and radiotherapy. Surgery and irradiation are regarded as local therapies; chemotherapy is generally indicated in the treatment of metastases, although it has been used before operation to reduce tumour size. Following total or partial excision, the rhabdomyosarcoma can be staged as proposed by the Intergroup Rhabdomyosarcoma Study[46]. The staging criteria[46,47] are given in Table 7.3.

As complete local resection of rhabdomyosarcoma often cannot be achieved, additional chemotherapy or irradiation becomes necessary. Fortunately, rhabdomyosarcoma responds well to chemotherapeutic agents such as vincristine, actinomycin D and cyclophosphamide. In addition, Adriamycin, cisplatin, etoposide and ifosfamide have been shown to be effective in treating this neoplasm[47]. Radiotherapy can control local disease in neonates, but radiotherapy to immature

Table 7.3 Staging of rhabdomyosarcoma: Intergroup Rhabdomyosarcoma Study

Group	Description
1	Localized disease, completely resected Regional nodes not involved a Confined to muscle or organ of origin b Contiguous involvement Infiltration outside the muscle or organ of origin, as though facial planes
II	a Grossly resected tumour with microscopic residual disease (nodes negative) b Regional disease, completely resected (nodes positive or negative) c Regional disease with involved nodes, grossly resected, but with evidence of microscopic residual disease
III	Incomplete resection or biopsy with gross residual disease
IV	Metastatic disease present at onset

From Freeman and Woods[47].

tissues such as brain, lung, liver and bone can induce major secondary pathologies in survivors[48]. Gale et al.[10] reported radiographic evidence of structural scoliosis in 70% following radiation treatment with a dose of 3380 cGy. Indirect effects on growth by interference with the endocrine system have also been mentioned with radiotherapy[10]. Depression of immune function may be induced indirectly, and the development of secondary malignancy is reported[49]. However, there is no evidence that neonates are especially vulnerable[48]. Lie et al.[49] computed a 17% cumulative probability for developing a second cancer in an irradiated field in patients surviving 20 years. Ragab et al.[41] recommended reducing the commonly applied dose of 5000–6000 cGy in older children to not more than 4000 cGy over a period of 5 weeks.

Chemotherapy in the neonate is associated with a higher incidence of complications, such as infection caused by depressing the immune system, or compromised somatic development[50]. A higher death rate related to chemotherapy has been reported in infancy and in neonates[41]. It has been recommended that the doses be reduced to 50% of that commonly administered in the older child: if this reduced dose is well tolerated without myelodepression it can be gradually increased to the full dose. Recent reports[16,41,51] indicate that this dose-reduced chemotherapy is not associated with life-threatening side-effects, and more importantly has not negatively affected the survival rate of patients[41]. The frequency of local recurrence is estimated to be approximately 30% despite adequate surgery and chemotherapy[46]. Early lymphatic spread has been reported, especially in tumours of the lower limb[52], although initial metastases are generally rare in infants[53]. Secondary haematogenous metastases appear later in life[7] and involve the lungs in 40% and the bones in 10%–20%. Ragab et al.[41] reported an overall survival rate of 63% in infants and neonates. Survival rate in patients with group I tumours was 90%, group II 66%, group III 41% and group IV only 33%. Rhabdomyosarcoma of the embryonal type is generally associated with a better prognosis than that of the alveolar form[44], therefore accurate differentiation is essential. Recent reports[19,54] stress the importance of biochemical and immunohistochemical analysis of muscular proteins for achieving this.

In summary, rhabdomyosarcomas in neonates carry a slightly better prognosis than those in older children; however, the risk and benefit of aggressive treatment has to be carefully calculated and discussed with the parents in advance.

Undifferentiated sarcoma

Unclassifiable undifferentiated sarcomas are the third important group of neonatal soft-tissue sarcomas, although they are only occasionally diagnosed. Twelve undifferentiated neonatal sarcomas were reported in four series[10–12,16]. The trunk (six patients) and head and neck (five) were the main sites involved. In only one case was the neoplasm found to be localized at the lower limb. Histologically, these tumours generally appear as small round-cell neoplasms with scant cytoplasm and hyperchromatic nuclei[1,2]. They may resemble embryonal rhabdomyosarcoma. Apart from the fact that they occur in neonates and children and that they are only partly responsive to irradiation and chemotherapy, little is known about these tumours.

Treatment of the above-mentioned 12 neonatal tumours was predominantly by surgery, alone (five patients) or in combination with chemotherapy (four). One patient was treated with surgery, chemotherapy and radiation, and one with chemotherapy and radiation alone. No treatment was initiated in the remaining patient. Of the 12 patients, eight died and four are alive and well. Of the four patients who were disease free, the lesion involved the chest wall in three and was treated by surgery alone (two patients) and surgery with chemotherapy (one). A further undifferentiated tumour was localized in the orbit of the neonate. Up to now, undifferentiated sarcomas have had the worst clinical course, and most fatalities are seen in this group of soft-tissue sarcomas. Electron microscopy, biohistochemistry immune assays and molecular biology now allow specific classification of these lesions, which assists in choosing the optimal treatment and predicting the prognosis.

Haemangiopericytoma

Haemangiopericytoma, first described by Stout and Murray[55], is a relatively rare vascular tumour in childhood and especially in neonates. The neoplasm develops mainly from pericytes, which are contractile cells surrounding the capillaries. Some structural and clinicopathological features are similar to those of congenital fibromatosis[11,35]. A particular form of haemangiopericytoma presents with multiple subcutaneous nodular lesions[56]. According to Maillet et al.[57], the diagnosis of haemangiopericytoma is based on the existence of a normal wall of the vessel, extravascular tumour-cell proliferation and a surrounding reticulin net. They also state that no histological sign is prognostic. Tumours having a histologically malignant appearance can evolve into benign lesions, and tumours classified as benign can become malignant, showing local recurrence and metastases[57]. For this reason it is suggested that these tumours be considered malignant until evolution proves otherwise. However, Enterline[58] states that tumours arising in neonates are essentially benign, irrespective of their appearance. Salloum et al.[16] go even further and state that malignancy is often overestimated, based on increased cellularity, the relatively immature aspect of the tumour cells, the tendency for infiltration and the high mitotic activity of the lesion[56,60]. In the series published by Kauffman and Stout[43], 9.2% of 120 congenital mesenchymal tumours were classified as haemangiopericytoma. In eight patients (6.7%) diagnosis was made in the neonatal period: the disease followed a favourable course in all eight. Maillet et al.[57], however, found in a literature search that, of 94 children with haemangiopericytoma, 23 (24%) were diagnosed in the neonatal period. A predominance of the male sex was reported. Of these tumours, 66% were found in subcutaneous tissues, predominantly in the extremities, the head and neck region and the trunk[43,57]. Maillet et al.[57] report an overall malignancy rate of 45% (42 out of 94) in children as opposed to 20% (five of 25) in neonates. Common sites of metastases were the lungs, bones, lymph nodes and liver. The treatment of choice for malignant haemangiopericytoma is wide local excision. If only partial resection is possible or the tumour is resected within an infiltrated margin, chemotherapy should be started immediately. Adriamycin seems to be the most effective drug; however, combination with vincristine, cyclophosphamide and actinomycin D allows a reduction in the amount of each drug, thus reducing toxicity[61].

In summary, haemangiopericytomas are tumours of uncertain malignancy and outcome. Malignant changes often become evident only a long time after the onset of the disease[62]. Primary therapy should be wide surgical excision. If this is not possible, adjuvant chemotherapy should be introduced.

Leiomyosarcoma

Leiomyosarcomas are malignant tumours arising from smooth muscle. They are rare in adults and represent approximately 15% of all soft-tissue sarcomas. Leiomyosarcomas are the most common soft-tissue sarcomas of the gastrointestinal tract[2]. Because of the intra-abdominal site of these tumours, they are often diagnosed only in an advanced state. The prognosis of these lesions in adults is poor. In a series of 36 adult patients, Krementz and Munchmore[2] found a 5 year survival rate of only 28%. Leiomyosarcomas infiltrate locally into the surrounding tissue and metastasize predominantly into the local lymph nodes, the liver and the lungs. Histologically, anaplastic, bizarre, often ovoid-looking cells with monomorphous blunt-ended nuclei are described[60]. Leiomyosarcoma has been reported in 16 children[12,63], of whom seven (44%) were newborns. In four neonatal patients the site of the tumour was the colon and in the other three the small bowel. Four were females and two males, and in one case the sex was not reported. This female predominance in the neonatal age group could also be found when analysing "all" known children with leiomyosarcoma[63]. In adults, however, a male predominance has been reported[64]. Therapy of choice seems to be wide surgical resection, often requiring small or large bowel resection. Adjuvant chemotherapy with vincristine, cyclophosphamide, actinomycin D and in particular adriamycin seem to have a positive effect on the disease[63,65]. Although radiotherapy has been used[66], it is generally considered to be ineffective. Analysing the ten children for whom follow-up was available, the survival rate[12,63] was 90%, and one child in whom a jejunal leiomyosarcoma was diagnosed in the neonatal period died. The survival rate dropped to 85.7% in neonates, still being much higher than that seen in adults. These findings are in accordance with Kriss's statement[67] that leiomyosarcomas are far less malignant in children than in adults.

References

1. Stout AP, Lattes RL (1966) Atlas of tumour pathology, second series, fascicle 1, Tumours of the soft tissues. Armed Force Institute of Pathology, Washington, DC p 14.
2. Krementz ET, Munchmore MD (1983) Soft tissue sarcomas. Behaviour and management. Adv Surg 16: 147–196.
3. Gorman PA, Malone M, Pritchard J, Sheer D (1990) Deletion of part of the short arm of chromosome 17 in a congenital fibrosarcoma. Cancer Genet Cytogenet 48: 193–198.
4. Speleman F, Dalcin P, De Potter K et al. (1989) Cytogenetic investigation of a case of congenital fibrosarcoma. Cancer Genet Cytogenet 39: 21–24.
5. Perk K, Maloney JB, Jenkins EG (1967) Further studies on the relationship of a rhabdomyosarcoma virus to muscle tissue. Int J Cancer 22: 43.
6. Pettit VE, Chamness JT, Ackermann LV (1954) Fibromatosis and fibrosarcoma following irradiation therapy. Cancer 7: 149.
7. Gatti RA, Good RA (1971) Occurrence of malignancy in immunodeficiency disease: a literature review. Cancer 28: 89–98.
8. Bader JL, Miller RW (1979) US cancer incidence and mortality in the first year of life. Am J Dis Child 133: 157–159.
9. Barson AJ (1978) Congenital neoplasia: the society's experience. Arch Dis Child 53: 436.
10. Gale GB, D'Angio GJ, Uri A, Chatten J, Koop CE (1982) Cancer in neonates: the experience at the Children's Hospital of Philadelphia. Pediatrics 7: 409–413.
11. Isaacs HJ (1985) Perinatal (congenital and neonatal) neoplasms: a report of 110 cases. Pediatr Pathol 3: 165–216.
12. Campbell AN, Chan HS, O'Brien A, Smith CR, Becker LE (1987) Malignant tumours in the neonate. Arch Dis Child 62: 19–23.
13. Fraumeni JF, Miller RW (1969) Cancer death in the newborn. Am J Dis Child 117: 186–189.
14. Davis CF, Carachi R, Young DG (1988) Neonatal tumours: Glasgow 1955–86. Arch Dis Child 63: 1075–1078.
15. Coffin CM, Dehner LP (1990) Soft tissue tumours in first year of life. A report of 190 cases. Pediatr Pathol 10: 509–526.
16. Salloum E, Flamant F, Caillaud JM et al. (1990) Diagnostic and therapeutic problems of soft tissue tumors other than rhabdomyosarcoma in infants under one year of age: a clinicopathological study of 34 cases treated at the Institute Gustave Roussy. Med Pediatr Oncol 18: 37–43.
17. Pautard B, Canarelli JP, Gontier MF, Risbourg B, Piussan C, Flamant F (1990) Rhabdomyosarcoma embryonnaire de découverte anténatale. Arch Fr Pediatr 47: 433–435.
18. Huth JF, Gupta RK, Morton DL (1981) Development of an enzyme immunoassay to detect and quantitate tumor-associated antigens in the urine of sarcoma patients. Cancer 47: 2856–2861.
19. Barbet JP, Kurzenne JY, Butler-Browne GS, Mouly V, Laurent M, Gubler JP (1989) Rhabdomyosarcoma de découverte néonatale. Etude des marqueurs de différenciation musculaire. Ann Pathol 9: 363–368.
20. Clinical conference (1994) Small-round-cell tumours of childhood. Lancet 344: 725–729.
21. Enneking WF, Spanier SS, Malawar MM (1981) The effect of the anatomic setting on the results of surgical procedures for soft parts sarcoma of the thigh. Cancer 47: 1005–1022.
22. Russel WD, Cohen J, Edmonson JH (1981) Staging system for soft tissue sarcoma. Semin Oncol 8: 156.
23. Soule EH, Pritchard DJ (1977) Fibrosarcoma in infants and children. A review of 110 cases. Cancer 40: 1711–1721.
24. Balsaver AM, Butler J, Martin RG (1967) Congenital fibrosarcoma. Cancer 20: 1607–1616.
25. Chung EB, Enzinger FM (1976) Infantile fibrosarcoma. Cancer 38: 729–739.
26. Gonzalez-Crussi F, Wiederhold MD, Sotelo-Avida C (1980) Congenital fibrosarcoma: presence of a histiocytic component. Cancer 46: 77–86.
27. Enzinger FM, Weiss SW (1983) Soft tissue tumors, 2nd edn. CV Mosby, St. Louis, pp 115–124.
28. Blocker S, Koenig J, Ternberg J (1987) Congenital fibrosarcoma. J Pediatr Surg 22: 665–760.
29. Iwasaki H, Enjoji M (1979) Infantile and adult fibrosarcomas of the soft tissues. Acta Pathol Jpn 29: 377–388.
30. Martell JR, Brusnardo MS, Barja RH, Gordon F (1986) Congenital fibrosarcoma of the forearm. A case report. J Bone Joint Surg 68: 620–623.
31. Tarsitano BF (1990) Oral infantile fibrosarcoma: report of a case. J Oral Maxillofac Surg 48: 1228–1230.
32. Desrousseaux B, Gourdin C, Atat I et al. (1989) Fibrosarcome pulmonaire néonatal. Chir Pédiatr 30: 295–296.
33. Stout AP (1962) Fibrosarcoma in infants and children. Cancer 15: 1028–1040.
34. Ninane J, Gosseye S, Panteon E, Claus D, Rombouts JJ, Cornu G (1986) Congenital fibrosarcoma. Preoperative chemotherapy and conservative surgery. Cancer 58: 1400–1406.
35. Dehner LP (1981) Neoplasms of the fetus and neonate. In: Naeye RL, Kissane JM, Kauffman N, eds. Perinatal disease. Monographs in pathology 22. Williams and Wilkins, Baltimore, 286–346.
36. Coffin CM, Jaszcz W, O'Shea PA, Dehner LP (1994) So called congenital infantile fibrosarcoma: does it exist and what is it? Pediatr Pathol 14: 133–150.
37. Flamant F, Hill C (1984) The improvement in survival associated with combined chemotherapy in childhood rhabdomyosarcoma: a historical comparison of 345 patients in the same center. Cancer 53: 2417–2421.
38. Hays DM, Mirabal VQ, Karlan MS, Patel HR, Landing BH

(1970) Fibrosarcomas in infants and children. J Pediatr Surg 5: 176–183.
39. Stout AP (1946) Rhabdomyosarcoma of the skeletal muscles. Ann Surg 123: 447–472.
40. Dias P, Kumar P, Marsden HB et al. (1987) Evaluation of desmin as a diagnostic and a prognostic marker of childhood rhabdomyosarcomas and embryonal sarcomas. Br J Cancer 56: 361–365.
41. Ragab AH, Heyn R, Tefft M, Hays DN, Newton WAJ, Beltangady M (1986) Infants younger than 1 year of age with rhabdomyosarcoma. Cancer 58: 2606–2610.
42. Li PF, Fraumeni JF (1969) Rhabdomyosarcoma in children: epidemiologic study and identification of familial cancer syndrome. J Natl Cancer Inst 43: 1365–1373.
43. Kauffman SL, Stout AP (1956) Congenital mesenchymal tumors. Cancer 18: 460–476.
44. Palmer NF, Foulkes MA, Sachs N, Newton WA (1983) Rhabdomyosarcoma: a cytological classification of prognostic significance. Proc Am Soc Clin Oncol 2: 229.
45. Kudet R, Newton WA Jr, Hamoudi AB, Asmar L, Jacobs DL, Maurer HM (1993) Childhood rhabdomyosarcoma with anaplastic (pleomorphic) features: a report of the Intergroup Rhabdomyosarcoma Study. Am J Surg Oncol 17: 443–453.
46. Maurer HM, Beltangady M, Gehan EA, Crist W, Hammond D (1988) The Intergroup Rhabdomyosarcoma Study-1. A final report. Cancer 61: 209–220.
47. Freeman AI, Woods G (1990) Genitourinary tumors. In: Ashcraft KW, ed. Pediatric urology. WB Saunders, Philadelphia, pp 449–456.
48. Littman P, D'Angio GJ (1981) Radiation therapy in the neonate. AM J Pediatr Hematol Oncol 3: 279–285.
49. Li FP, Cassady JR, Jaffe N (1975) Risk of second tumour in survivors of childhood cancer. Cancer 35: 1230–1235.
50. Siegel SE, Moran RG (1981) Problems in the chemotherapy of cancer in the neonate. Am J Pediatr Hematol Oncol 3: 287–296.
51. Koscielniak E, Harms D, Schmidt D et al. (1989) Soft tissue sarcomas in infants younger than 1 year of age: a report of the German soft tissue sarcoma study group (CWS-81). Med Pediatr Oncol 17: 105–113.
52. Shimada H, Newton WA, Soule EH, Beltangady MS, Maurer HM (1987) Pathology of fatal rhabdomyosarcoma. Report from the Intergroup Rhabdomyosarcoma Study. Cancer 59: 459–465.
53. Ruymann BF, Maddux RH, Ragab A (1988) Congenital anomalies associated with rhabdomyosarcoma: an autopsy study in 115 cases. Med Pediatr Oncol 16: 33–39.
54. Molenaar WM, Oosterhuis JW, Ramakaers FCS (1985) Mesenchymal and muscle-specific intermediate filaments (vimentin and desmin) in relation to differentiation in childhood rhabdomyosarcomas. Hum Pathol 16: 838–843.
55. Stout AP, Murray MR (1942) Hemangiopericytoma. A vascular tumor featuring Zimmerman's pericyte. Ann Surg 116: 26–33.
56. Seibert JJ, Seibert RW, Weisenburger DS, Allsbrook W (1978) Multiple congenital hemangiopericytomas of the head and neck. Laryngoscope 88: 1006–1012.
57. Maillet P, Lamesch A, Dawagne MP (1985) L'hémangiopéricytome congénital: à propos de deux cas personnels. Revue de la littérature. Chir Pediatr 26: 22–25.
58. Enterline HT (1981) Histopathology of sarcomas. Semin Oncol 8: 133.
59. Chen KTK, Kassel SH, Medrano VA (1986) Congenital hemangiopericytoma. J Surg Oncol 31: 127–129.
60. Atkinson JB, Mahour GH, Issacs H, Ortega JA (1984) Hemangiopericytoma in infants and children. A report of six patients. Am J Surg 48: 372–374.
61. Wong PP, Yagoda A (1978) Chemotherapy of malignant hemangiopericytoma. Cancer 41: 1256–1260.
62. Hollmann G, Heopner F, Daum R, Stuhlinger M (1972) Beitrag zur Klinik des Hämangioperizytoms. Langenbecks Arch Klin Chir 330: 128.
63. Angerpointer TA, Weitz H, Haas RJ, Hecker WC (1981) Intestinal leiomyosarcoma in childhood – case report and review of the literature. J Pediatr Surg 16: 491–495.
64. Akwarei OE, Dozois RR, Weiland LH, Beahrs OH (1978) Leiomyosarcoma of the small and large bowel. Cancer 42: 1375–1384.
65. Pinedo HM (1977) Chemotherapy of advanced soft tissue sarcomas in adults. Cancer Treat Rev 4: 67–86.
66. Sztankay C (1959) Geheiltes Rektumsarkom im Kindesalter. Zentralbl Chir 84: 826–830.
67. Kriss N (1960) Leiomyosarcoma of the colon in an infant. Am J Roentgenol Radiat Ther Nucl Med 84: 540–545.

Ovarian Tumours

Jean Gaudin

8

Introduction

The presence of an abdominal mass in a female neonate should suggest the diagnosis of an ovarian tumour. Ovarian cysts are the commonest ovarian tumours during this period. Before antenatal ultrasonography was available, these tumours were usually detected during routine abdominal examination or when serious complications (rupture or haemorrhage) ensued. Now, ultrasonography permits both antenatal and postnatal detection, assessment and follow-up of these cases. The possibility of complications developing justifies management being carried out in a surgical unit.

The pathophysiology of the neonatal follicular cyst is yet to be determined and probably results from hormonal hyperstimulation. The high gonadal steroid levels in the follicular cystic fluid and the luteinization of the cyst lining probably reflect this hormonal stimulation. Small ovarian cysts (a few millimetres in diameter) are therefore frequently seen in neonates[1]. The development of pathological follicular cysts may be the consequence of a precocious peak of follicle-stimulating hormone between the 20th and 30th weeks or of an abnormal peak of human chorionic gonadotrophin (for example in maternal diabetes and placental senescence, but recent reports do not support these associations). They may also be caused by an abnormal ovarian follicle or a disorder of enzymatic activity in the internal theca.

Embryology and pathogenesis

The gonad remains undifferentiated till the 50th gestational day. The process of ovarian differentiation is then marked by the proliferation and migration of the coelomic epithelium in the underlying mesenchyma. The presence in the ovarian cortex of crypts lined by the surface epithelium and then of cystic inclusions in the coelomic epithelium seems almost constant in the 12th week. The follicles appear in the 4th month and evolve towards the antral follicular stage. From the 21st week onwards, antral follicles with crowns of granulosa cells are present. Follicle-stimulating hormone and luteinizing hormone trigger follicular development, and then human chorionic gonadotrophin stimulates development up to the diploid stage.

Pathology

The majority of neonatal tumours detected on ultrasonography, if not all, are ovarian cysts. These cysts bulge through the cortex of the ovary and have a bluish smooth surface with a fine vascular architecture. They are unilocular, thin walled and filled with yellowish serous fluid. Pathological examination confirms their benign nature and differentiates a follicular from a simple cyst. Histologically a follicular cyst is lined by a layer of granulosa cells and surrounded by a connective tissue capsule, whereas a simple cyst is lined by simple epithelium with no distinguishing characteristics.

In torsion, necrosis makes classification impossible because the ovarian parenchyma is damaged. However, the histopathologist may find some more or less well preserved follicles. The absence

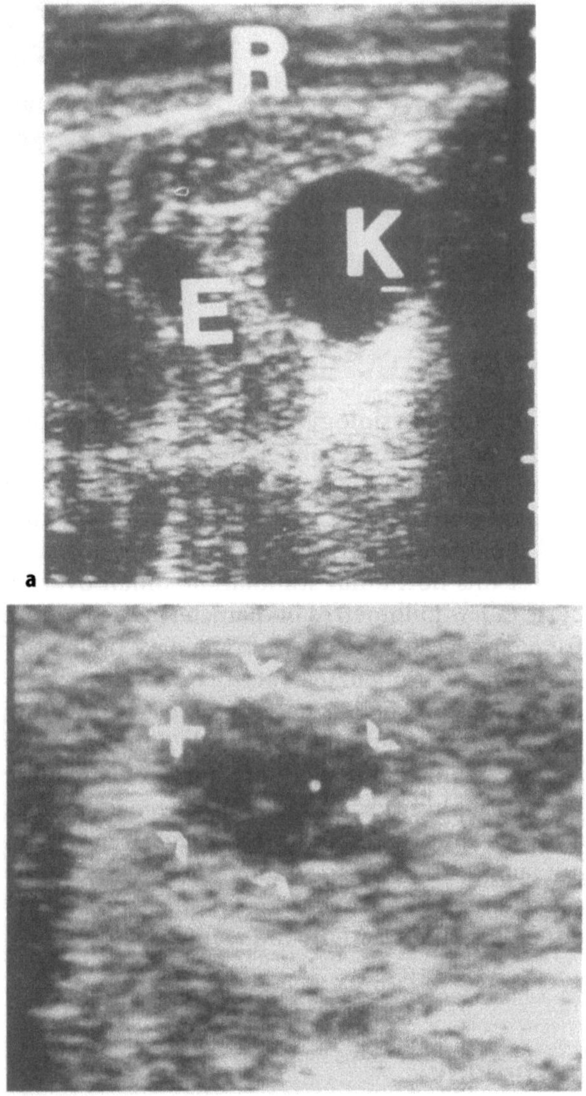

a

b

Figure 8.1 **a** Antenatal ultrasonography at 34 weeks' gestation revealed an ovarian cyst – a fluid-filled mass. K, cyst; R, kidney; E, stomach. **b** Postnatal ultrasonography on day 2 of life of the same infant showed spontaneous regression in cyst size to 15 mm. On day 7 there was no evidence of the cyst by ultrasonography.

of identifiable ovarian follicles and the presence of cystic calcium deposits and signs of resorption (giant cells) are evidence of an old ischaemic torsion.

Malignant ovarian tumour in a neonate is rare and the reported cases are few[2], and benign ovarian tumours (teratoma, cystadenoma, granulosa cell tumour, parovarian tumour) constitute less than 20% of ovarian tumours. With the more frequent use of antenatal ultrasonography more ovarian cysts are being identified, and the percentages of both benign and malignant tumours have decreased[3–6].

Prenatal diagnosis

These cysts are now usually diagnosed during routine antenatal ultrasonography, usually after the 28th week, as a rounded intra-abdominal fluid-filled mass in a female fetus (Figure 8.1*a*). The scan shows a fluid mass of homogeneous content, often found in the hypochondrium or the mid-abdomen. It is flexible and mobile during examination, or from one examination to the next. A cyst is considered pathological when more than 20 mm in diameter. These can reach 120 mm in size[5,7]. The quantity of amniotic fluid is normal. The image of a divided cyst may be seen. Ultrasonography also helps to detect urinary tract malformations, which are not uncommon.

Sonographic follow-up of these cysts will reveal their antenatal development. They may spontaneously regress, remain static with no sign of complication, or proceed to develop complications in utero. Spontaneous regression of these cysts, which is not due to rupture, seems to be quite common: it can occur in up to 50% of cysts discovered antenatally and is more often encountered in cysts measuring less than 40 mm in diameter. This regression often begins towards the end of pregnancy or sometimes during the first few days of independent life (Figure 8.1*b*).

Torsion of these ovarian cysts mostly occurs antenatally. Its frequency is about one in two[8–10]. In utero torsion is diagnosed sonographically by the presence of intracystic floculation, in which the sediment is deposited in the most dependent part of the cyst, giving a characteristic fluid level (Figure 8.2). At the end of development, a rare image is that of a solid mass, moderately echogenic and homogeneous (Figure 8.3), or of a double-level aspect if the cystic cavity is divided[11] (Figure 8.4). Floculation is pathognomonic of torsion, whereas some torsions do not reflect ultrasonic beams. Torsion may develop secondary complications such as pericystic adhesions (causing obstruction[12], perforation of the bowel[13] or adhesions to the opposite fallopian tube) or cystic rupture (causing peritonitis or haemoperitoneum)[14]. The discovery of bilateral cysts is infre-

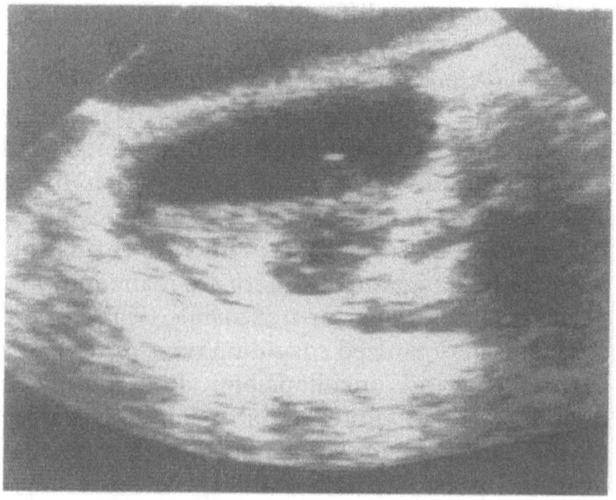

Figure 8.2 Antenatal ultrasonography showing intracystic floculation, indicating in utero torsion of an ovarian cyst.

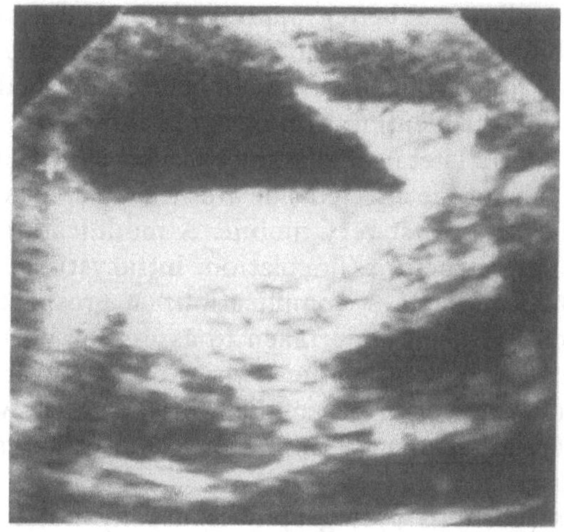

Figure 8.4 Antenatal torsion of an ovarian cyst. Ultrasonography showed a cystic cavity divided by fluid level.

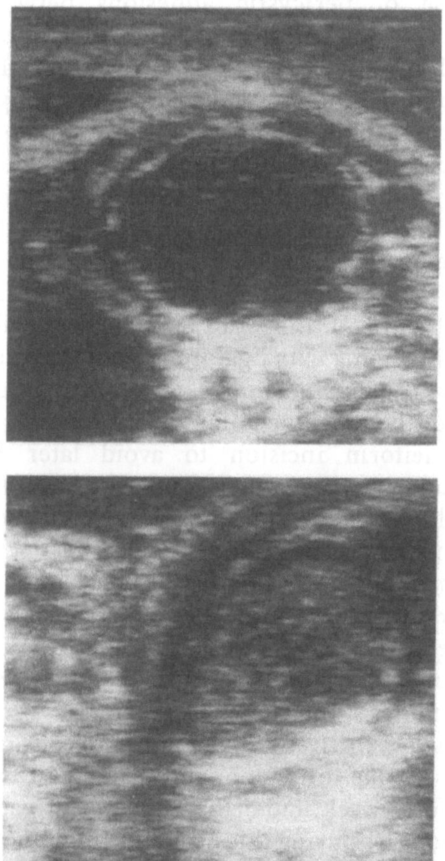

a

b

Figure 8.3 Antenatal torsion of an ovarian cyst. The sediment gradually filled the entire cystic cavity. **a** 35 weeks' gestation. **b** 40 weeks'gestation.

quent and is an acute problem as it may affect ovarian function in later life[15,16].

Clinical presentation

In recent years, with routine prenatal ultrasonography, increasing numbers of ovarian cysts have been detected. Only 50% of these cases are detectable as an abdominal mass during routine examination or present with complications such as obstruction, peritonitis, haemorrhage, torsion or ascites.

Differential diagnosis

It is usually easy to exclude a renal or bladder abnormality – endopelvic sacrococcygeal teratoma, anterior meningocele or encysted meconium peritonitis – by ultrasonography. Ovarian cysts should also be differentiated from other intra-abdominal fluid masses – the infrequent antenatal choledochal cyst, pancreatic cyst, mesenteric cyst or gastrointestinal duplication, which can usually be excluded by postnatal assessment.

Abdominal plain radiography can show the mass displacing the intestinal loops. Postnatal scan allows a better appreciation of the size, mobility and of the cyst. The exact localization of a cyst to the right or left can only be established by the correct identification of the healthy ovary on the contra lateral side, as the vascular pedicle and the tube of the affected side are stretched, making the ovarian cyst very mobile. A modification of the echostructure (floculation, intracystic level) should indicate a complication. A prospective study has been undertaken to assess the normal ovaries in infants under 2 years of age. Ovarian cysts were seen in 84% of the ovaries imaged, with cysts larger than 9 mm in 18% of all cystic ovaries[17].

Intravenous pyelography is usually not indicated if the ultrasound diagnosis is certain. On rare occasions, a tumour is revealed by ultrasonography as a heterogeneous mass, near a cyst with vegetations, or by the presence of calcification on plain radiography.

Management

Delivery should take place according to obstetric criteria only. The possibility of spontaneous regression towards term contraindicates in utero therapy. Close collaboration between obstetricians and paediatric surgeons ensures that neonatal assessment will be carried out in the first few days of life and under optimal conditions.

Treatment

Treatment depends on the nature of the cyst, its possible evolution (regressing, stationary or complicated) and knowledge of the exact nature of the tumour. The aim for treatment of uncomplicated cysts is to avoid torsion and to preserve as much parenchyma as possible, and in antenatal cystic torsion to avoid gastrointestinal, peritoneal and gynaecological complications.

Choice of treatment will depend on the progress, aspect and size of the cyst: the decision is simple for cysts which are regressing or are in torsion, but more difficult for simple unchanging cysts[7,9,11,18–20].

A cyst that diminishes *significantly in size* before birth or during the first few days of life without any peritoneal effusion must be followed ultrasonographically to check its return to an accepted size (20 mm) and then its disappearance.

Torsion requires surgery. Puncture is possible but may be dangerous (if there are many multiple pericystic adhesions) or impossible (if the cystic content is of organized coagulum type, or the walls mummified and uncollapsible). Laparotomy is done through a Pfannenstiel incision. Exploration of the affected side to determine the state of ovarian parenchyma, viability of the cyst (necrosed or not) and state of the tube (necrosis of the distal part, atrophy, pedicle rupture with wandering tumour)[21] follows. The opposite ovary frequently contains minor cysts and must be examined. This exploration may necessitate the release of pericystic adhesions between the necrosed cyst and the opposite tube and ovary, small intestine or colon. Delivery of the cyst through the incision is usually easy owing to the pedicle's length (Figure 8.5). However, large cysts can be punctured after protecting the abdominal cavity and determining the benign nature of the cyst. The surgical manoeuvre depends on the state of the ovary. Detorsion is undertaken. The discovery of old torsion, frequently with necrosis of the distal part of the adnexa, demands salpingo-oophorectomy with ligature of both the round and ovarian ligaments and resection of the proximal part of the tube, including the intramural part, by a cuneiform incision to avoid later risk of extrauterine pregnancy. However, every effort should be made to conserve as much ovarian parenchyma as possible.

Unchanged cysts must be kept under close observation, as a surgical decision may have to be made early: these cysts are liable to postnatal torsion. Most authors consider that the size of cyst determines surgical management.

Small cysts (less than 40 mm) are considered to be less liable to torsion, and we suggest observation for a week under the guidance of paediatric surgeons, as during this period regression is noted in a number of cases. In the absence of regression, ultrasonic-guided puncture is performed either by the transperitoneal or by the transvaginal route. Hormonal analysis of the aspirated fluid should allow assessment of the ovarian nature of the

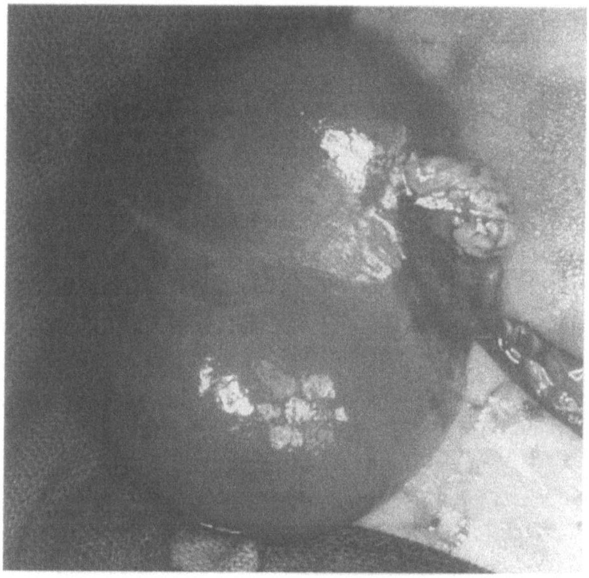

Figure 8.5 Torsion of an ovarian cyst at laparotomy.

punctured cyst[22]. Puncture can be repeated, avoiding laparotomy, but recurrences are not uncommon. Presence of blood in the aspirated fluid (a sign of a complicated cyst), failure to collapse the cyst and recurrence are indications for surgery. Laparotomy allows the evaluation of both ovaries and the performance of conservative surgery in the absence of torsion.

Cysts *larger* than 40 mm must be punctured or operated on before complications occur. Laparotomy allows enucleation of the cyst with maximum preservation of the parenchyma. It occasionally reveals a torsion not detected by ultrasonography.

Bilateral ovarian cysts are not frequent, but they are liable to bilateral torsion. Thus antenatal ultrasound-guided puncture is justified and, in the postnatal period, the decision for surgical intervention should not be delayed if the cysts persist.

If the ultrasonographer cannot ensure the benign nature of a neonatal ovarian mass, aspiration should not be undertaken because of low sensitivity and poor predictive value to differentiate between benign and malignant tumours[23,24]. Laparotomy should be undertaken after measurement of chorionic embryonic antigen and α-fetoprotein in blood. Frozen section should be done if the benign nature remains uncertain. Benign tumours ought to be treated by enucleation with preservation of the normal compressed parenchyma and tube. A plane of cleavage is generally found. If no parenchyma is identifiable, oophorectomy is performed. These benign tumours are also liable to torsion, and the presence of ischaemic lesions makes salpingo-oophorectomy necessary. The rare malignant tumours will necessitate more extensive resection by salpingo-oophorectomy, according to their nature and extent.

Although neonatal ovarian tumours are almost always benign cystic lesions, the incidence of long-term recurrence remains unknown. Thus, the follow-up of these children is necessary during infancy and puberty. Doubt about the future is another reason for trying to conserve ovaries at all cost.

References

1. De Sa DJ (1975) Follicular ovarian cysts in stillbirths and neonates. Arch Dis Child 50: 45–50.
2. Ziegler EE (1945) Bilateral carcinoma in a 30 week fetus. Arch Pathol 40: 279.
3. Gauthier F, Valayer J, Bienayme J (1979) Tumeurs et kystes de l'ovarie du nouveau-né, du nourrisson et de l'enfant. Chir Pédiatr 20: 75–83.
4. Grapin C, Montagne JP, Sirinelli D, Silberman B, Gruner M, Faure C (1987) Diagnosis of ovarian cysts in the perinatal period and therapeutic implications (20 cases). Ann Radiol 30: 497–502.
5. Henrion R, Helardot PG (1987) Le diagnostic des kystes de l'ovarie in utéro. Ann Pédiatr 34: 65–69.
6. Vaillant F, Ganichaud P, Denis A, Duverne C, Coupris L, Grosieux P (1984) Les kystes ovariens neonatals. A propos de quatre cas. J Gynecol Obstet Biol Reprod 13: 663–669.
7. Fekete CLN, Henrion R, Bessis R, Thibaud E (1986) Conduite à tenir devant la découverte échographique d'une image kystique ovarienne de plus de 2 cm. Séminaire Médico-chirurgical de Gynécologie Pédiatrique, Paris.
8. Ahmad S (1971) Neonatal and childhood ovarian cyst. J Pediatr Surge 6: 702–708.
9. Bourgeot P, Cockenpot P (1985) Les kystes de l'ovaire du noveau-né. Aspects échographiques pré et postnataux. A propos de 9 observations. Journal d'Echographie et de Médecine par Ultrasons 6: 285–292.
10. Gaudin J, le Treguille C, Parent P et al. (1988) Neonatal ovarian cysts. Twelve cysts with antenatal diagnosis. Pediatr Surg Int 3: 158–164.
11. Sandler MA, Smith SJ, Pope SG, Madrozo BL (1985) Prenatal diagnosis of a septicated ovarian cyst. JCU J Clin Ultrasound 13: 55–57.
12. Dieter RA Jr, Kindrachuk W, Muller RP (1980) Neonatal intestinal obstruction due to torsion of an ovarian cyst. J Fam Pract 10: 533–534.
13. Scholz PM, Key L, Filston HC (1982) Large ovarian cyst causing cecal perforation in a newborn infant. J Pediatr Surg 17: 91–92.
14. Vyas ID, Variend S, Dickson JA (1984) Ruptured ovarian cyst as a cause of ascites in a newborn infant. Z Kinderchirgie

39: 143–144.
15. Alvear DT, Rayfields MM (1976) Bilateral ovarian cysts in early infancy. J Pediatr Surg 11: 992–995.
16. Jouppila P, Kirkinen P, Tounonen S (1982) Ultrasonic detection of bilateral cysts in the fetus. Eur J Obstet Gynaecol Reprod Biol 13: 87–92.
17. Cohen HL, Shapiro MA, Mandel FS, Shapiro ML (1993) Normal ovaries in neonates and infants: a sonographic study of 77 patients, 1 day to 24 months old. AJR Am J Roentgenol 160: 583–586.
18. Fremond B, Guibert L, Jouan H et al. (1986) Les kystes de l'ovarie à diagnostic antenatal. Chir Pediatr 27: 128–133.
19. Holzgreve W, Winde B, Willital GH, Beller FK (1985) Prenatal diagnosis and perinatal management of fetal ovarian cyst. Prenat Diagn 5: 155–158.
20. Ikeda K, Suita S, Nakano H (1988) Management of ovarian cyst detected antenatally. J Pediatr Surg 23: 432–435.
21. Avni EF, Godart S, Israel C, Schmitz C (1983) Ovarian torsion cyst presenting as a wandering tumor in a newborn: antenatal diagnosis and postnatal assessment. Pediatr Radiol 13: 169–171.
22. Montag TW, Auletta FJ, Gibson M (1983) Neonatal ovarian cyst: prenatal diagnosis and analysis of the cyst fluid. Obstet Gynecol 61: 38–41.
23. Moran O, Menezer J, Bon Baruch G, Lipitz S, Goor E (1993) Cytologic examination of ovarian cyst fluid for the distinction between benign and malignant tumors. Obstet Gynecol 82: 444–446.
24. Trimbos JB, Hacker NF (1993) The case against aspirating ovarian cysts. Cancer 72: 828–831.

Brain Tumours

C. C. Bailey

9

Introduction

Brain tumour in an infant is extremely rare. Kumar et al.[1] have reviewed the records held in the Manchester Children's Tumour registry, which is a population-based registry of childhood tumours, and have calculated that one in 25 000 live births developed intracranial tumour within the first 18 months of life.

The pattern of distribution within the brain and the distribution of histological subtypes of brain tumour in very young infants is different from that seen in older children. Reports by Asai et al.[2] and Buetow et al.[3] show that two-thirds of the brain tumours occurring during the first year of life are located in the supratentoral region of the brain, whereas in older children the majority of tumours occur in the infratentoral regions. This shift probably occurs[4] between the ages of 2 and 4 years. There were malignant tumours in 85% of the 92 children reviewed by Kumar et al.[1] and in 28 of the 45 children reviewed by Buetow et al.[3] (62%).

Table 9.1 Intracranial tumours in infants less than 18 months of age 1953–1987

Histology	No. of cases
Medulloblastoma	21
Ependymoma	18
Juvenile astrocytoma	11
Astrocytoma	8
Choroid plexus tumour	6
Optic nerve glioma	4
Meningioma	4
Gliosarcoma	3
Glioblastoma	3
Pineal tumour	1
Ganglioglioma	1
Meningeal sarcoma	1
Pituitary tumour	1
Malignant melanoma	1
Neuroepithelioma (primitive neuroectodermal tumour, PNET)	1
Unclassified	5
Unverified	3
Total	92

With permission of Dr J.M. Birch.

Histological distribution

Table 9.1 shows the distribution of tumour types recorded by the Manchester Children's Tumour Registry in children under the age of 18 months. Gerlach et al.[5] collected data on 742 cases of microscopically confirmed central nervous system tumours with symptoms occurring during the first year of life. Of these, 173 tumours time-related to the perinatal period, i.e. tumours in stillbirths, tumours histologically verified during the first week of life and tumours symptomatic during the first week of life but with later histological verification. The commonest tumour in this group of patients was intracranial teratoma, accounting for over half the cases. Tumours histologically confirmed during the first year of life totalled 589. Their histological distribution is shown in Table 9.2.

Table 9.2 589 histologically verified tumours of the central nervous system in the first year of life

Tumour types	No. of cases	%
Choroid plexus papilloma	113	19.2
Teratoma	80	13.6
Astrocytoma/spongioblastoma	76	12.9
Medulloblastoma	57	9.7
Ependymoma	39	6.6
Glioma, not specified	30	5.1
Glioblastoma	23	3.9
Other	171	29.0

From Gerlach et al.[6].

Clinical presentation

The symptom complex presented in an infant with brain tumour is most commonly that of raised intracranial pressure rather than specific localizing neurological signs. Vomiting and increasing head circumference are the commonest signs, with developmental delay reported in some infants. The ability of the skull to expand in the infant with unfused sutures means that papilloedema is seen in less than 30% of infants. Bulging of the fontanelle, sutural separation and the "cracked pot" percussion sound of the skull may all be demonstrated. After clinical examination, the definitive diagnostic study is computed tomography with contrast enhancement, although some authorities recommend ultrasonography of the brain utilizing the open fontanelle, which can be performed quickly and without the need for immobilization or anaesthesia and may be of advantage to an ill infant. Magnetic resonance imaging may give better information than computed tomography when the tumour is situated in the brain stem or in the posterior fossa and has the advantage of allowing spinal imaging to be obtained. Thallium-201 single photon emission tomography is also helpful in the assessment of children with brain tumours[6].

Infants in whom a primitive neuroectodermal tumour is found will require examination of the cerebrospinal fluid for cytology and of the spine for drop metastases. These investigations should, however, be carried out after the raised intracranial pressure has been controlled by tumour removal or shunting.

Therapy

The planning of therapy for an infant with a brain tumour must take into account the immediate problems caused by the tumour, the possibility of tumour eradication and the likely long-term sequelae for the infant of damage to the brain caused both by the tumour and by any therapy delivered to it.

The first step of therapy is the careful correction of any electrolyte disturbance caused by the child's fluid and electrolyte loss associated with vomiting and of any acid-base disturbance. Only when these have been achieved can anaesthesia be safely contemplated. Raised intracranial pressure should be controlled during this period using dexamethasone and/or diuretics. Of the 41 infants reported by Asai et al.[2], 66% required cerebrospinal fluid shunting. Galassi et al.[7] reported that, although 22 of their 28 patients had hydrocephalus, tumour excision relieved the hydrocephalus in the majority of patients who survived surgery.

The aim of surgery should be total removal of the tumour. If this is impossible without unacceptable damage, removal of as much of the tumour bulk as possible with restoration of the cerebrospinal fluid pathway should be attempted. In a small number of infants biopsy is the only surgery possible; this will be of considerable value to the therapist, however, as a knowledge of the histology will allow more logical treatment planning.

An operative mortality rate of 12% was reported by Tomita and McLowe[8] and 7% by Asai et al.[2]. The correlation between completeness of tumour removal and survival has been extensively documented in older children with medulloblastoma and glioma. This correlation is not yet so clear in infants[2]. It is, however, logical to suppose that in the future lower operative mortality rates and more effective adjuvant therapies will correlate with better survival for those whose tumour can be removed.

The completeness, or otherwise, of surgical removal should be assessed within 72 h after operation by postoperative computed tomography. After this time, postoperative neovascularization causes enhancement in the operative field, and the assessment of residual tumour becomes impossible[9].

Radiotherapy has in the past been the major mode of therapy after surgery. The well known late effects of radiotherapy on the developing brain have led to a dose reduction of approximately 20% in the radiation delivered to children under 2 years old compared with older children. This, however, is an unsatisfactory compromise as even with such a dose reduction the effects caused by radiation in an infant will be considerable, and several studies have shown that doses less than 50–55 Gy are associated with increased incidence of local tumour recurrence[10,11].

This may in part account for the low survival rates of infants with brain tumours and for the poor quality of survival of those who have been cured[12]. The goal for treatment must therefore be to reduce the toxicity caused by radiotherapy by restricting its use to cases in which it is essential, or by devising alternative treatment strategies. Radiotherapy in patients who have progressive or residual disease treated with multiagent chemotherapy and maximal surgical resection produces long-term disease-free survival in almost half the patients, but neurodevelopmental deficits are frequent among survivors[13]. Chemotherapy may allow the delivery of radiotherapy to be delayed until myelinization is complete at the age of 3 years, and may be able to eradicate the tumour in some cases. A further alternative which has been explored in a small number of cases is the use of interstitial radiotherapy using stereotactically placed implants, which allows the radioactive sources to be placed such that a high dose is delivered to the tumour with sparing of the surrounding normal tissue.

Benign astrocytoma and optic glioma

Children with low-grade completely removed astrocytoma in the supratentorial or infratentorial area can safely be allowed to enter a period of conservative management. Further therapy may not be necessary for many of these infants. In the event of local recurrence, further operative removal of the tumour will be the treatment of choice. Low-grade astrocytomas that cannot be completely removed and optic gliomas, may be very slow growing, and a period of observation is advisable to establish the rate of growth and, by using visual evoked responses in optic glioma, to assess the threat to visual function. In tumours that are obviously growing and/or causing visual impairment, radiotherapy using a localized field to the tumour-bearing area should be used. This will have a high risk of long-term intellectual or neuroendocrine sequelae. In an attempt to avoid this, infants with residual or recurrent low-grade astrocytic tumours have recently been treated using chemotherapy. Lefkowitz et al.[14] reported ten children with recurrent low-grade gliomas treated with vincristine and lomustine, of whom six remained in continuous remission at the time of the report. Packer et al.[15] reported 24 infants with hypothalamic or chiasmatic gliomas treated with vincristine and actinomycin D without radiotherapy, 15 of whom remained free of progressive disease and received no further therapy. It must be emphasized that these are early reports and must be interpreted as such; however, this clearly is an area worth further exploration. Such cases should therefore be discussed with a paediatric oncology centre.

Malignant tumours

Malignant tumours present a much more difficult challenge. These tumours are often rapidly growing aggressive lesions, which attain large size before diagnosis and can disseminate through the cerebrospinal fluid pathways. Two large therapeutic trials have been completed for children with medulloblastoma. These studies included infants under the age of 2 years and both emphasized the relatively poor outcome for these infants, who had a 38.5% survival rate[16] compared with 50% 5-year survival for older children[17]. The studies were identical in structure, with all children having surgical removal of the tumour and craniospinal radiotherapy. In the European trial, they were randomly assigned to receive either vincristine and lomustine or no further therapy. In the American trial, prednisone was added to vincristine and lomustine, and was also compared with no further therapy. The infants receiving chemotherapy appeared in both trials to derive some benefit.

The standard follow-up care of these children should include regular clinical evaluations and surveillance of the central nervous system with computed tomography or magnetic resonance imaging. Long-term follow-up of these patients, however, reveals a disturbing pattern. In a series of 120 patients operated on at the Hôpital des Enfants Malades[18] between 1967 and 1987, the IQ of 58% of the survivors was above 80 at 5 years after therapy, but was only greater than 80 in 15% of the children 10 years after treatment; these psychological sequelae were related to age – the younger the child at the time of treatment, the lower the final IQ.

This damage may be caused by the tumour itself, by the associated hydrocephalus, by neurosurgical intervention or by radiotherapy or chemotherapy. In studies comparing children who have received radiotherapy to the posterior fossa only and those receiving the whole-brain radiation necessary for medulloblastoma, those receiving whole-brain therapy have always had the poorest outlook in terms of quality of survival[16], with the greatest damage seen in children treated at the youngest age[19].

Chemotherapy is now being explored in infants with brain tumours to ascertain whether its use will allow the delay, or even avoidance, of radiotherapy for very young children. Baram et al.[20] treated nine infants with medulloblastoma with surgery followed by chemotherapy utilizing nitrogen mustard, procarbazine, prednisolone and vincristine (MOPP). At the time of the report, six were alive without having received any radiotherapy. One further child was alive having suffered a relapse at the age of 37 months and been given craniospinal radiation. Six of these survivors were tested for neurological and neuropsychological function and four were found to be normal. The other chemotherapeutic options include eight drugs in one day or carboplatin and etoposide with high response rate but severe toxicity[21].

Horowitz et al.[22] reported 12 consecutively diagnosed infants who were treated with chemotherapy after surgery. Two children had low-grade astrocytoma, one high-grade astrocytoma, one ependymoma, five medulloblastoma and three primitive neuroectodermal tumour. Nine of these children received the MOPP regimen and three a regimen containing cisplatin, vincristine, cyclophosphamide and prednisone. At the time of the report, both children with low-grade astrocytoma remained without evidence of disease. The child with ependymoma had suffered disease progression 35 months after diagnosis and had then received further surgery and irradiation. Five of the eight children with either medulloblastoma or primitive neuroectodermal tumour remained free of disease and three had suffered disease progression.

Kretschmar et al.[23] treated 21 children, all with high-risk medulloblastoma, with pre-irradiation chemotherapy consisting of vincristine and cisplatin for 9 weeks. Six infants aged 6–18 months were then maintained using nitrogen mustard, procarbazine and vincristine until the age of 2 years, when they were referred for irradiation. Four of the six infants remained disease free for between 19 and 57 months from diagnosis.

This shows that malignant brain tumours in infants are sensitive to chemotherapy and suggests that its use to delay radiotherapy, allowing the brain more time for maturation, could be explored. A cautionary note, however, needs to be sounded in that children treated using this approach may not experience enhanced quality of survival; indeed, the children treated by Horowitz et al.[22] have been shown on long-term follow-up to have significant neuropsychological problems[24]. An intensive chemotherapeutic regimen with eight drugs in 1 day (vincristine, carmustine, procarbazine, hydroxyurea, cisplatin, cytarabine, prednisone and cyclophosphamide) was used in 82 children under 18 months of age with primitive neuroectodermal tumours and ependymomas, after surgery and postoperative staging on Children's Cancer Group (CCG) protocol. Of these patients, 50% had complete excision and 23% had metastatic disease at diagnosis. Objective tumour response was seen in 28% of accessible patients after two cycles of chemotherapy. Five children died of chemotherapy-related complications. The 3 year progression-free survival rate was 29% in patients without metastatic disease compared with 11% for those with metastatic disease[25].

This avenue of investigation now needs to be pursued in the context of large-scale controlled clinical trials. Such trials are currently at an advanced stage of preparation, by the Children's Cancer Study Group and Pediatric Oncology Group in the USA and by the International Society for Paediatric Oncology in Europe.

Choroid plexus tumours

Choroid plexus papillomas often present with massive hydrocephalus, which requires urgent therapy. This may be tumour removal to restore the cerebrospinal fluid pathway or possibly shunting. However, the best approach remains an area of debate[26]. Primary therapy for the tumour is surgical removal, with vigorous attempts being made to achieve total tumour removal. The outlook is good for infants with benign papilloma that is completely removed[27]. Children with residual or recurrent papilloma have in the past been treated with radiotherapy.

Choroid plexus carcinomas have a poorer outlook. Treatment is surgical removal and radiotherapy. In view of the severe late effects associated with radiotherapy, attempts have been made to treat them with chemotherapy, and there are reports of good response being obtained[28–30]. The author has treated one such case with good tumour response but progression after 1 year.

Acknowledgements

The Manchester Children's Tumour Registry is supported by Cancer Research Campaign.

References

1. Kumar R, Jones RA, Tekk OKIH (1990) Has modern management improved the outcome of infants with intracranial tumours? Childs Nerv Syst 6: 327–330.
2. Asai A, Hoffman HJ, Hendrick EB, Humphreys RP, Becker LE (1989) Primary intracranial neoplasms in the first year of life. Childs Nerv Sys 5: 230–233.
3. Buetow PC, Smirniotopoulos JG, Done S (1990) Congenital brain tumours. A review of 45 cases. Am J Neuroradiol 11: 793–799.
4. Tomita T, McLowe DG (1986) Medulloblastoma in childhood. Results of radical resection and low dose neuraxis radiation therapy. J Neurosurg 64: 238–242.
5. Gerlach H, Janisch W, Schreiber D (1982) Intracranial and spinal tumours in newborns and infants. In: Voth D, Gutjahr P, Langmaid C, eds. Tumours of the central nervous system in infancy and childhood. Springer-Verlag, Berlin, pp 53–57.
6. Maria BL, Drane WE, Dursling RG et al. (1994) Value of thallium 201 SPECT imaging in childhood brain tumours. Pediatr Neurosurg 20: 17–18.
7. Galassi E, Godano U, Cavallo M, Donati R, Nasi MT (1989) Intracranial tumours during the first year of life. Childs Nerv Syst 5: 288–298.
8. Tomita T, McLowe DG (1985) Brain tumours during the first twenty-four months of life. Neurosurgery 176: 913–919.
9. Cairncross JG, Pexman JH, Rathbone MP, Del Maestro RF (1985) Postoperative contrast enhancement in patients with brain tumours. Ann Neurol 17: 570–572.
10. Hughes EN, Shillito J, Salan SE, Loeffler JS, Cassady JR, Tarbel NJ (1988) Medulloblastoma at the Joint Center for Radiation Therapy between 1968 and 1984. Cancer 61: 1992–1998.
11. Levin VA, Kodriguel LA, Edwards MSB et al. (1988) Treatment of medulloblastoma with procarbazine, hydroxyurea and reduced doses whole brain and spine. J Neurosurg 68: 383–387.
12. Duffner PK, Cohen ME (1985) Treatment of brain tumors in babies and very young children. Pediatr Neurosci 112: 304–310.
13. Gajjar A, Bulhern RK, Heiderman RL et al. Medulloblastoma in very young children: outcome of definitive craniospinal irradiation following incomplete response to chemotherapy. J Clinical Oncol 12: 1212–1216.
14. Lefkowitz IB, Packer RJ, Sutton LN et al. Results of the treatment of children with recurrent gliomas with lomustine and vincristine. Cancer 61: 896–902.
15. Packer RJ, Sutton LN, Bilaniuk LT et al. (1988) Treatment of chiasmatic/hypothalamic gliomas of childhood with chemotherapy: an update. Ann Neurol 23: 79–85.
16. Evans AE, Jenkin RDT, Sposto R et al. (1990) The treatment of medulloblastoma. Results of a prospective randomized trial of radiation therapy with and without CCNU, vincristine and prednisolone. J Neurosurg 72: 572–582.
17. Tait DM, Thornton-Jones H, Bloom HJG, Lemerle J, Morris-Jones P (1990) Adjuvant chemotherapy for medulloblastoma: the first multicentre control trial of the International Society of Paediatric Oncology (SIOP). Eur J Cancer 26: 464–469.
18. Hoppe-Hirsch E, Renier D, Lellouch-Tubiana A, Sainte-Rose C, Pierre-Kahn A, Hirsch JF (1990) Medulloblastoma in childhood: progressive intellectual deterioration. Childs Nerv Syst 6: 60–65.
19. Hirsch JF, Renier D, Czernichow R et al. (1979) Medulloblastoma in childhood: survival and functional results. Acta Neurochir 48: 1–15.
20. Baram TZ, Van Eys J, Dowell RE, Cangir A, Pack B, Bruner JM (1987) Survival and neurologic outcome of infants with medulloblastoma treated with surgery and MOPP chemotherapy: a preliminary report. Cancer 60: 173–177.
21. Genler JC, Doz F, Bouffet F et al. (1994) Carboplatin and VP16 in medulloblastoma: a phase II study of the French Society of Pediatric Oncology (SFOP). Med Pediatr Oncol 23: 422–427.
22. Horowitz ME, Mulhearn RK, Kun LE et al. Brain tumours in the very young: postoperative chemotherapy in combined modality treatment. Cancer 61: 428–434.
23. Kretschmar CS, Tarbell NJ, Kupsky W et al. (1989) Pre-irradiation chemotherapy for infants and children with medulloblastoma, a preliminary report. J Neurosurg 71: 820–825.
24. Mulhearn RK, Horowitz ME, Kounar EH, Langston J, Sanford RA, Kun LE (1989) Neurodevelopmental states of infants and young children treated for brain tumours with pre-irradiation chemotherapy. J Clin Oncol 7: 1660–1666.
25. Geyer JR, Zettzer PM, Boych JM et al. (1994) Survival of infants with primitive neuroectodermal tumours or malignant ependymomas of the CNS treated with eight drugs in one day: a report from the Children's Cancer Group. J Clin Oncol 12: 1607–1615.
26. Ellenbogan RG, Winston KR, Kupsky WJ (1989) Tumours of the choroid plexus in children. Neurosurgery 25: 327–335.
27. Boyd MC, Steinbok P (1987) Choroid plexus tumours. Problems in diagnosis and management. J Neurosurg 66: 800–805.
28. Arico M, Raiteri E, Bessi G et al. (1994) Choroid plexus carcinoma: report of one case with favorable response to treatment. Med Pediatr Oncol 22: 274–278.
29. Maria BL, Graham ML, Strauss LC, Wharam MD (1985) Response of a current choroid plexus tumour to combination chemotherapy. J Neurooncol 3: 259–262.
30. Pierga JY, Kalifa C, Terrier-Lacombe MJ, Habarand JR, LeMorle J (1993) Carcinoma of the choroid plexus: a pediatric experience. Med Pediatr Oncol 21: 480–487.

Retinoblastoma

Michael O'Keefe

10

Introduction

Retinoblastoma was first described in 1597, and until the late nineteenth century was a fatal tumour of childhood. It is the commonest intraocular tumour of childhood, with a frequency of one in 20 000 live births[1]. The average age at diagnosis is 12 months, and 90% are diagnosed before the age of 4. The tumour arises from primitive retinal cells and occurs in hereditary and non-hereditary forms. Current survival rates have improved from 5% in 1869 to 95% in recent series.

Inheritance

It is inherited as autosomal dominant[2,3] with incomplete penetrance and variable expressivity. Some 10% of tumours are familial and 90% sporadic. Among the sporadic cases, 25% arise as germinal mutations and will become heritable. The rest of the cases arise as a result of somatic cell mutation and are not heritable. Bilateral retinoblastomas as well as multiple tumours in one eye are inherited. Of patients with retinoblastoma, 1%–3% have a chromosome abnormality, 13q14, and are mentally retarded with other abnormalities[4,5]. Genetic counselling is based on clinical evaluation. About 6% of new cases have a family history, and offspring of patients with a family history of retinoblastoma or bilateral tumours have a 50% chance of inheriting the abnormal gene and developing tumour. Musarella and Gallie[6] have calculated the risks of various relatives of the proband and compiled tables for counselling. Recent advances have resulted in a method of identification of individuals carrying the retinoblastoma gene, and this will allow more accurate genetic counselling in families with two or more affected individuals[7].

Presentation

The presenting features in retinoblastoma are:

- White reflex
- Strabismus
- Glaucoma
- Poor vision
- Hyphaemia

The most common presentation is leucocoria or white reflex[8,9] (Figure 10.1). The second most common presentation is strabismus[8,9]. Less common presenting symptoms include red inflamed eye, hyphaemia and hypopyon. Examination of the eye reveals a white or cream colour to the pupil, with or without vessels on the iris surface. Diagnosis is based on fundal examination with a widely dilated pupil and the child sedated or under general anaesthesia. A creamy-coloured pink mass may be evident, with blood vessels on the surface of the tumour, and calcification is evident by white cottage cheese apppearance (Figure 10.2).

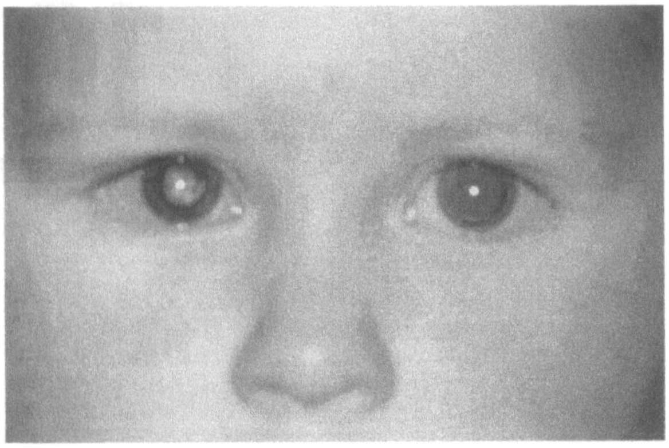

Figure 10.1 White pupil or leucocoria in an infant.

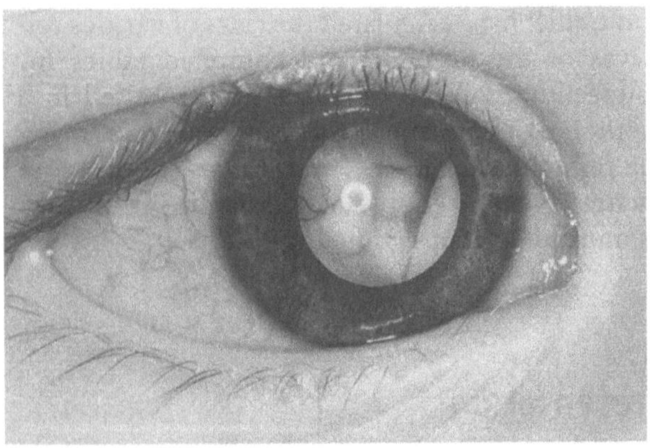

Figure 10.2 Cream-coloured pink mass with blood vessels on the surface.

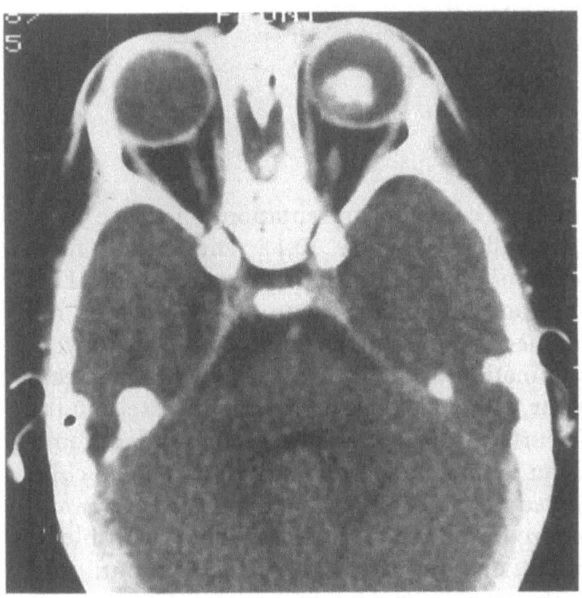

Figure 10.3 Ocular calcification on computed tomography.

Differential diagnosis

A number of conditions mimic retinoblastoma and may present with leucocoria or white reflex[10]. These include:

- Persistent hyperplastic primary vitreous
- Coats' disease
- Retinopathy of prematurity
- Toxocariasis
- Retinal dysplasia
- Dominent exudative vitreoretinopathy
- Norrie's disease

Persistent hyperplastic primary vitreous is usually congenital and unilateral, present in a microphthalmic eye. Toxocariasis causes inflammation resulting in granuloma formation or vitreous opacity: it usually presents in older healthy children. There is rarely calcification, and enzyme-linked immunosorbent assay may be positive.

Coats' disease is unilateral, mostly occurring in males. Examination reveals an exudative detachment with dilated telangiectatic vessels and subretinal lipid and cholesterol. Retinal dysplasia presents at birth with bilateral retrolental masses without calcification. Retinopathy of prematurity occurs shortly after birth in infants with a history of severe prematurity. The history and eye examination usually confirm the diagnosis.

Investigations

Specialized investigations to confirm the diagnosis include orbital and brain computed tomography[11], which demonstrates the presence of calcification (Figure 10.3). Other useful investigations include ultrasonography, which helps to distinguish retinoblastoma from other causes of leucocoria. Management involves a multidisciplinary approach involving ophthalmologist, oncologist, radiotherapist and geneticist.

The presence of calcification demonstrated by computed tomography usually confirms the diagnosis of retinoblastoma. Computed tomography also helps to exclude any spread outside the eye, and scanning of the brain will demonstrate a

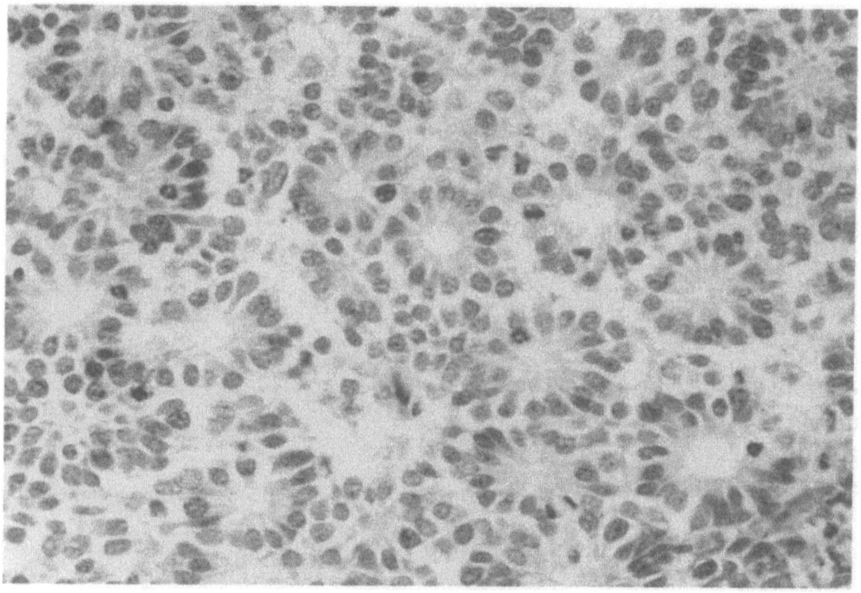

Figure 10.4 Presence of rosettes.

midline intracranial neoplasm. The association of a bilateral retinoblastoma with an intracranial tumour has been termed trilateral retinoblastoma[12]. In selected cases where diagnosis is in doubt, aqueous aspiration to measure lactate dehydrogenase may be attempted. Rarely, if ever, should a biopsy of the tumour be performed because of the risk of extraocular spread[13]. Magnetic resonance imaging may be used, as it has a greater ability to differentiate subretinal fluid from tumour, conferring high accuracy in measuring tumour size. It also helps to differentiate other diseases, such as Coats' disease[14].

Pathology

There is no clear agreement concerning the pathogenesis of hereditary and non-hereditary tumour[15,16]. At the cellular level the tumour arises from primitive retinal cells. They form rosettes (Figure 10.4) such as Flexner–Wintersteiner and Homer Wright rosettes as well as fleurettes. Flexner–Wintersteiner rosettes consist of a central lumen lined by cubodial cells that have nuclei positioned away from the lumen. Homer Wright rosettes contain cobweb-like material. Fleurettes are flower-like groupings of tumour cells. Tumours with abundant Flexner–Wintersteiner rosettes have a better prognosis than patients without rosettes. The presence of fleurettes also indicates a good prognosis. Retinoblastoma may grow from the external retinal layers (exophytic growth) or from the inner layers of the retina (endophytic growth) into the vitreous, or in both directions. The tumour may invade the choroid, extend to the lamina cribrosa and invade the optic nerve. An uncommon type of retinoblastoma occurring in older children is the diffuse infiltrating type[17], which can lead to difficulty in diagnosis. Metastatic spread occurs via the optic nerve, the scleral forminae, the blood or the lymphatic system[18]. Once the tumour spreads outside the eye it is highly malignant, with metastatic spread occurring early; metastasis is rare more than 3 years after treatment[19]. Metastasis occurs when there is invasion beyond the lamina cribrosa, and uveal, trans-scleral and orbital involvement. When metastasis occurs it proves fatal within the first 2 years after diagnosis. Late metastatic deaths are rarely observed after treatment of retinoblastoma.

Retinoma[20] is a non-malignant tumour originating in childhood, and is non-progressive. It has lost its potential for malignant change. Its importance is that its presence indicates that the individual carries the retinoblastoma gene.

Treatment

This depends on the stage of the tumour at diagnosis. Longer term follow-up includes genetic counselling, examination of relatives and periodic examination of the child. Treatment options vary, and include:

- Enucleation
- Total irradiation
- Focal irradiation
- Cryotherapy
- Photocoagulation
- Chemotherapy

The presence of metastatic spread heralds a poor prognosis.

The staging or classification was first devised by Reese and Ellsworth in 1958, and is based on the site, size, number and spread of the tumour (Table 10.1).

Table 10.1 Reese-Ellsworth classification of retinoblastoma

Group		Description
I	(a)	Solitary tumour, less than 4 disc diameters DD in at or behind the equator.
	(b)	Multiple tumours, less than 4 DD size all at or behind the equator
II	(a)	Solitary tumour, 4–10 DD in size, all at or behind the equator
	(b)	Multiple tumours, 4–10 DD in size at or behind the equator
III	(a)	Any lesion anterior to the equator
	(b)	Solitary tumours larger than 10 DD behind the equator
IV	(a)	Multiple tumours some larger than 10 DD
	(b)	Any lesion extending anterior to the ora serrata
V	(a)	Massive tumours involving more than half the retina
	(b)	Vitreous seeding

Enucleation of the eye is still the commonest form of treatment and may result in complete cure. Most patients with unilateral tumours present late, with more than half the globe involved, and enucleation is the only option[21] (Figure 10.5). Where less than half the globe is involved and there is no optic nerve involvement, radiotherapy may be used. In bilateral retinoblastoma, the worst eye is enucleated. However, if there is bilateral extensive disease, bilateral enucleation is the only option. It is important not to rupture the globe during enucleation and to obtain a long stump of the nerve.

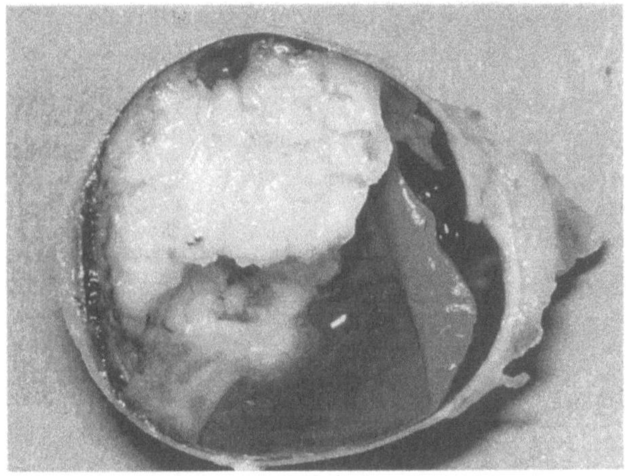

Figure 10.5 More than half the globe full of tumour.

External beam radiation has been used since 1903. It is indicated where the tumour involves less than half the globe, in multiple tumours, in vitreous seeding, in tumours near the macula or optic disc, and to the orbit after enucleation where there is possible spread outside the globe. The effects of radiation are seen about 3 weeks after starting treatment, and three types of regression are seen[22]. Type 1 is the cottage cheese appearance, type 2 reduction in size and a fish-flesh appearance, and type 3 a combination of types 1 and 2. Complications of radiation include a sicca syndrome, corneal ulceration, perforation, cataract, radiation retinopathy, optic nerve infarction and orbital growth problems[23,24]. Improvement in delivery, reduction of the total dose and fractionation have reduced these effects. Irradiation is completed over 5–6 weeks and a total dose of 3500–4500 cGy is given[21]. Focal radiation involves the use of colbalt plaques: these are used in solitary tumours less than 15 mm in diameter that are not near the macula or the disc in tumour recurrences.

Cryotherapy was first used in 1967. It destroys the tumour and underlying choroid by cell lysis, vascular destruction and denaturation of protein[25,26]. It is used in tumours anterior to the equator, which appear after irradiation. Photocoagulation or laser therapy is useful in small posterior tumours: it is applied around the tumour to coagulate the blood supply. Tumours with retinal pigment atrophy, eyes with opaque media, are poor candidates for laser therapy.

Chemotherapy is generally used in patients with orbital, intracranial and metastatic disease. Following initial management frequent follow-up to monitor response to therapy and to detect new tumours is required[27]. Regular follow-up under general anaesthesia is essential until 4 years of age, and after this, follow-up occurs on an outpatient basis. In many patients, follow-up should be lifelong.

Second tumours

Retinoblastoma patients who survive are at risk of subsequent development of other tumours[28-30]. Those most at risk have germinal mutations for retinoblastoma. Tumours arise out of field and in the field of radiation. The most common tumours reported are osteosarcoma and fibrosarcomas. Others have reported high maternal age as significant risk factors for sporadic hereditary retinoblastoma[31].

Recent advances

Retinoblastoma cells in tissue culture have specific high-affinity receptors for calcitriol[32]. Vitamin D_2 inhibits growth of retinoblastoma in tissue culture, although at dose levels that produce in vivo toxicity[33]. At present, genetic counselling is based on clinical assessment. Identification of individuals carrying the retinoblastoma gene may help to change counselling in the future. Improvements in both delivery and type of radiotherapy including possible combination of some chemotherapeutic drugs, such as carboplatin, with laser therapy may substantially improve the visual prognosis in tumours near the optic disc. Review of 15 years' experience in management of 324 cases of retinoblastoma by Shields et al.[34] show a definite trend away from enucleation in both unilateral and bilateral cases. They have suggested that earlier diagnosis of retinoblastoma and refinements in conservative methods of management are the main reasons. The hope for the future is that more children will preserve the affected eye with some or all of its vision and with minimal side-effects from treatment.

References

1. Sanders BM, Draper GJ, Kingston JE (1988) Retinoblastoma in Great Britain, 1969–80. Incidence, treatment and survival. Br J Ophthalmol 72: 516–583.
2. Migdal C (1976) Retinoblastoma occurring in four successive generations. Br J Ophthalmol 60: 151–152.
3. Francois B, De Bie S, Meton Van Liven MT (1979) Genesis and genetics in retinoblastoma. Paediatr Ophthalmol Strabismus 16: 85–100.
4. Cowell JK, Rutland P, Jay M, Hungerford J (1986) Deletions on the Esteraseo locus from a survey of 200 retinoblastoma patients. Hum Genet 72: 164–167.
5. Musarella MA, Gallie BL (1984) Retinoblastoma. In: Renie WA, ed. Goldberg's genetics and metastatic eye disease, 2nd edn. Little Brown, Boston, pp 423–438.
6. Musarella MA, Gallie BL (1987) A simplified scheme for genetic counselling in retinoblastoma. J Paediatr Ophthalmol Strabismus 24: 124–125.
7. Wiggs JL, Dryga TP (1988) Predicting the risk for hereditary retinoblastoma. Am J Ophthalmol 106: 346–351.
8. Ellsworth RM (1969) The practical management of retinoblastoma. Trans Am Ophthalmol Soc 67: 462–534.
9. Shields JA (1983) Diagnosis and management of intraocular tumours. CV Mosby, St Louis.
10. Char DH, Hedges TR, Norman D (1984) Retinoblastoma, CT diagnosis. Ophthalmology 91: 1347–1350.
11. Shields JA, Augsberger JJ (1981) Current approaches to the diagnosis and management of retinoblastoma. Survey Ophthalmol 25: 347–371.
12. Pesin SR, Shields JA (1989) Seven cases of trilateral retinoblastoma. Am Ophthalmol 107: 121–126.
13. Char DH, Millar TR (1984) Fine needle biopsy in retinoblastoma. Am Ophthalmol 97: 686–690.
14. Bects-Tan RA, Hendricks MJ, Ramos LM, Tam KB (1994) Retinoblastoma – CT and MRI. Neuroradiology 36: 59–62.
15. Knudson AG, Meadows AY, Nichols WW, Hill R (1976) Chromosomal deletions in retinoblastoma. N Engl J Med 295: 1120–1123.
16. Murphee AL, Benedict WF (1985) Retinoblastoma clues to human oncogenesis. Science 223: 1028–1033.
17. Morgan G (1971) Diffuse infiltrating retinoblastoma. Br J Ophthalmol 55: 600–606.
18. Zimmerman LE (1985) Retinoblastoma and retinocytoma. In: Spencer WH, ed. Ophthalmic pathology. An atlas and textbook, 3rd edn. WB Saunders, Philadelphia, pp 1292–1351.
19. Saunders BM, Draper GJ, Kingston JE (1988) Retinoblastoma in Great Britain 1969–80: incidence, treatment and survival. Br J Ophthalmol 72: 516–583.
20. Margo C, Hidayata A, Kopelman JE, Zimmerman LE (1983) Retinocytoma; a benign variant of retinoblastoma. Arch Ophthalmol 101: 1519.
21. Shields JA, Augsberger JJ (1981) Current approaches to diagnosis and management of retinoblastoma. Surv Ophthalmol 25: 347–371.
22. Ellsworth RM (1969) The practical management of retinoblastoma. Trans Am Ophthalmol Soc 67: 462–534.
23. Reese AG, Merriam GL, Martin HE (1949) Treatment of bilateral retinoblastoma by irradiation and surgery. Report on 15 years results. Am J Ophthalmol 32: 175.

24. Martin HE, Reece AB (1936) Treatment of retinal gliomas by fractionated or divided dose principal of Roentgen radiation. Preliminary report. Arch Ophthalmol 16: 733.
25. Abramson DH, Ellsworth RM, Rozakis GW (1982) Cryotherapy for retinoblastoma. Arch Ophthalmol 100: 1253.
26. Abramson DH (1984) Cryotherapy in retinoblastoma. In: Jacobiec, ed. Technique in ophthalmic surgery. WB Saunders, Philadelphia, p 433.
27. Salmousen PC, Ellsworth R, Kitchin FD (1979) The occurrence of new retinoblastoma after treatment. Ophthalmology 86: 840–843.
28. Abramson DH, Ellsworth RM, Zimmerman LE (1976) Non ocular cancers in retinoblastoma survivors. Trans Am Acad Ophthalmol Otolaryngol 81: 454–457.
29. Abramson DH, Ellsworth RM, Kitchen FD, Ting G (1984) Second non ocular tumours in retinoblastoma survivors: are they radiation induced? Ophthalmology 91: 1351–1355.
30. Draper GJ, Saunders BM, Kingston JE (1986) Retinoblastoma and second primary tumours. Br J Cancer 53: 661–671.
31. Derkinderen DJ, Willemkoten J, Karl EWP, Jan MD, Beemer FA, Van Pomunde LKJ, Den Otter W (1990) Parental age in sporadic hereditary retinoblastoma. Am J Ophthalmol 100: 605–609.
32. Saulens AM, Cohen SM, Key L (1988) Vitamin D and retinoblastoma. The presence of receptors and inhibition of growth in vitro. Arch Ophthalmol 106: 533–535.
33. Albert DM, Saulenas AM, Cohen SM (1988) Verhoeff's query: is vitamin D effective against retinoblastoma? Arch Ophthalmol 106: 536–540.
34. Shields JA, Shields CL, Sivalingam V (1989) Decreasing frequency of enucleation in patients with retinoblastoma. Am J Ophthalmol 108: 185–188.

Cystic Hygroma

Jacob C. Langer

11

Introduction

Cystic hygromas are common tumours, which usually present in the neonatal period[1]. They range from small clinically insignificant masses to huge debilitating or disfiguring lesions that penetrate widely into surrounding structures. Although they are usually found in the neck and shoulder regions, they may also occur in the mediastinum, retroperitoneum, groin and other areas.

Pathology

The terms "cystic hygroma" and "lymphangioma" are often used interchangeably, and describe a spectrum of benign cystic tumours of the lymphatic system[2]. These lesions consist of cystic cavities filled with clear or straw-coloured fluid, which grow slowly, often surrounding and infiltrating adjacent structures. The cysts are lined by endothelium, and the fluid is often identical with lymph. The reason for growth in cystic hygromas has been debated. Some authors suggest that they are neoplasms with potential for new tissue formation[3]; others have felt that increase in size is a result of thrombosis and organization within the tumour[4].

Embryology and aetiology

According to Sabin, the lymphatic system arises from the formation of the five primitive "lymph sacs": paired jugular sacs lateral to the jugular vein, a retroperitoneal sac at the root of the small bowel mesentery, and paired sacs posterior to the sciatic veins[5]. These sacs produce buds, which arborize centrifugally to form the peripheral lymphatic system. Later work by Kampmeier[6] suggested that the lymphatic cavities form from slits in the reticulum of the large venous plexuses in the neck. Cyst formation would result from failure of the lymphatic spaces to join with the venous system[7]. Cystic hygromas may therefore be caused by sequestration of a sac or part of a sac[8], failure of fusion with the venous system[9], or secondary obstruction of lymphatic drainage[5]. The recently recognized association of cystic hygroma with cardiovascular and venous malformations has led to a number of further theories involving abnormalities of extracellular matrix and neural crest migration during early embryonic development[10,11]. Clinical work examining the pathology of these tumours[12], as well as observations on prenatally diagnosed cases[13], has called some of these theories into question, and suggest that a number of different mechanisms may result in a cystic hygroma.

Prenatal diagnosis

Cystic hygromas are often diagnosed sonographically before birth[14]. The differential diagnosis of a cystic lesion in the fetus is extensive[15], but in experienced hands the correct diagnosis can be made in most cases[16]. Although most paediatric surgeons think of cystic hygroma as having an excellent prognosis, prenatal ultrasonography has revealed a high "hidden mortality rate" among

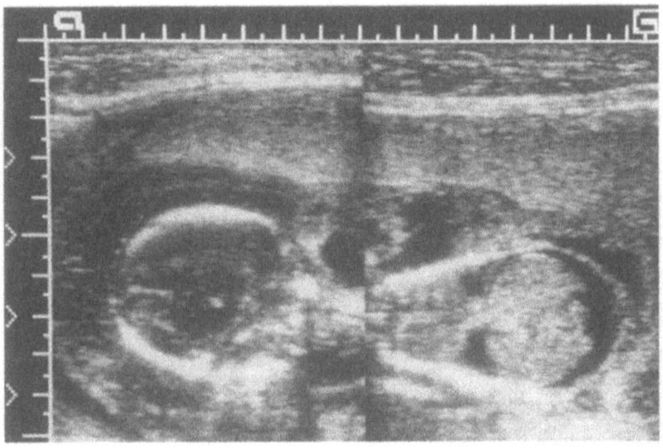

a

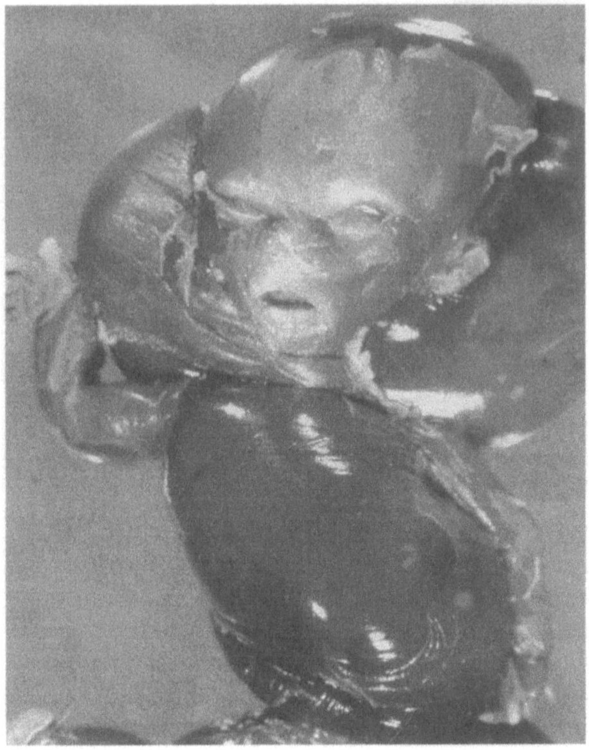

b

Figure 11.1 **a** Prenatal ultrasonography shows a large posterior cervical cystic hygroma in a fetus with Turner's syndrome. **b** The same fetus after spontaneous abortion, showing a large hygroma and hydrops.

fetuses with this condition[17–20]. The majority of fetuses with cystic hygroma develop hydrops fetalis or diffuse lymphangiomatosis prior to fetal demise (Figure 11.1). There is usually either an associated chromosomal abnormality (usually Turner's syndrome[9], although many others have been reported[21]) or a familial syndrome associated with other structural anomalies (such as multiple pterygium syndrome[22] or Robert's syndrome[23]). Although most of these fetuses die in utero, spontaneous regression has occasionally been seen in fetuses with Turner's and Noonan's syndromes[13,24,25].

We recently reviewed our experience with 29 prenatally diagnosed cystic hygromas at two perinatal centres over a 4 year period (Figure 11.2)[13]. Of 27 fetuses diagnosed before 30 weeks' gestation, only one survived. Twenty-five of the 27 were aborted; severe hydrops was present in 21 of these 25. Two of the 27, both with stigmata of Noonan's syndrome, underwent spontaneous regression during the second trimester: one died at 2 weeks of age from associated anomalies, and the other survived. Karyotype analysis appeared to be important for genetic counselling, in that fetuses with abnormal chromosomes tended to be sporadic cases, with a low risk of recurrence in future pregnancies. Normal chromosomes were correlated with a history of consanguinity, multiple structural anomalies, polyhydramnios, and familial syndromes, with a higher recurrence risk.

The two fetuses diagnosed after 30 weeks'gestation had a much different outcome. Neither had hydrops, polyhydramnios, associated anomalies or an abnormal karyotype. One was completely normal on ultrasonography at 17 weeks' gestation, which suggested that the cystic hygroma had developed later in gestation. Both were operated on within the first 4 days of life: one did well without complications, and the other required a permanent tracheostomy because of extensive hypopharyngeal involvement. We have since had several additional cases, one of which was diagnosed at 32 weeks' gestation and resolved before birth. The child remained well until the age of $2\frac{1}{2}$ years, when she presented with an expanding cervical mass. On exploration the mass was found to be a cystic hygroma (Figure 11.3). From our data and from similar reports in the literature, it appears that cystic hygroma presenting in the fetus has a different natural history and prognosis from one presenting postnatally[26]. The natural

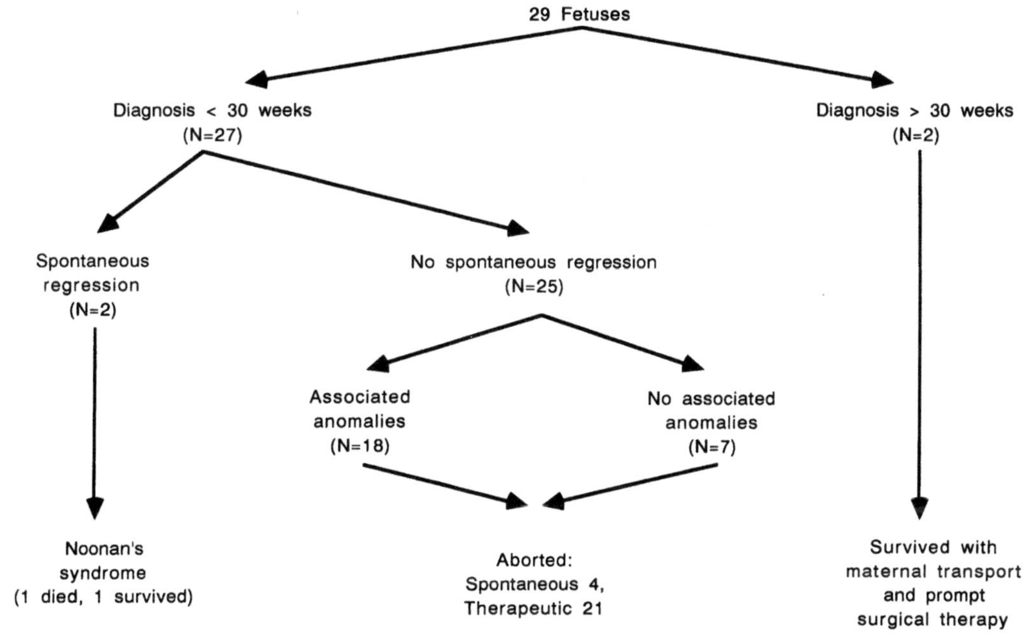

Figure 11.2 Outcome in 29 fetuses with prenatal diagnosis of cervical cystic hygroma.

a 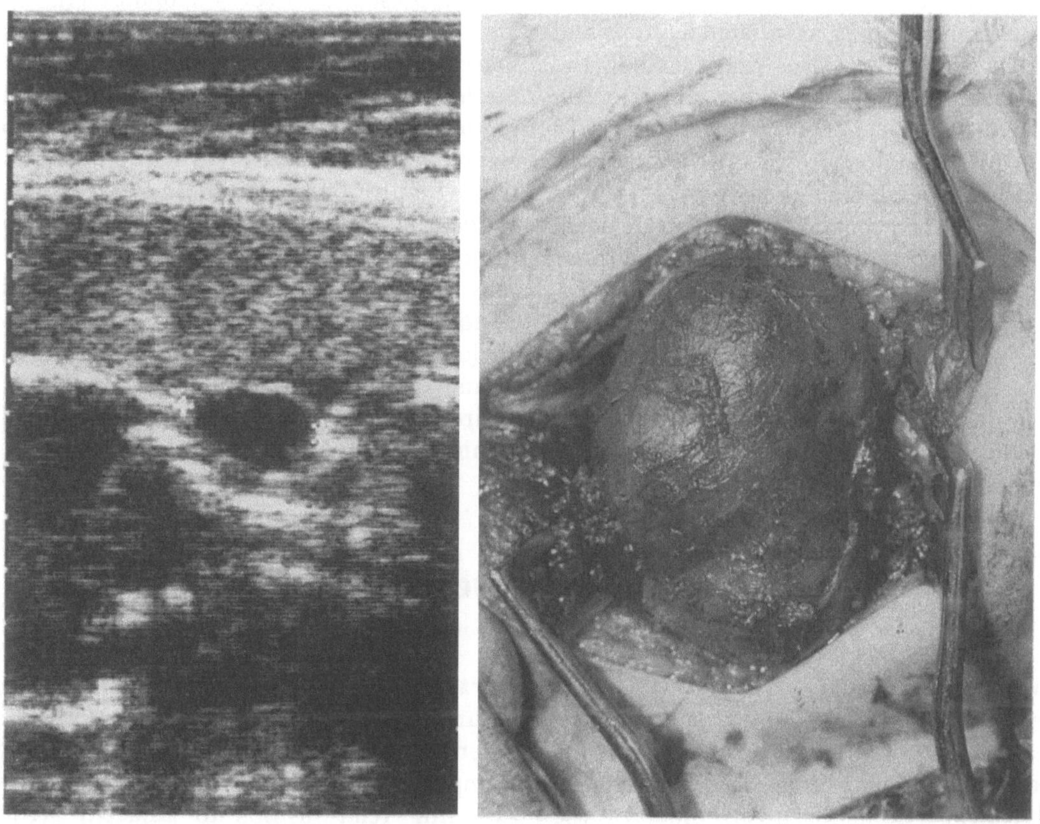 b

Figure 11.3 **a** Prenatal ultrasonography at 32 weeks' gestation revealed a large cystic hygroma on the right lateral aspect of the neck. Follow-up ultrasonography revealed that the lesion had resolved, and the child was well at birth. **b** At age $2\frac{1}{2}$ years, the child presented with a cervical mass on the right side, which proved to be a cystic hygroma.

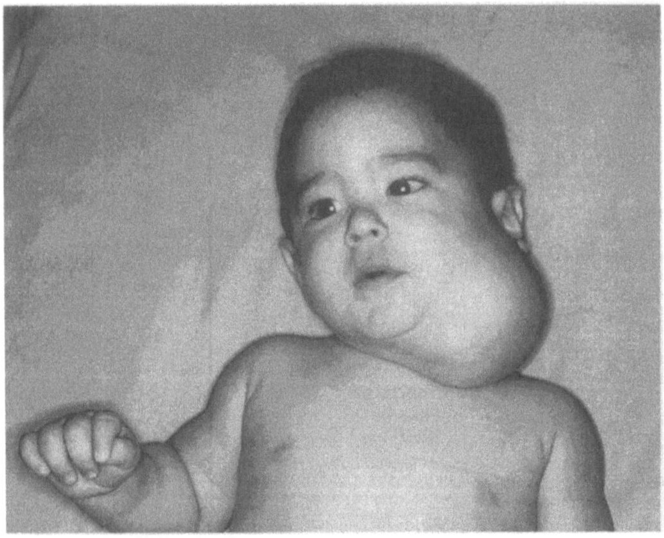
a

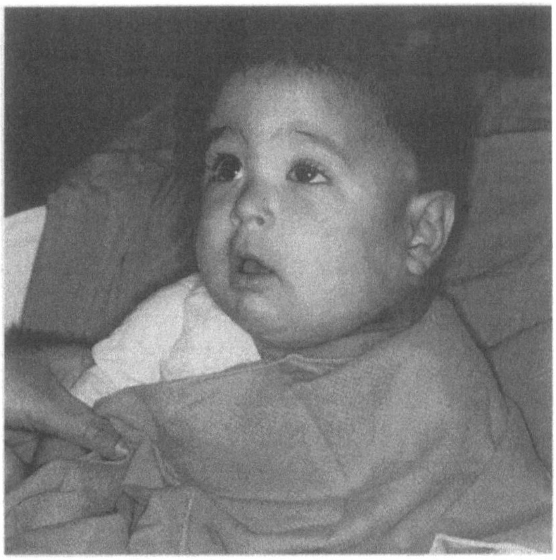
b

Figure 11.4 A 5-month-old child with a moderate-sized hygroma, which was relatively asymptomatic, **a** before and **b** after operation. (Courtesy of Dr R.M. Filler)

history of cystic hygromas detected prenatally varies according to the gestational age at which nuchal thickening appears, associated hydrops and abnormal karyotyping. Cases diagnosed in the first trimester without any other abnormality usually have good prognosis, with spontaneous resolution in the majority[27,28,29]. However, those with hydrops and abnormal karyotype have a poorer outlook. The prognosis of patients detected in the second trimester is usually poor[30], but those in whom cystic hygroma is diagnosed in late gestation form a different group. Cases diagnosed late in gestation are comparatively rare[31–33], and are likely to represent an aetiological mechanism occurring during the latter half of pregnancy. Prognosis in this group is much more favourable, and prenatal diagnosis should be followed by delivery and aggressive surgical management at a perinatal centre.

Clinical presentation

The majority of cystic hygromas occur in the neck, axilla or retroperitoneum; involvement of the mediastinum, groin, extremities and face are much less common[34,35]. Approximately 80% are diagnosed before the age of 5 years, and over half present in the neonatal period. Typically, these lesions present as a soft fluctuant swelling in the lateral or anterior neck, which may or may not increase in size with age and are often asymptomatic (Figure 11.4). Occasionally, huge lymphangiomas involving the floor of the mouth or the larynx will present at birth with airway obstruction (Figure 11.5). Rapid increases in size or sudden pain may be due to haemorrhage into the tumour or to infection. Abdominal cystic hygromas usually present as an asymptomatic abdominal mass (Figure 11.6), or occasionally chyloperitoneum. Cystic hygromas of the extremity may be small and localized, or may involve the entire extremity in an infiltrative and debilitating fashion (Figure 11.7).

Investigations

Ultrasonography is useful for defining the cystic nature of the lesion[36,37], and Doppler studies can determine whether there is flow within it[38]. Computed tomography is extremely useful for assessing relationships to adjacent structures, especially within the mediastinum and retroperitoneum[39,40]. Coronal computed tomography has been described for better visualization of the neck

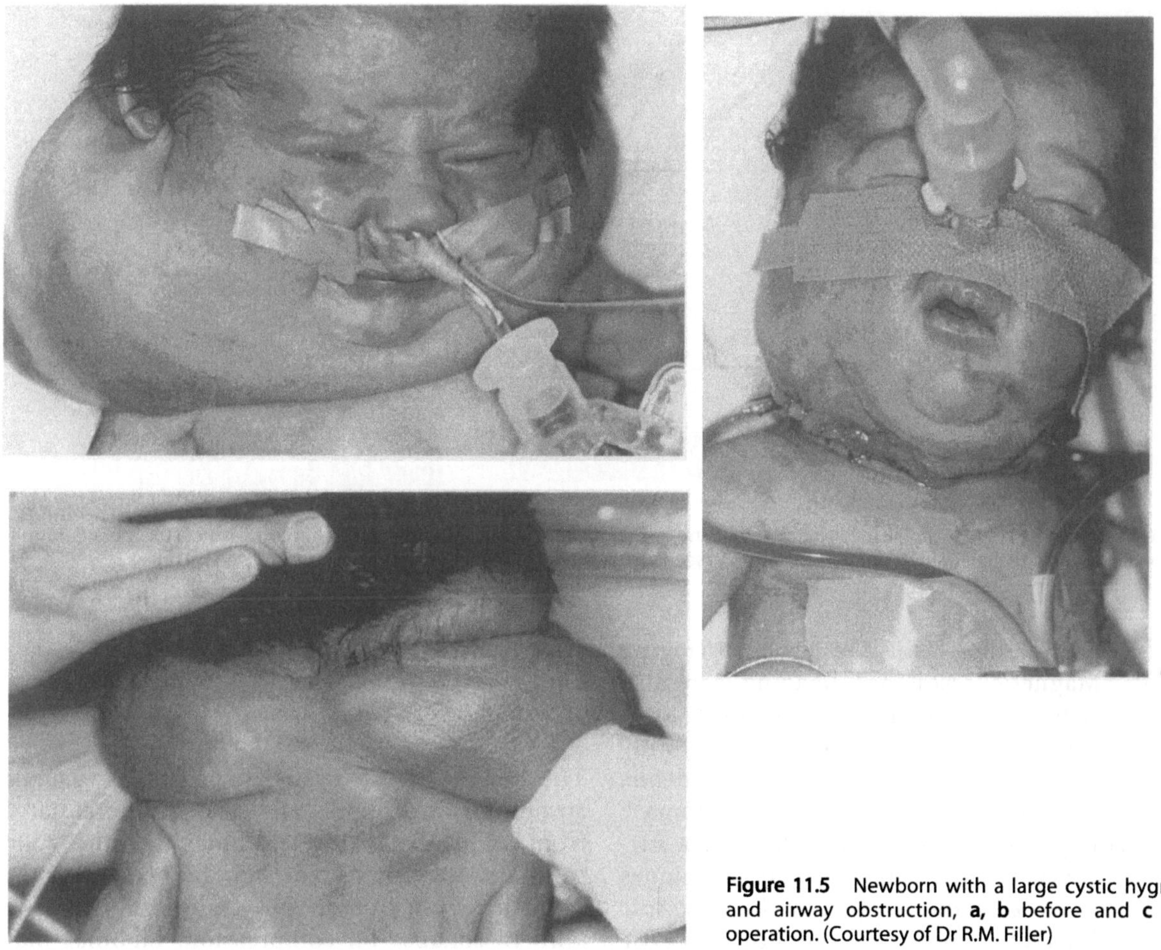

Figure 11.5 Newborn with a large cystic hygroma and airway obstruction, **a, b** before and **c** after operation. (Courtesy of Dr R.M. Filler)

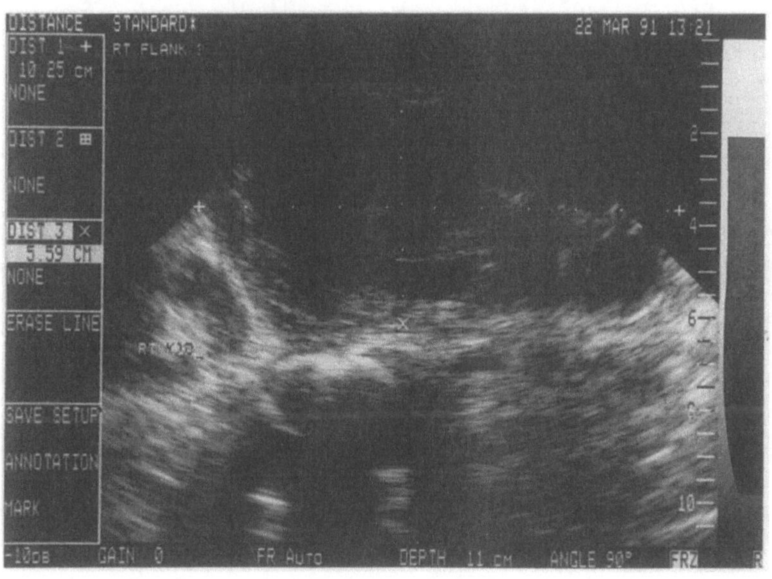

Figure 11.6 Ultrasound image of a retroperitoneal cystic hygroma presenting as an asymptomatic abdominal mass in a newborn male.

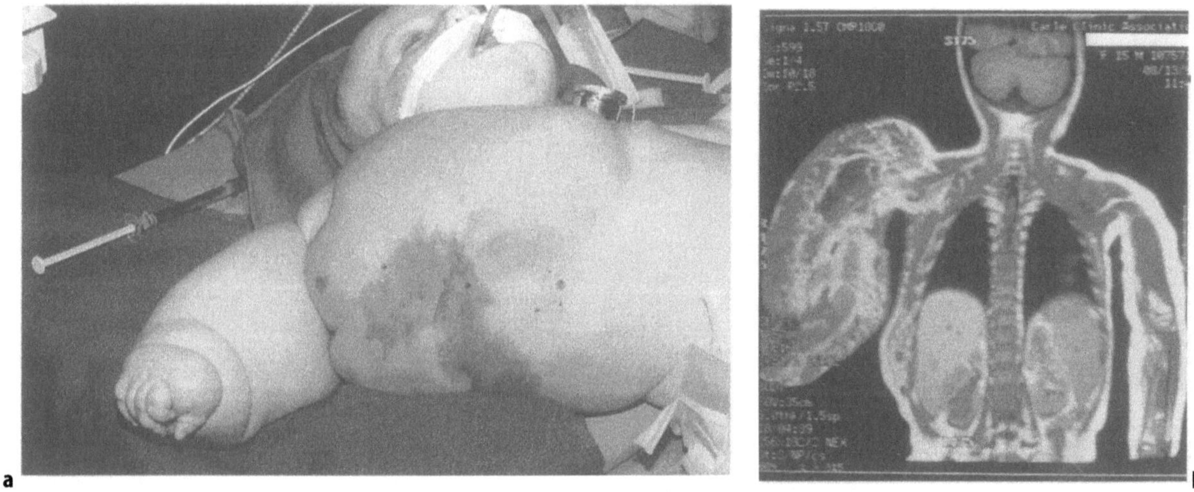

Figure 11.7 A large cystic hygroma involving the right arm and shoulder and the right side of the chest wall. Note **a** the gross deformity and oedema, and **b** the infiltrative nature of the lesion as seen on magnetic resonance imaging. (Courtesy of Dr R.P. Foglia)

and mediastinal masses in the newborn (Figure 11.8)[41]. Magnetic resonance imaging can also supply further information about anatomic location in complicated cases[42,43]. Boxen et al. recently described the use of lymphoscintigraphy to define the lymphatic supply of a large cystic hygroma[44]; this technique may be useful for planning a surgical approach. Often a combination of techniques must be used to define completely the anatomic relationships of a large or complicated cystic hygroma (Figure 11.9).

Differential diagnosis

The diagnosis of cystic hygroma is usually straightforward, and it can be easily differentiated from lymphadenopathy, teratomas and other solid tumours. Haemangiomas may be present in the same location, but do not transilluminate and tend to collapse on compression. Lipomas may also be confused with superficial lymphangiomas,

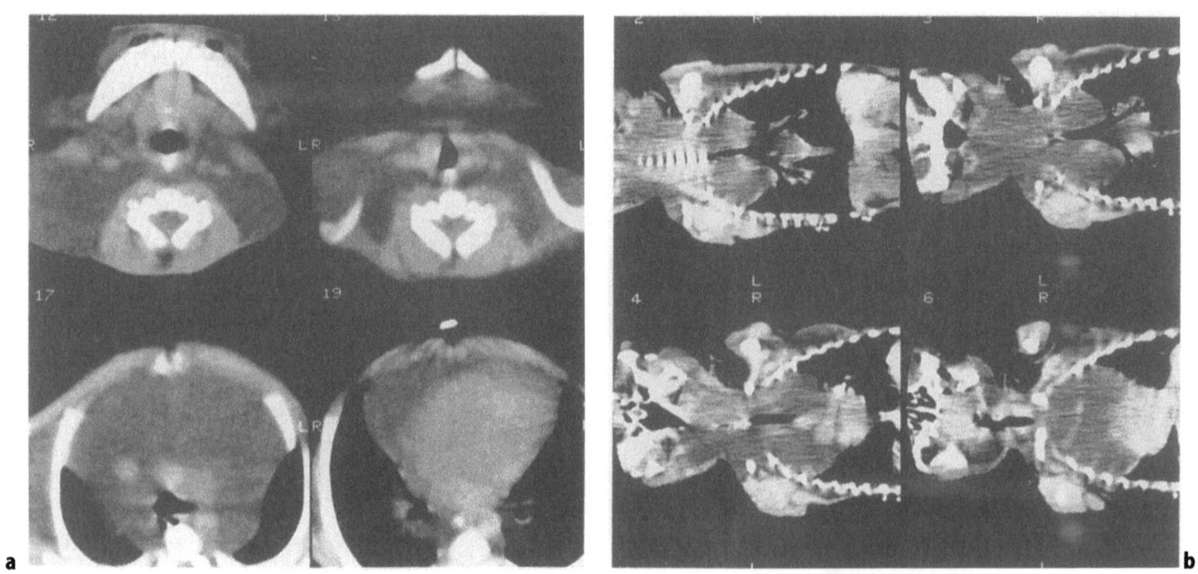

Figure 11.8 **a** Axial and **b** coronal computed tomography of a newborn showed a cervical cystic hygroma extending into the anterior mediastinum. (Courtesy of Dr L. Friedman)

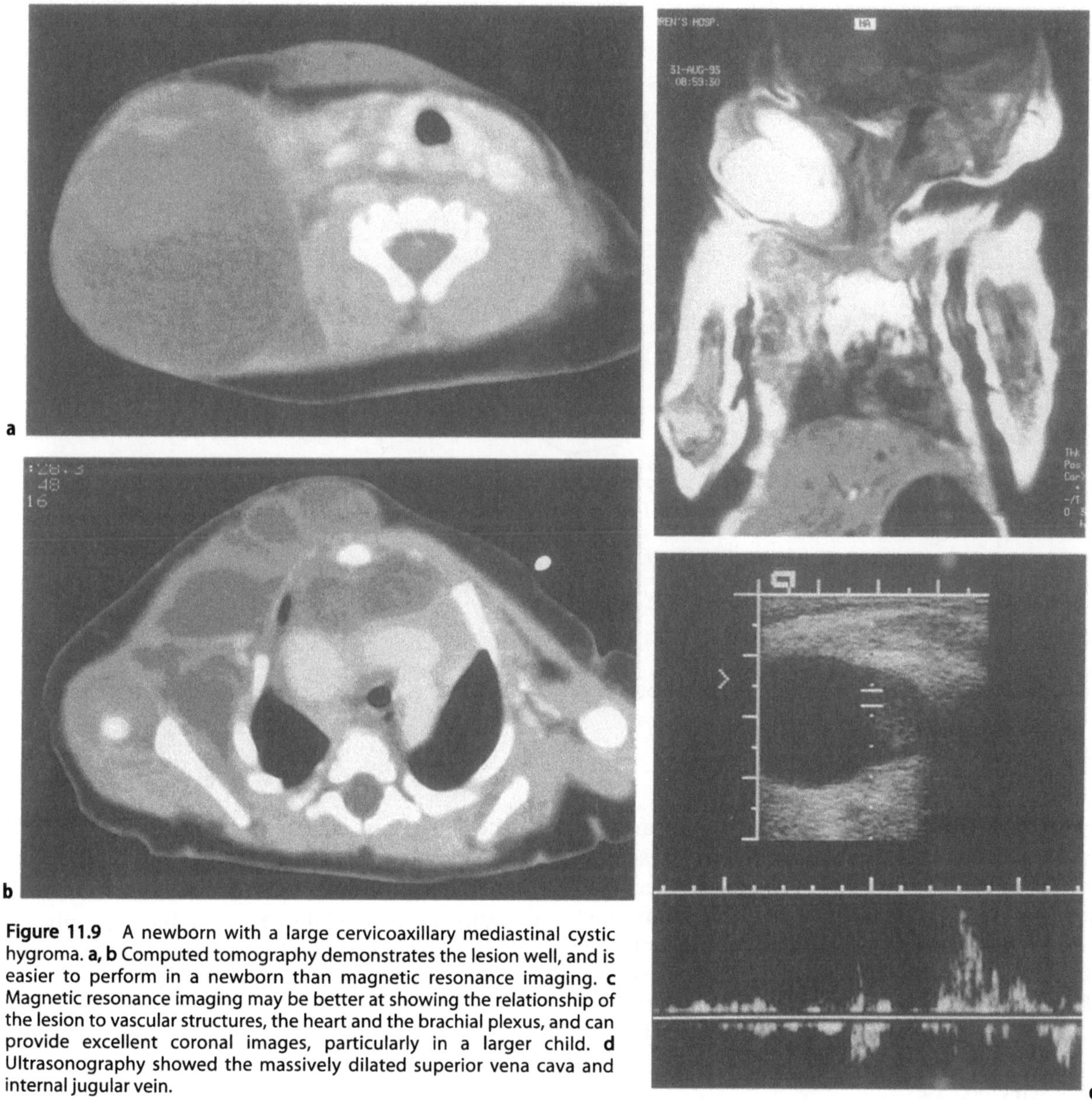

Figure 11.9 A newborn with a large cervicoaxillary mediastinal cystic hygroma. **a, b** Computed tomography demonstrates the lesion well, and is easier to perform in a newborn than magnetic resonance imaging. **c** Magnetic resonance imaging may be better at showing the relationship of the lesion to vascular structures, the heart and the brachial plexus, and can provide excellent coronal images, particularly in a larger child. **d** Ultrasonography showed the massively dilated superior vena cava and internal jugular vein.

but will not have a cystic appearance on ultrasonography.

Non-operative management

Most authors advise early surgical excision of cystic hygromas, to avoid the complications of infection, haemorrhage and continued growth with further infiltration of surrounding tissues[12]. Spontaneous regression of these lesions after birth is thought to be rare[34,45]. In the past, the high mortality rate associated with resection stimulated the development of non-surgical techniques using irradiation[46], incision and drainage, and injection of sclerosing agents[47] or boiling water[12]. In recent years, there has been a revival of the concept of injection sclerotherapy for tumours located in

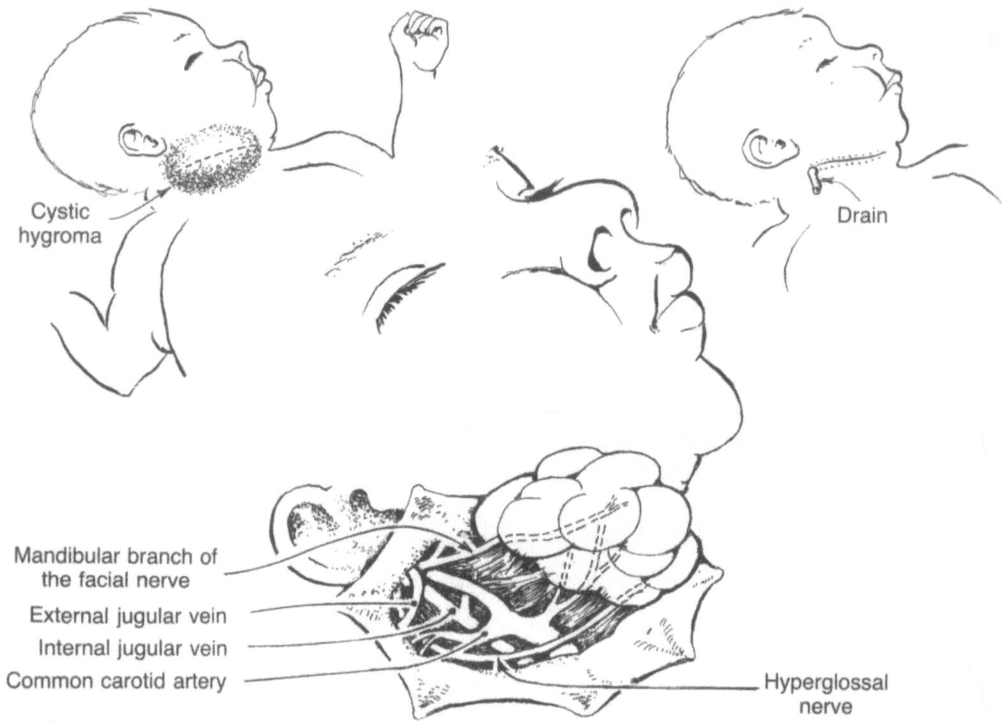

Figure 11.10 Exposure of a cervical cystic hygroma. Note the location of vital neurovascular structures, which must not be damaged during the dissection.

regions where resection would be too hazardous, for those that have been incompletely resected, and for recurrent tumours. The agents used with the most success are OK-432 (a bacterial product from *Streptococcus pyogenes*[48,49]) and antineoplastic agents such as bleomycin[50] and cyclophosphamide[51]. Although safe surgical excision is possible in most cases, it appears that injection sclerotherapy has an important role for appropriately selected cases[52].

Surgical management

Most cystic hygromas are easily resected without undue mortality rate or morbidity, as long as the following principles are adhered to:

1. Adequate exposure must be obtained.
2. Meticulous dissection must be used to preserve vital structures, including nerves, vessels, trachea, and oesophagus.
3. Because this is a benign disease, it is not justifiable to sacrifice a vital structure to excise the lesion completely.
4. Whenever possible, the lymphatic supply to the hygroma should be ligated to prevent postoperative accumulation of lymph.

Cystic hygromas of the neck can usually be approached through a transverse cervical incision under general intratracheal anaesthesia. Perioperative antibiotics are usually employed. After division of the platysma muscle, the mass is carefully dissected from all surrounding structures (Figure 11.10). The hygroma is usually well encapsulated, and every attempt should be made not to rupture the cysts. The fluid within the cyst aids the surgeon in defining the cyst wall, and therefore in finding the correct plane in which to dissect. Particular care must be taken to avoid injury to the carotid artery and its branches, or to the jugular vein. A number of nerves are often closely associated with the lesion, including the facial nerve, the spinal accessory nerve, the vagus nerve, and the brachial plexus. Although pathological studies have shown that microscopic tumour is often left behind[3], recurrence is rare when all gross tumour is removed. Once the hygroma has been removed, and if possible the lymphatic supply to the hygroma ligated, a closed-suction drain should be left in the tumour bed for several days to prevent early accumulation of fluid.

A small number of cervical cystic hygromas extend into the axilla or the mediastinum. For axillary extension, the child should be elevated 15–20° on the involved side, with the arm draped free, and both cervical and axillary crease incisions should be used[12]. The cervical component is approached first, separating the lesion away from the brachial plexus until the hygroma is seen to pass below the clavicle. The axillary portion is then dissected out. The most difficult aspect of the operation is removing the lesion from the brachial plexus behind the clavicle, where it is often densely adherent. Only careful meticulous dissection will permit complete removal of the hygroma without injury to the nerves.

Extension into the mediastinum also presents a difficult technical challenge. The best approach is one-stage resection through an "inverted hockey-stick" incision, as described by Grosfeld et al.[53], where a transverse neck incision is extended inferiorly into a midline sternotomy. This approach provides adequate exposure to dissect the lesion safely away from the jugular, carotid and subclavian vessels and the aortic arch, oesophagus and pericardium, with preservation of the phrenic, vagus and recurrent laryngeal nerves. Cystic hygromas confined to the mediastinum, which are rare, can be approached either through a lateral thoracotomy or through a midline sternotomy[54].

Perhaps the most difficult cystic hygromas to approach surgically are the massive lesions involving the tongue, floor of the mouth and larynx. These are usually present at birth, and may result in early airway obstruction, either by sheer mass effect or as a result of haemorrhage into the tumour. In many cases, tracheostomy is necessary as a life-saving procedure, followed by multiple extensive operative procedures[55]. For prenatally diagnosed cases, access to the airway can be achieved at the time of caesarian section before clamping the umbilical cord[56]. The same surgical principles are employed as outlined above, but the strategy for each patient must be individualized. Recurrence rates in these patients are higher, but do not seem to correlate with the removal of all macroscopic tumour[57]. Repeated or staged surgical approaches seem to offer the best hope for palliation. The use of laser technology for controlling airway obstruction from laryngeal or tracheal involvement has been highly successful in this group of patients[57,58]. Finally, cystic hygromas in this location may lead to bony malformations of the growing mandible, which may require subsequent surgical correction[59].

Complications

The mortality rate associated with surgical resection of a cystic hygroma should approach zero. Early intervention before infectious complications or airway obstruction, and strict adherence to the principles described above, permit safe removal with little morbidity in the majority of cases. The complications of surgery include seroma, infection and neurological sequelae such as Horner's syndrome, facial nerve palsy and spinal accessory nerve injury. Although these problems are usually transient, surgical intervention may occasionally be required[60].

Recurrence can occur after surgical excision, especially if the first resection has been incomplete. Ultrasonography, computed tomography and magnetic resonance imaging may all be useful for demonstrating these recurrent lesions[60]. Options for management include further resection or injection sclerotherapy, depending on the anatomic location and the likelihood of injury to neurovascular structures.

References

1. Coffin CM, Dehner LP (1990) Soft tissue tumours in first year of life: a report of 190 cases. Pediatr Pathol 10: 509–526.
2. Bill AH, Sumner DS (1965) A unified concept of lymphangioma and cystic hygroma. Surg Gynecol Obstet 120: 79–86.
3. Goetsch E (1938) Hygroma colli cysticum and hygroma axillare. Arch Surg 36: 394.
4. Willis RA (1953) Pathology of tumors, 2nd edn. Butterworths, London.
5. Sabin FR (1909) The lymphatic system in human embryos with a consideration of the morphology of the system as a whole. Am J Anat 9: 43.
6. Kampmeier OF (1931) Ursprung und Entwicklungsgeschichte

des Ductus thoracicus nebst Saccus lymphaticus jugularis und Cysternachyli beim Menschen. Morphologisches Jahrbuch 67: 157.
7. Godart S (1966) Embryological significance of lymphangioma. Arch Dis Child 41: 204–206.
8. Levine C (1989) Primary disorders of the lymphatic vessels – a unified concept. J Pediatr Surg 24: 233–240.
9. Chervenak FA, Isaacson G, Blakemore KJ et al. (1983) Fetal cystic hygroma: cause and natural history. N Engl J Med 309: 822–825.
10. Joseph AE, Donaldson JS, Reynolds M (1989) Neck and thorax venous aneurysm: association with cystic hygroma. Radiology 170: 109–112.
11. Miyabara S, Sugihara H, Maehara N et al. (1989) Significance of cardiovascular malformations in cystic hygroma: a new interpretation of pathogenesis. Am J Med Genet 34: 489–501.
12. Ravitch MM, Rush BF (1986) Cystic hygroma. In: Welch KJ, Randoph JG, Ravitch MM, O'Neill JA, Rowe MI, eds. Pediatric surgery. Year Book Medical, Chicago, pp 533–539.
13. Langer JC, Fitzgerald PG, Desa D et al. (1990) Cervical cystic hygroma in the fetus: clinical spectrum and outcome. J Pediatr Surg 25: 58–62.
14. Edwards MJ, Graham JM (1990) Posterior nuchal cystic hygroma. Clin Perinatol 17: 611–640.
15. Rempen A, Feige A (1985) Differential diagnosis of sonographically detected tumours in the fetal cervical region. Eur J Obstet Gynecol Reprod Biol 20: 89–105.
16. Rahmani MR, Fong KW, Connor TP (1986) The varied sonographic appearance of cystic hygromas in utero. J Ultrasound Med 5: 165–168.
17. Byrne J, Blanc WA., Warburton D, Wigger J (1984) The significance of cystic hygroma in fetuses. Hum Pathol 15: 61–67.
18. Marchese C, Savin E, Dragone E et al. (1985) Cystic hygroma: prenatal diagnosis and genetic counselling. Prenat Diagn 5: 221–227.
19. Garden AS, Benzie RJ, Miskin M, Gardner HA (1986) Fetal cystic hygroma colli: antenatal diagnosis, significance, and management. Am J Obstet Gynecol 154: 221–225.
20. Pijpers L, Reuss A, Stewart PA, Wladimiroff JW, Sachs ES (1988) Fetal cystic hygroma: prenatal diagnosis and management. Obstet Gynecol 72: 223–224.
21. Cowchock ES, Wapner RJ, Kurtz A, Chatzkel S, Barnhart JS, Lesnick DC (1982) Not all cystic hygromas occur in the Ullrich–Turner syndrome. Am J Med Genet 12: 327–331.
22. Chen H, Immken L, Blumberg B et al. (1982) Lethal form of multiple pterygium syndrome. Presented to the 1982 March of Dimes Birth Defects Conference, Atlanta, Georgia.
23. Graham JM, Stephens TD, Shepard TH (1983) Nuchal cystic hygroma in a fetus with presumed Robert's syndrome. Am J Med Genet 15: 163–167.
24. Chodirker BN, Harman CR, Greenberg CR (1988) Spontaneous resolution of a cystic hygroma in a fetus with Turner syndrome. Prenat Diagn 8: 291–296.
25. Macken MB, Grantmyre EB, Vincer MJ (1989) Regression of nuchal cystic hygroma in utero. J Ultrasound Med 8: 101–103.
26. Tannirandorn Y, Nicolini Y, Nicolaidis PC, Fisk NM, Arulkumaran S, Rodeck CH (1990) Fetal cystic hygromata: insights gained from fetal blood sampling. Prenat Diagn 10: 189–193.
27. Nadel A, Bromley B, Benacerraf BR (1993) Nuchal thickening or cystic hygromas in first or early second trimester fetuses: prognosis and outcome. Obstet Gynecol 82: 43–48.
28. Johnson MP, Johnson A, Holzgreve W et al. (1993) First trimester simple hygroma: cause and outcome. Am J Obstet Gynecol 168: 156–161.
29. Shulman LP, Emerson DS, Grevengood C, Felker RE, Phillips OP, Elias S (1994) Clinical course and outcome of fetuses with isolated cystic nuchal lesions and normal karyotypes detected in the first trimester. Am J Obstet Gynecol 171: 1278–1281.
30. Thomas RL (1992) Prenatal diagnosis of giant cystic hygromas: prognosis, counselling and management: case presentation and review of the recent literature. Prenat Diagn 12: 919–923.
31. Lyngbye T, Haugaard L, Klebe JG (1986) Antenatal sonographic diagnoses of giant cystic hygroma of the neck. Acta Obstet Gynecol Scand 65: 873–875.
32. Benacerraf BR, Frigoletto FD (1987) Prenatal sonographic diagnosis of isolated congenital cystic hygroma, unassociated with lymphedema or other morphologic abnormality. J Ultrasound Med 6: 63–66.
33. Goldstein I, Jakobi P, Shoshany G, Filmer S, Itskoviz I, Maor B (1994) Late-onset isolated cystic hygroma: the obstetrical significance, management, and outcome. Prenat Diagn 14: 757–761.
34. Ninh TN, Ninh TX (1974) Cystic hygroma in children: a report of 126 cases. J Pediatr Surg 9: 191–195.
35. Bhattacharyya NC, Yadav K, Mitra SK, Pathak IC (1974) Lymphangiomas in children. Aust N Z J Surg 9: 191–195.
36. Sheth S, Nussbaum AR, Hutchins GM, Sanders RC (1987) Cystic hygromas in children: sonographic–pathologic correlation. Radiology 162: 821–824.
37. Orrison WW, Sty JR (1989) Ultrasound in the diagnosis of lymphangioma. Wis Med J 80: 30–32.
38. Dates CP, Wilson AW, Ward-Booth RP, Williams ED (1990) Combined use of Doppler and conventional ultrasound for the diagnosis of vascular and other lesions in the head and neck. Int J Oral Maxillofac Surg 19: 235–239.
39. Mahboubi S, Potsic WP (1989) Computed tomography of cervical cystic hygroma in the neck. Int J Pediatr Otorhinolaryngol 18: 47–51.
40. Davidson AJ, Hartman DS (1990) Lymphangioma of the retroperitoneum: CT and sonographic characteristics. Radiology 175: 507–510.
41. Friedman L, Halls SB (1990) Coronal computed tomography. Can Assoc Radiol J 41: 287–290.
42. Cutillo DP, Swayne LC, Cucco J, Dougan H (1989) CT and MR imaging in cystic abdominal lymphangiomatosis. J Comput Assist Tomogr 13: 534–536.
43. Siegel MJ, Glazer HS, St Amour TE, Rosenthal DD (1989) Lymphangiomas in children: MR imaging. Radiology 170: 467–470.
44. Boxen I, Zhang ZM, Filler RM (1990) Lymphoscintigraphy for cystic hygroma. J Nucl Med 31: 516–518.
45. Saigo M, Munro IR, Mancer K (1975) Lymphangioma – a long term follow up study. Plast Reconstr Surg 56: 642.
46. Figi FA (1929) Radium in the treatment of multilocular lymph cysts in the neck in children. AJR Am J Roentgenol 21: 473–480.
47. Harrower G (1933) Treatment of cystic hygroma of the neck by sodium morrhuate. Br Med J ii: 148–155.
48 Ogita S, Tsuto T, Tokiwa K, Takahashi T (1987) Intracystic injection of OK-432: a new sclerosing therapy for cystic hygroma in children. Br J Surg 74: 690–691.
49. Ogita S, Tsuto T, Nakamura K, Deguchi E, Iwai N (1994) OK-432 therapy in 64 patients with lymphangioma. J Pediatr Surg 29: 784–785.
50. Okada A, Kubota A, Fukuzawa M, Imura K, Kainata S (1992) Injection of bleomycin as a primary therapy of cystic lymphangioma. J Pediatr Surg 27: 440–443.
51. Dickerhoff R, Bode VU (1990) Cyclophosphamide in nonresectable cystic hygroma. Lancet 335: 1474–1475.
52. Ogita S, Tsuto T, Deguchi E, Tokiwa K (1989) Treatment of lymphangiomas arising around cervico-facial region: surgery, bleomycin therapy and OK-432 therapy. Nippon Geka Gakkai Zasshi 90: 1389–1391.
53. Grosfeld JL, Weber TR, Vane DW (1982) One-stage resection for massive cervicomediastinal hygroma. Surgery 92:

693–699.
54. Moore TC, Cobo JC (1984) Massive symptomatic cystic hygroma confined to the thorax in early childhood. J Thorac Cardiovasc Surg 89: 459–468.
55. Seashore JH, Gardiner LJ, Arlyan S (1985) Management of giant cystic hygromas in infants. Am J Surg 149: 459–465.
56. Langer JC, Tabb T, Thompson P, Paes BA, Caco C (1992) Management of prenatally diagnosed tracheal obstruction: access to the airway in utero prior to delivery. Fetal Diagn Ther 7: 12–16.
57. Cohen SR, Thompson JW (1986) Lymphangiomas of the larynx in infants and children: a survey of pediatric lymphangioma. Ann Otol Rhinol Laryngol Suppl 127: 1–20.
58. Apfelberg DB, Maser MR, Lash H, White DN (1989) Sapphire tip technology for YAG laser excisions in plastic surgery. Plast Reconstr Surg 84: 273–279.
59. Osborne TE, Levin LS, Tilghman DM, Haller JA (1987) Surgical correction of mandibulofacial deformities secondary to large cervical cystic hygromas. J Oral Maxillofac Surg 45: 1015–1021.
60. Hancock BJ, St Vil Y, Luks FI et al. (1992) Complications of lymphangiomas in children. J Pediatr Surg 27: 220–224.

Sacrococcygeal Teratoma

Rajendra Surana and Prem Puri

12

Introduction

Willis defined teratoma as a tumour composed of multiple tissues of kinds foreign to the part in which they arise[1]. Sacrococcygeal teratoma is the commonest extragonadal teratoma arising from the caudal end of the spine. The incidence is approximately 1 in 40 000 live births[2,3]. These tumours are most commonly found in the neonatal period.

Embryology

It is now generally accepted that the teratomas are not a variant of fetus in fetu or twins, but originate from totipotent cells from Hansen's node[1,4,5] or primitive germ cells during their migration from the yolk sac to the genital ridge[6]. Ashcraft and Holder reported 23 patients with a hereditary group of presacral teratomas occurring in a Mendelian dominant genetic pattern[7].

Pathology

Macroscopically, sacrococcygeal teratoma are lobulated. The consistency of the tumour varies according to the structures present. It may be cystic, solid or both. Robbins defined a teratoma as a tumour composed of cells representing more than one germ layer[8]. By definition, therefore, the teratoma is composed of several types of tissue derived from two or three germ layers. The common components of the teratoma include skin, teeth, endocrine structures, central nervous tissue, and respiratory and alimentary mucosa.

Within any one tumour, the cells can vary from totally benign to cells that appear frankly malignant. However, many sacrococcygeal teratoma contain "immature" cells, which resemble malignant cells. If these tumours are completely excised they do not recur.

The extent of the tumour and age at operation have been associated with risk of malignancy. In the American Academy of Pediatrics (AAP) Survey, malignancy was noted in 7% of neonatal patients and in 37% by 1 year of age; almost half were malignant by 2 years of age[9].

Altman et al.[10] classified sacrococcygeal teratoma into four groups. Type I tumours are almost exclusively exterior, with a minimal pelvic component (Figure 12.1): these are rarely malignant. Type II tumours have a significant pelvic component (Figure 12.2): 6% of the type II tumours in AAP survey were malignant. Type III tumours have an intrapelvic and intra-abdominal component greater than the external component: 20% of these were malignant in AAP survey. Type IV tumours are exclusively presacral, with 8% malignant. Malignant teratomas either invade locally or have metastasis to regional nodes, lungs, liver and/or vertebrae.

Prenatal diagnosis

With the advent of routine ultrasonography, the prenatal diagnosis of sacrococcygeal teratoma has

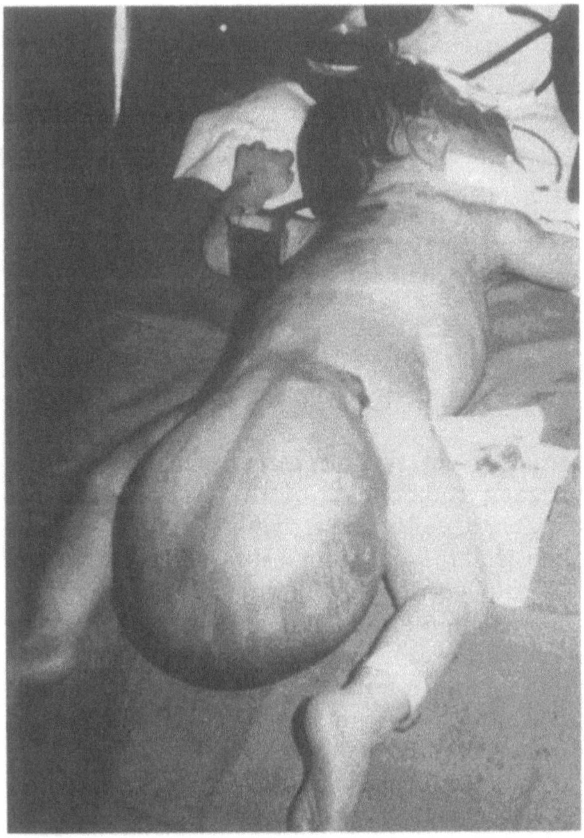

Figure 12.1 A newborn with type I sacrococcygeal teratoma. The tumour is confined exclusively to the exterior.

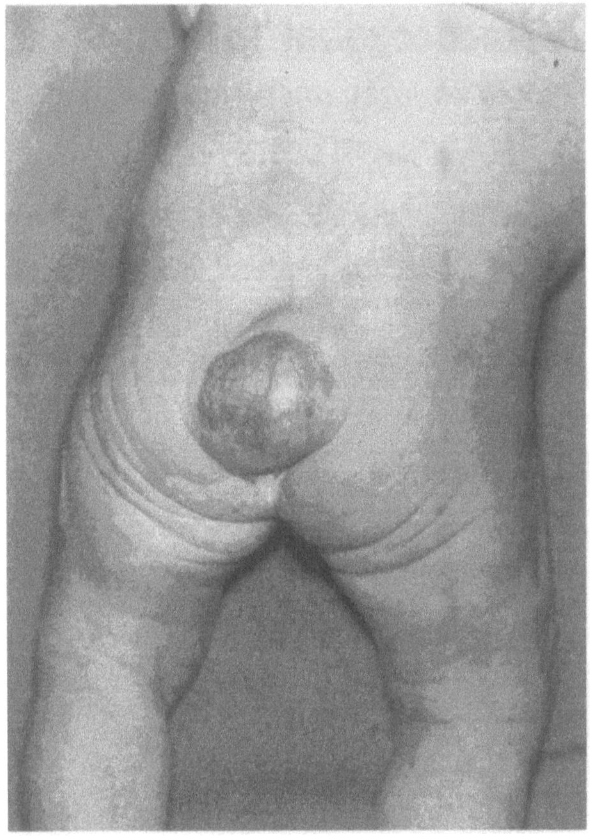

Figure 12.2 Sacrococcygeal teratoma. In this newborn, two-thirds of the tumour was in the pelvis.

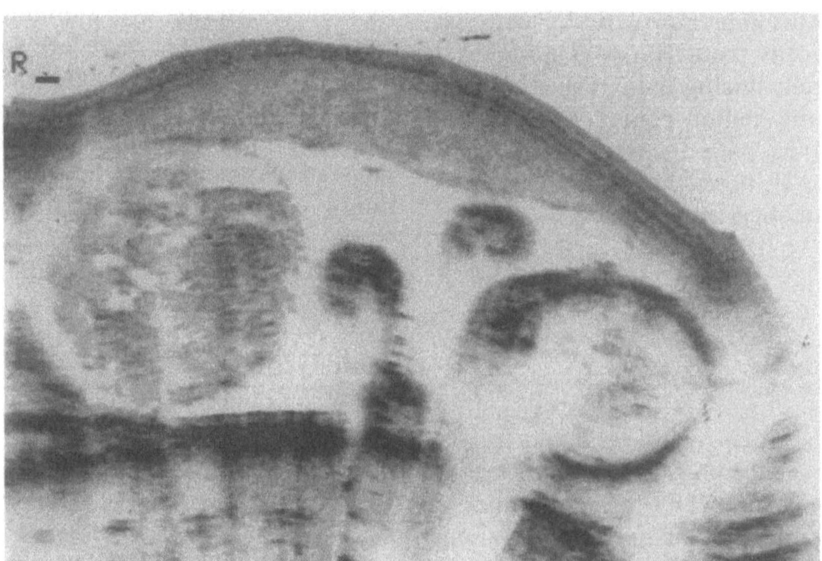

Figure 12.3 A large sacrococcygeal teratoma discovered by antenatal ultrasonography. (Courtesy of Dr Elshafie, Toledo, Ohio)

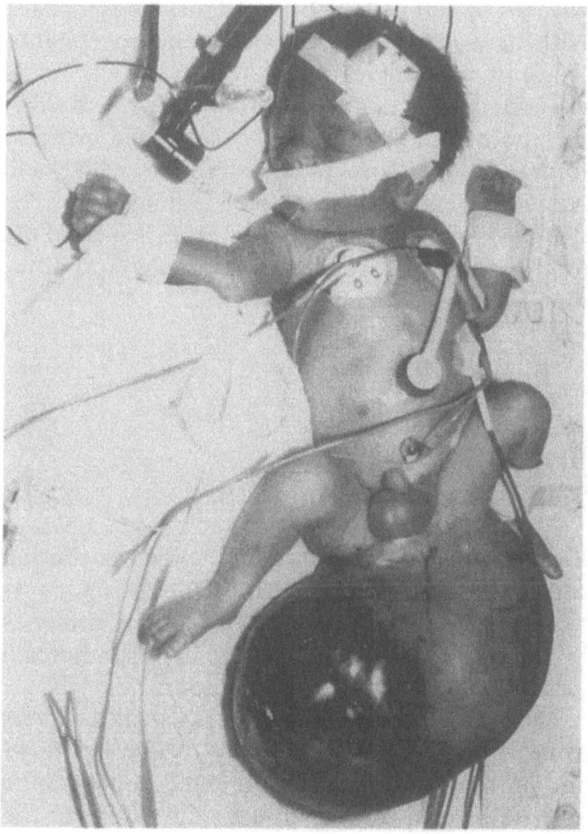

Figure 12.4 A large sacrococcygeal teratoma with necrotic skin. (Courtesy of Dr Elshafie, Toledo, Ohio)

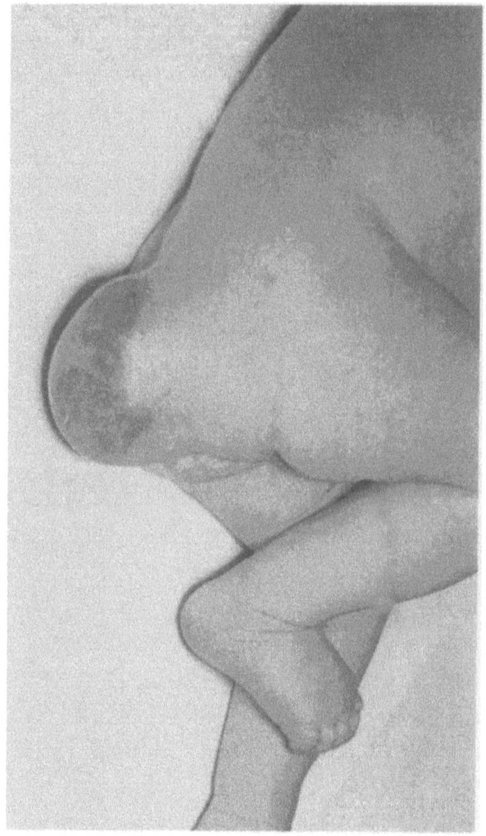

Figure 12.5 Sacrococcygeal teratoma with overlying haemangioma.

increasingly been made (Figure 12.3)[9]. The obvious severity criteria include tumour size greater than biparietal diameter of the fetus, rapid tumour growth and presence of hydrops[11,12]. Series reporting the antenatal diagnosis of sacrococcygeal teratoma have revealed that fetuses diagnosed as having sacrococcygeal teratoma are likely to die before delivery[13–15]. Most of the fetuses reported to have died following antenatal diagnosis had tumours with a mass as great as or greater than the rest of the fetus. In most of the antenatal series reported, fetal non-immune hydrops is very common[13,16–18]. Ikeda et al.[19] reported characteristics of 20 cases of prenatally diagnosed sacrococcygeal teratoma. Six infants delivered at gestational ages of 25–32 weeks died prematurely; 14 delivered after 32 weeks survived. Prenatal diagnosis in a subset of patients may therefore offer a hope of survival with surgical intervention in utero[20]. Because large sacrococcygeal teratomas cause dystocia, these cases may benefit from abdominal delivery[21]. However, the decision about prenatal and postnatal management should include discussion between neonatologists, paediatric surgeons and obstetricians.

Presentation

The most common presentation is the presence of a large sacral mass that is obvious at birth[5,9,22–26]. Girls are more commonly affected than the boys. The mass may be in the midline or paramedian. The size of the mass varies from a small lesion to a mass the size of the baby. The overlying skin is usually normal, but may be necrotic (Figure 12.4) and there may be overlying haemangioma (Figure 12.5). In patients with intrapelvic extension, the anus is pushed anteriorly. Digital rectal examination will reveal this. Rupture of the tumour is

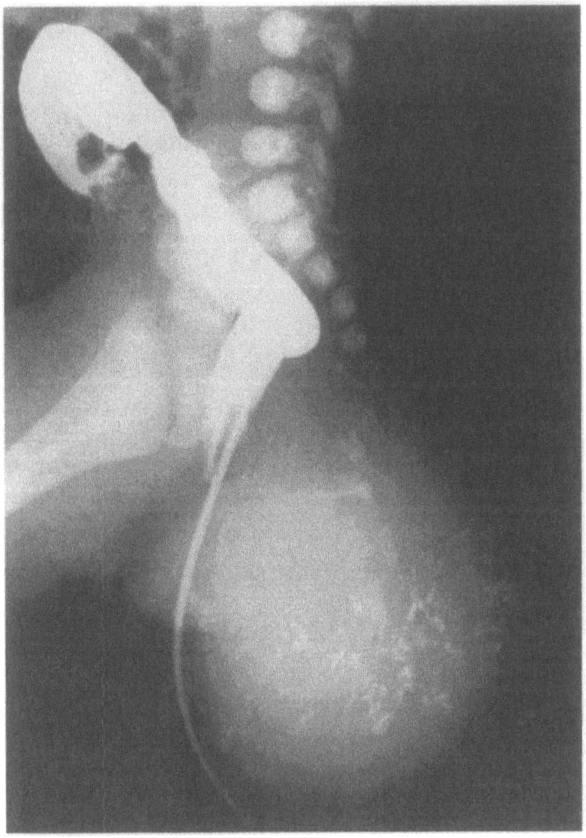

Figure 12.6 Radiograph showing extensive calcification in a large sacrococcygeal teratoma.

unusual but may occur during delivery. Intrapelvic tumours are often not diagnosed until later in life when they may present with symptoms due to pressure on the rectum or bladder. Malignant tumours present with a rapidly growing buttock mass[27,28]. Distant metastases are usually present at the time of diagnosis.

Associated anomalies are found in one-fifth of cases and include vertebral, renal, cardiac and gastrointestinal anomalies[9,29].

Differential diagnosis

Lesions that can cause diagnostic difficulties include myelomeningocele, chordoma and other rare lesions[30]. Myelomeningocele is usually at a higher level than sacrococcygeal teratoma and is covered by serous membrane. It may be associated with neurological deficit and/or hydrocephalus. Anterior meningocele will feel cystic on rectal examination, with anterior bony defect. Dillard et al.[25] point out the need to observe the anterior fontanelle during rectal examination, which will bulge on pressing the anterior meningocele. The diagnosis can be established by radiography of the lumbosacral region. Ultrasonography and computed tomography may be helpful.

Investigations

Radiography of the pelvis and spine may reveal calcification (Figure 12.6) or structures such as teeth and bones, or there may be a bony defect as in neural tube defect. These may also indicate intrapelvic extensions of the tumour.

Abdominal ultrasonography is useful to determine the size and consistency of any pelvic or abdominal component. Computed tomography may be helpful in determining the extent of the mass and the presence of intraspinal extension. Magnetic resonance imaging will clearly distinguish between sacrococcygeal teratoma and anterior meningocele, and may be able to detect the occasional extension of the tumours into the spinal canal.

α-Fetoprotein is a useful serum marker in sacrococcygeal teratoma. Elevated levels are observed in malignant lesions, but its main importance is in postoperative serial monitoring to detect malignant recurrence.

Treatment

The treatment of sacrococcygeal teratoma is complete excision as soon as possible.

If the lesion is intact, surgery should be planned as soon as possible. Blood is crossmatched. Adequate intravenous access and arterial line are established. Blood is collected for baseline α-fetoprotein determination for comparison with postoperative values to ensure that they decline at a normal rate[27,31,32]. If the tumour is ruptured, a pressure bandage may reduce blood loss, but there is a theoretical risk of squeezing immature cells into the venous drainage from the tumour. Emergency surgery will be required in these patients.

An inverted V incision is made in the skin over the dorsum of the mass. The apex of the V is placed over the lower sacrum. The dissection is continued in the midline directly down to the fourth or fifth sacral vertebra. A clamp is passed from one edge of the sacrum to the other, keeping the forcep flush to the central surface of the sacrum to avoid middle sacral vessels. The sacrum is divided and the tumour displaced inferiorly to expose, ligate and divide middle sacral vessels to control the blood loss.

The tumour is dissected outside the capsule from thinned out levator and gluteus muscle. The pelvic component is displaced anteriorly until its upper extent is reached. The tumour is dissected out from the pelvis and rolled inferiorly. The upper end of the rectum is identified by a vaseline gauze pack or by passing a Hegar dilator through the anus. The tumour is dissected off the rectum and the anal canal. The inferior skin flap is dissected and divided from the tumour and the tumour removed. The pelvic floor reconstruction is undertaken by muscle and fascial reconstruction and the anus sited at the proper place.

Abdominal exploration is necessary if there is any large abdominal component[33,34], or occasionally if the tumour is ruptured and actively bleeding[35]. The abdomen is opened via a transverse infra-umbilical incision to allow ligation and division of the middle sacral vessels. The mass is tied from the pelvic area and rolled inferiorly. The abdomen is then closed and the patient positioned prone. The tumour is then resected as previously described.

Postoperative management

α-Fetoprotein levels should be determined immediately after operation, on discharge, at monthly intervals for 3 months and then at 3 monthly intervals for a year. Follow-up should continue for at least 3–5 years. Rectal examination will detect any local recurrence.

Prognosis

In the absence of distant metastases at presentation, and if excision is complete, the overall outlook is good. Voiding dysfunction is not uncommon after surgical excision of large sacrococcygeal teratoma, and recent investigations have reported neurogenic bladder in 12%–80% of patients. These include detrusor instability, pelvic overactivity and bladder sphincter dysfunction[36,37]. Faecal continence is usually normal. However, only 27% of patients at a mean age of 30 years had completely normal bowel habits[38]. Recurrence in cases of benign sacrococcygeal teratoma with complete excision including removal of the coccyx is unusual. In a 4–43 year follow-up of 45 patients, three recurrences (two benign and one malignant mucinous adenocarcinoma) were noted in adulthood 21–43 years after the original operation. In a patient with malignant recurrence, the coccyx was not removed at original operation[39]. The prognosis for patients presenting with a malignant sacrococcygeal teratoma must be guarded. Modern chemotherapy has produced some improvement in survival rate, although the regimens are toxic and the tumour tends to be resistant to therapy.

References

1. Willis RA (1962) The borderland of embryology and pathology. Butterworths, London.
2. Calbet JR (1983) Contribution a L'étude des tumeurs congenitales d'origine parasitaire de la région sacrococcygienne. G Steinheil, Paris.
3. McCune WS (1964) Management of sacrococcygeal tumours. Ann Surg 159: 911.
4. Vaez-Zadeh K, Sieber WK, Sherman FE, Kiesewetter WB (1972) Sacrococcygeal teratomas in children. J Pediatr Surg 7: 152.
5. Gross RE, Clatworthy HW, Meeker IA (1951) Sacrococcygeal teratomas in infants and children: a report of 40 cases. Surg Gynecol Obstet 92: 341.
6. Teilium G (1959) Endodermal sinus tumours of the ovary and testis: comparative morphogenesis of the so called mesonephroma ovarii (Schiller) and extraembryonic (yok-sac allantoic) sutures of the rat's placenta. Cancer 12: 1092–1105.
7. Ashcraft KW, Holder CM (1974) Hereditary presacral teratoma. J Pediatr Surg 9: 691–697.
8. Robbins SL (1976) Pathology neoplasia. WB Saunders, Philadelphia, p 92.
9. Irving IM (1990) Sacrococcygeal teratoma. In: Lister J, Irving IM, eds. Newborn surgery. 3rd edn. Butterworths, London, pp 142–152.

10. Altman RP, Randolph JG, Lilly JR (1974) Sacrococcygeal teratoma: American Academy of Pediatrics Surgical Section Survey-1973. J Pediatr Surg 9: 389.
11. Veschambre P, Wartanian R, Lebouvier B, Rosenau L, Lepinard C, Denis A (1993) Rev Fr Gynecol Obstet 88: 325–330.
12. Walton JM, Rubin SZ, Soucy P, Berizie R, Ash K, Nimmod C (1993) Fetal tumours associated with hydrops: the role of the pediatric surgeon. J Pediatr Surg 28: 1151–1153.
13. Flake AW, Harrison MR, Adzick NS et al. (1986) Fetal sacrococcygeal teratoma. J Pediatr Surg 21: 563.
14. Holzgreve W, Mahony BS, Glick PL et al. (1985) Sonographic demonstration of fetal sacrococcygeal teratoma. Prenat Diagn 5: 245.
15. Holzgreve W, Miny P, Anderson R, Golbus MS (1987) Experience with 8 cases of prenatally diagnosed sacrococcygeal teratomas. Fetal Therapy 2: 88.
16. Kuhlmann RS, Warsof SL, Levy DL et al. (1987) Fetal sacrococcygeal teratoma. Fetal Therapy 2: 95.
17. Pringle KC, Weiner CP, Soper RT, Kealey P (1987) Sacrococcygeal teratoma. Fetal Therapy 2: 80.
18. Sheth S, Nussbaum AR, Sanders RC et al. (1988) Prenatal diagnosis of sacrococcygeal teratoma: sonographic–pathologic correlation. Radiology 169: 131.
19. Ikeda H, Okumura H, Nagashima K et al. (1990) The management of prenatally diagnosed sacrococcygeal teratoma. Pediatr Surg Int 5: 192–194.
20. Flake AW (1993) Fetal sacrococcygeal teratoma. Semin Pediatr Surg 2: 113–120.
21. McCurdy CM Jr, Seeds JW (1993) Route of delivery of infants with congenital anomalies. Clin Perinatol 22: 81–106.
22. Bale PM (1975) Teratomas in childhood. Pathology 7: 209.
23. Berry CL, Keeling J, Hilton C (1969) Teratomata in infancy and childhood: a review of 91 cases. J Pathol 98: 241.
24. Billmire DF, Grosfeld JL (1986) Teratomas in childhood: analysis of 142 cases. J Pediatr Surg 21: 548.
25. Dillard BM, Mayer JH, McAlister WH et al. (1970) Sacrococcygeal teratoma in children. J Pediatr Surg 5: 53.
26. Donnellan WA, Swenson O (1968) Benign and malignant sacrococcygeal teratomas. Surgery 64: 834.
27. Chretien PB, Milam JD, Foote FW, Miller TR (1970) Embryonal adenocarcinomas (a type of malignant teratoma) of the sacrococcygeal region: clinical and pathologic aspects of 21 cases. Cancer 25: 522.
28. Ein SH, Mancer K, Adeyami SD (1985) Malignant sacrococcygeal teratoma - endodermal sinus, yolk sac tumour - in infants and children. A 32 year review. J Pediatr Surg 20: 473.
29. Lehdenne P, Heikinheimo M, Juaskekimes J, Merikanto J, Heikkila J, Siimes MA (1991) Vertebral abnormalities associated with congenital sacrococcygeal teratomas. J Pediatr Orthop 11: 603–607.
30. Lemire RJ, Graham CB, Beckwith JB (1971) Skin covered sacrococcygeal masses in infants and children. J Pediatr 79: 948.
31. Johnston PW (1988) The diagnostic value of α-fetoprotein in an infant with sacrococcygeal teratoma. J Pediatr Surg 23: 862.
32. Tsuchida Y, Endo Y, Saito S et al. (1979) Evaluation of α-fetoprotein in early infancy. J Pediatr Surg 13: 155.
33. Smith B, Passaro E, Clatworthy HW (1961) The vascular anatomy of sacrococcygeal teratomas: its significance in surgical management. Pediatr Surg 49: 534.
34. Hendren WH, Henderson BM (1970) The surgical management of sacrococcygeal teratomas with intrapelvic extension. Ann Surg 171: 77.
35. Lindahi H (1988) Giant sacrococcygeal teratoma: a method of simple intraoperative control of hemorrhage. J Pediatr Surg 23: 1068.
36. Boemers TM, van Gool JD, de Jong TP, Bax KM (1994) Lower urinary tract dysfunction in children with benign sacrococcygeal teratoma. J Urol 151: 174–176.
37. Reinberg Y, Long R, Manivel JC, Resnick J, Simonton S, Gonzalez R (1993) Urological aspects of sacrococcygeal teratoma in children. J Urol 150: 948–949.
38. Rintala R, Lahdenno P, Lindahe H, Sijmes M, Heikinkeimo M (1993) Anorectal function in adults operated for a benign sacrococcygeal teratoma. J Pediatr Surg 28: 1165–1167.
39. Lahdenne P, Heikinheimo M, Nikkanen V, Klemi P, Slimer MA, Rapola J (1993) Neonatal benign sacrococcygeal teratoma may recur in adults and give rise to malignancy. Cancer 72: 3727–3731.

Haemangiomas and Vascular Malformations

Prem Puri and George Ninan

13

Introduction

Haemangiomas are the most common benign tumour of infancy, occurring in approximately 10% of all infants during the first year of life[1–6]. Only 2% of haemangiomas are present at birth in full-term infants, but most appear during the first few weeks of life[2]. Haemangiomas are more common in premature infants weighing less than 1000 g, with a reported[1] incidence as high as 30%. Some 20%–75% of newborns have some vascular mark present at birth[7,8]. Girls are affected two to three times more commonly than boys[1,4–6]. Functional complications occur in 20% of all haemangiomas, and life-threatening complications develop in 3%–5% of children with haemangioma[3,9].

Pathology

Traditionally, haemangiomas are classified as "capillary", "cavernous" or "mixed", depending on the size of the vessels involved[10,11]. Histologically, capillary haemangiomas are composed of small thin-walled vessels of capillary size, lined by a single layer of flattened or plump endothelial cells that are usually surrounded by a discontinuous layer of pericytes, and reticulular fibres. These pericytes produce transforming growth factor β, which controls the growth rate of endothelial cells[3]. In cavernous haemangiomas, tangles of thin-walled cavernous vessels and spaces are seen, which are separated by a scanty connective tissue stroma. Mixed haemangiomas show histological features of both types.

The pathogenesis and natural history of haemangiomas are poorly understood, but are comparable to the developing blood supply of an embryonic limb bud. Instead of the usual orderly development of arteries, veins and capillaries, an arteriovenous fistula persists[12]. Thus a typical capillary angioma represents a localized arteriovenous fistula.

Controversy exists as to whether haemangiomas are hamartomas or true neoplasms[13]; the majority opinion is in favour of considering them as hamartomas[1,4,5,14,15]. By defining the cellular features of cutaneous vascular lesions in relation to their history and clinical outcome, Mulliken has suggested that childhood vascular lesions should be classified as haemangiomas or vascular malformations[16,17]. The underlying pathology of haemangiomas and vascular malformations is similar, both representing mesodermal rests of vasoformative tissue from which the vascular tree develops[9]. Haemangiomas contain a significantly higher number of calcitonin gene-related peptide (CGRP), substance P and metenkephalin positive fibres. The most significant rise in number is that of CGRP-positive fibres. This neuropeptide is a known mitogen, which could be responsible for the growth of the haemangiomatous blood vessels. Substance P is a nociceptive neurotransmitter and its presence can explain the pain that often accompanies even tiny intramuscular haemangiomas[18].

Haemangiomas grow rapidly during the first few months of life and then begin to involute. Rapid growth proceeds over the first 3–6 months, with a plateau and cessation of growth noted between 6 and 18 months of age[1]. During the growth period there is increased endothelial cell activity, demonstrable by hyperplasia and incorporation of [^{3}H]thymidine into the cells. There is also an increase in the number of mast cells during this period. In this involution phase fibrosis and fat deposition are seen, with an absence of [^{3}H]thymidine-labelled endothelial cells[12,17].

Vascular malformations grow pari passu with the child, fail to regress, show no evidence of endothelial mitotic activity and are not hypercellular. They are lined by flat mature endothelium, demonstrate no [^{3}H]thymidine incorporation and have normal ultrastructural characteristics. Any combination of capillary, arterial, venous and lymphatic elements may exist in these lesions[11,12,17,19].

Port-wine stains, traditionally classified as haemangiomas, should be included under vascular malformations. They are derived from a progressive ectasia of the superficial vascular plexus, and there is marked decrease in the sympathetic autonomous nerves associated with these vessels. This leads to failure in regulation of blood flow with progressive vascular ectasia[7].

An abnormally high population of cytosol-specific oestrogen-binding receptors is seen in strawberry haemangiomas[20].

Both haemangiomas and vascular malformations are benign lesions. Malignant transformation is exceedingly rare, but haemangiosarcoma is reported to occur after irradiation of a haemangioma.

Table 13.1 Classification of haemangioma

Type	Description
1	Neonatal staining
2	Intradermal capillary haemangioma A Salmon patch B Port-wine stain C Spider angioma
3	Juvenile capillary haemangioma A Strawberry mark B Strawberry capillary haemangioma C Capillary cavernous haemangioma
4	Arteriovenous fistula A Arterial haemangioma B Haemangiomatous goganism
5	Cirsoid angioma (racemose aneurysm)

From Edgerton[21].

Table 13.2 Classification of vascular lesions in infants and children

Haemangiomas	Vascular malformations
Proliferating phase Involuting phase	Capillary Venous Arterial Lymphatic Fistula

From Mulliken and Glowacki[17].

Clinical features and classification

The clinical presentation depends on the type of lesion, its site and the development of complications. Edgerton, in 1976, proposed a logical classification based on their appearance, anatomic features and physiology (Table 13.1)[21]. Although this has been superseded by the classification based on endothelial characteristics by Mulliken[17] (Table 13.2), from a clinical point of view Edgerton's classification is more useful.

Edgerton's type 1 (neonatal staining) are present at birth and appear as light pink-staining patterns on the midline base of the neck and near the glabella. They almost always disappear within a few months of birth, and therefore no therapy is necessary.

Type 2 (intradermal capillary haemangiomas) are usually present at birth and are located in the deep dermal layers. Their patterns correspond to the skin distribution of sensory nerves in the area. The *salmon patch* (type 2A) is a variety of intradermal capillary haemangioma. Lesions varying from light pink to rust in colour and blanche on pressure. They are most frequently found on the nape of the neck, eyelids, glabella and mid-forehead. They remain constant over a period of many years. The *port-wine stain* (type 2B) is deeper in colour than the salmon patch and usually involves a larger surface area. It does not regress spontaneously; treatment options are laser therapy or surgical excision with skin grafting. *Spider angiomata* (type 2C) are small and multiple lesions. They consist of a small central dermal arteriole with a network of capillaries radiating out in a stellate fashion. They appear at 3 or 4 years of age and take several years to regress. Definitive therapy consists of applications of fine-needle diathermy cautery to the central arteriole.

Type 3 (juvenile capillary haemangiomas) are the only type of haemangioma in which spontaneous resolution occurs. *Strawberry marks* (type 3A) are pale halos of skin surrounding radiatory telangiectasias. Because spontaneous resolution is the rule, observation and reassurance are sufficient. *Strawberry capillary haemangiomas* (Figure 13.1) (type 3B) are the most common type. They are present at birth or appear as tiny red spots in the first few days of life. The lesions are bright red or purple in colour with well defined margins, lobulated, and blanche with pressure. Spontaneous regression occurs in most cases. *Capillary cavernous haemangiomas* (Figure 13.2) (type 3C) are poorly defined haemangiomas involving cutaneous vessels and occasionally larger venous sinusoids. They are easily reduced by digital pressure. Spontaneous regression usually takes place but is never complete. Other therapeutic options are dealt with in the section on treatment.

Type 4 (arteriovenous fistulae) are found almost exclusively in adults, and have a predilection for the lips and perioral skin.

Type 5 (cirsoid angioma) is primarily a venous haemangioma and is uncommon. Surgical excision is the preferred treatment.

Haemangiomas at special sites

Head and neck

Haemangiomas have a predilection towards the head and neck region (Figures 13.3 and 13.4), with 38%–60% occurring in the head and neck region[4,6,22] although this is only 14% of the total body surface area.

Parotid haemangiomas

Haemangiomas are the most common tumour in the parotid region. They account for 50% of all parotid tumours in infants, compared with 2% in adults[23]. Compression therapy has been advocated as an alternative to conservative management[24].

Orbital haemangiomas

These occur in approximately one in 200 live births[22]. Upper lid haemangiomas can cause occlusion or refractive amblyopia[25]. The incidences of amblyopia and anisometropia were 43% and 68%, respectively, in one reported series[26]. Intralesional steroid injections have been successfully used in such cases[27], but eyelid necrosis[25] and depigmentation[22] can complicate such therapy.

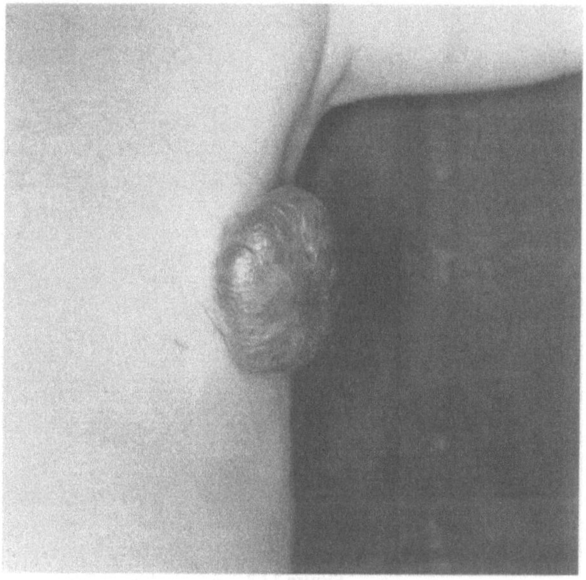

Figure 13.1 A typical strawberry capillary haemangioma.

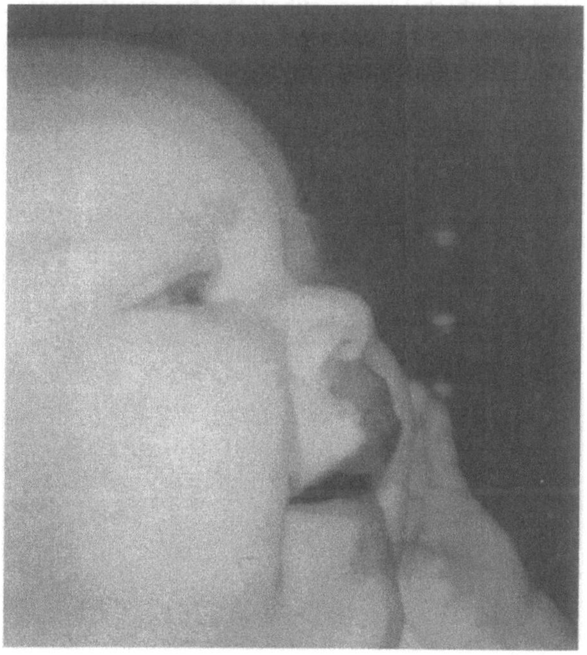

Figure 13.2 Haemangioma of the upper lip.

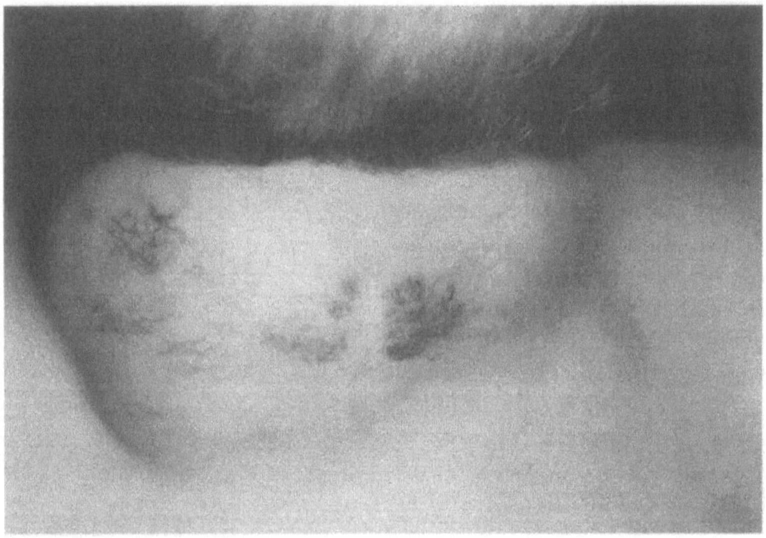

Figure 13.3 A large haemangioma in the back of the neck in a 3-week-old infant.

Laryngeal haemangiomas

These are the most common visceral haemangiomas. Among all the clinical manifestations of haemangiomas, airway obstruction secondary to a subglottic haemangioma is the most life-threatening symptom. The true incidence of subglottic haemangioma is not known. Hollinger and Brown described 846 cases of congenital laryngeal anomalies, of which 13 were subglottic haemangiomas[28]. Symptoms are usually present at birth; however, 85%–90% of affected children develop symptoms within the first 3 months of life. Some 50% of infants with subglottic haemangiomas will have associated cutaneous haemangiomas[29]. Confirmation of diagnosis usually requires laryngoscopy and bronchoscopy, and most symptomatic cases will need tracheostomy. Intralesional steroid injection has been used successfully[30].

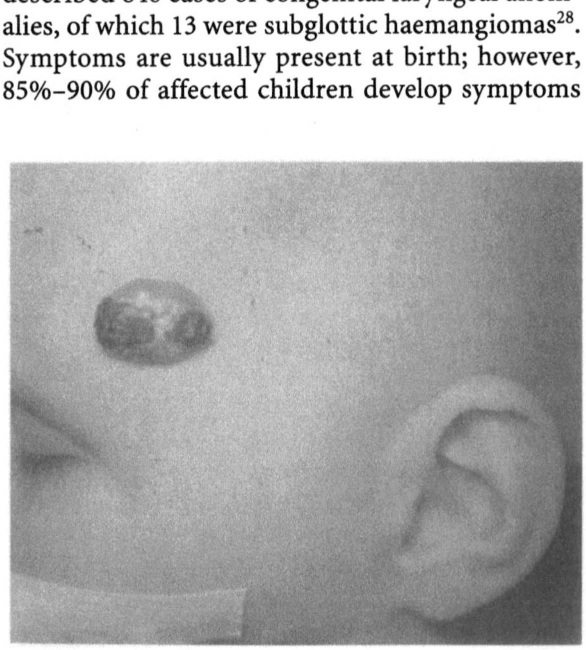

Figure 13.4 Haemangioma of the face needing surgical excision because of recurrent bleeding.

Intracranial haemangiomas

Cutaneous haemangiomas may have associated intracranial angiomatous malformation and arteriovenous malformations of the great vein of Galen[8]. In the newborn, such cases present with congestive cardiac failure, whereas in older children the presenting symptoms may include headache, hydrocephalus, focal neurological signs or subarachnoid haemorrhage[6]. An unusual case of von Hippel–Lindau disease characterized by almost total replacement of the spinal cord and medulla by capillary haemangioblastoma has been reported[31].

Thoracic haemangiomas

Intrathoracic haemangiomas are rare and the symptoms, when present, are unusual. One case presented with pulmonary hypertension[32], others as pulmonary pseudocyst[33] or respiratory distress and hyperinflation of one lung[34].

Hepatic haemangiomas

Haemangioma of the liver usually presents with hepatomegaly and congestive cardiac failure[35]. The greatest risk is in the first 6 months of life when, treated medically alone, the congestive cardiac failure has a mortality rate of around 70%. Early identification of these lesions is important; scintigraphy using ^{99}Tc-labelled red cells offers an accurate method of identification of these lesions[36]. Multinodular haemangiomatosis of the liver is a clinical syndrome, the features of which are hepatomegaly, congestive cardiac failure and cutaneous haemangioma. It may cause thrombocytopenia and consumptive coagulopathy[6].

Gastrointestinal haemangiomas

These are rare lesions. They may present as part of the blue rubber-bleb naevus syndrome[37] or with massive intestinal bleeding from isolated colonic haemangioma[38,39] (Figure 13.5).

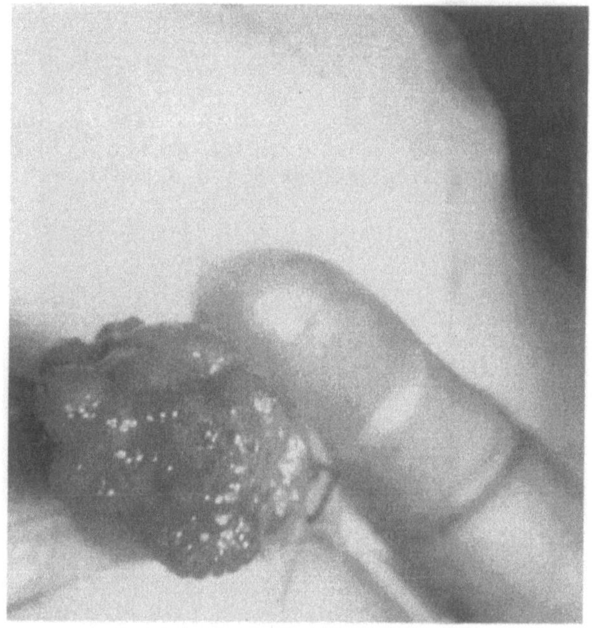

Figure 13.5 Surgical specimen of a colonic haemangioma from an infant who presented with massive bleeding.

Umbilical and placental haemangiomas

These are extremely rare[40]. Umbilical haemangiomas may be diagnosed by antenatal ultrasonography[35,41], and if undetected it can present with severe bleeding at birth[42]. Fetal anaemia from fetomaternal transfusion caused by placental haemangioma is a very unusual presentation[43].

Complications of haemangiomas

The minor complications of haemangiomas are ulceration, infection and bleeding of cutaneous haemangiomas (Figure 13.6). Perineal haemangiomas are more likely to develop these complications; treatment by conservative measures alone is difficult and is associated with high morbidity rates. Laser therapy has been used successfully in such cases[44]. Occasionally, bleeding into a haemangioma can be severe, necessitating surgery (Figure 13.7).

The life-threatening complications of haemangiomas are the development of congestive cardiac

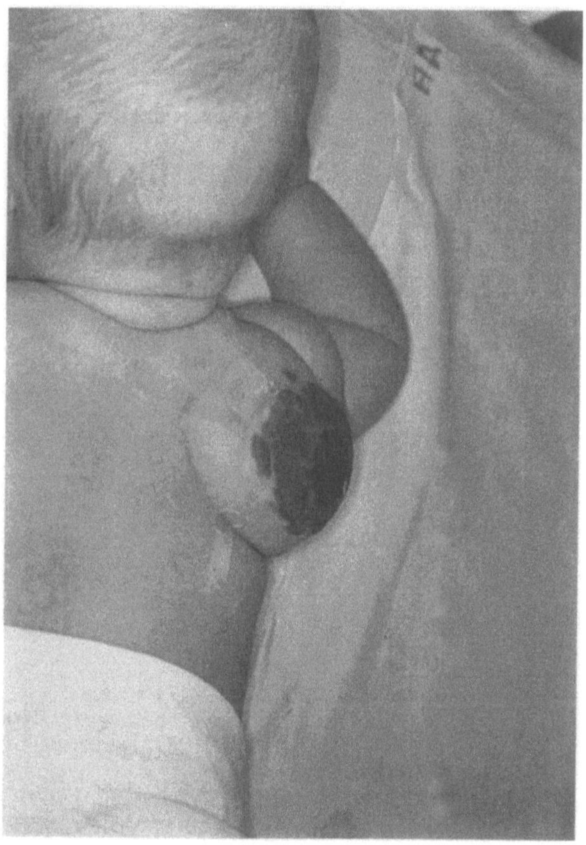

Figure 13.6 Haemangioma over the right scapula with central ulceration, infection and bleeding.

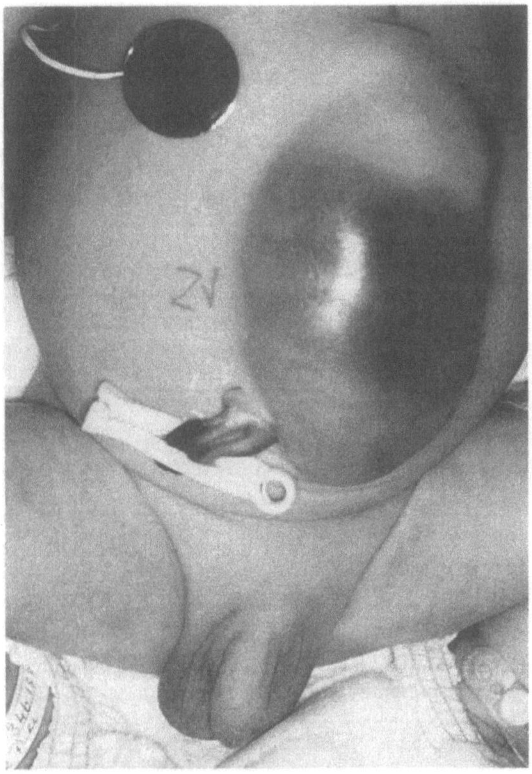

Figure 13.7 Haemangioma of the abdominal wall in a 1-day-old infant. The baby developed haemorrhage into the haemangioma during delivery. At exploration, the haemangioma involved skin, abdominal muscles and omentum.

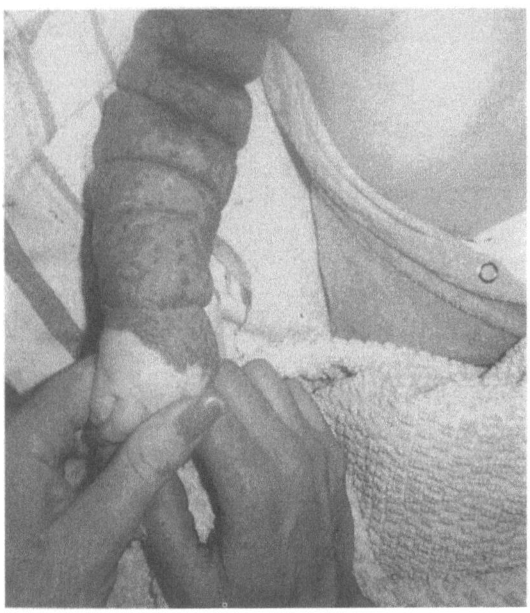

Figure 13.8 This infant with a large haemangioma of the right arm developed congestive cardiac failure.

failure and Kasabach–Merritt syndrome. Congestive cardiac failure is a complication of hepatic haemangiomas[2,36] and giant cutaneous haemangiomas[6,45,46] (Figure 13.8). It is caused by arteriovenous shunting leading to a high-output state. The mortality rate in congestive cardiac failure from medical treatment alone is high[2], therefore other therapeutic measures designed to treat the haemangioma aggressively should be instituted at the earliest opportunity.

Kasabach–Merritt syndrome

This syndrome, first described by Kasabach and Merritt[47] in 1940, features platelet trapping by haemangiomas, causing thrombocytopenia and consumptive coagulopathy. The sequestration of platelets in the haemangiomas in such cases has been confirmed by investigations demonstrating increased uptake of platelets tagged with chromium-51 within the haemangioma. The exact trigger mechanism that initiates platelet trapping is not fully understood[16]. Two-thirds of cases present in the first 3 months of life during active growth of the lesion; only 12% occur after 1 year of age[48]. The mortality rate is high, about 40%. Initial treatment consists of heparin, aspirin, fresh blood, platelet transfusion and steroids. If the infant becomes stable on this regimen, surgical excision should be attempted. If surgery is not feasible, long-term treatment with steroids, compression therapy or embolization of the feeder vessels should be attempted[45].

Syndromes associated with haemangioma

There are a number of syndromes involving various combinations of cutaneous and visceral haemangiomas.

Benign neonatal haemangiomatosis (BNH)

In this syndrome there are multiple skin haemangiomas without visceral involvement. They usually

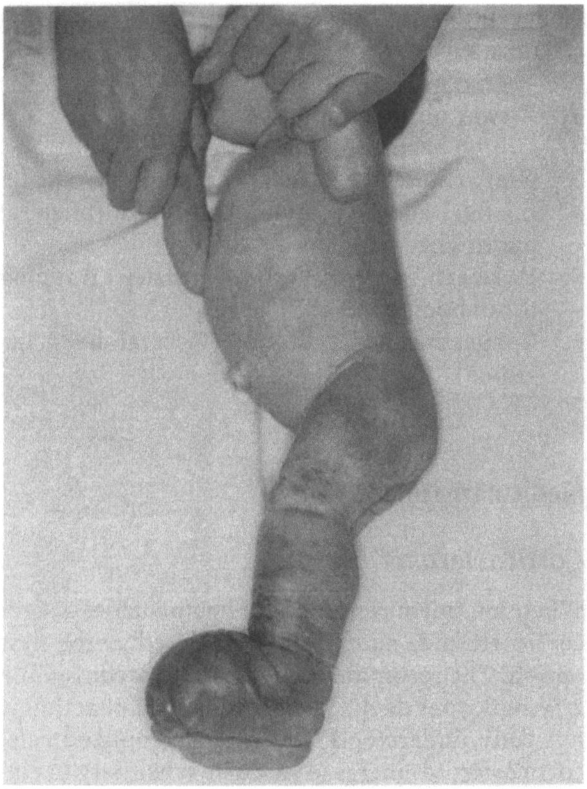

Figure 13.9 A newborn with Klippel–Trenaunay–Weber syndrome.

follow a benign course[10], but in some cases the skin lesions do not regress and new ones appear[49].

Diffuse neonatal haemangiomatosis

This is a rare entity in which cutaneous and visceral haemangiomas coexist[10,50]. The outlook may be improved by early diagnosis; therefore, any infant presenting with multiple skin haemangiomas should be investigated for visceral involvement[51]. Magnetic resonance imaging can be very useful in such cases[52]. Unusual presentation with infantile spasms has been reported[53]. High-dose corticosteroids can be effective in treatment[49], and interferon α_{2a} has been successfully used[54].

Sturge–Weber syndrome

This syndrome consists of port-wine-type malformations distributed along the ophthalmic division of the trigeminal nerve and haemangiomas of the meninges and choroid plexus, on one side of the body. Cortical damage, convulsions, mental defects, hemiparesis and hemianosmia affecting the contralateral side of the body may occur.

Blue rubber-bleb naevus syndrome

This is an autosomal dominant syndrome featuring multiple cutaneous haemangiomas with similar lesions in the gastrointestinal tract[15,37].

Von Hippel–Lindau syndrome

Angiomatous changes in the retina and cerebellum in association with haemangiomas, cysts or tumours of other organs are the features of this syndrome[55].

Klippel–Trenaunay–Weber syndrome

This syndrome is associated with port-wine stain, varicose veins, arteriovenous fistula and limb hypertrophy (Figure 13.9).

Investigations

Most haemangiomas are diagnosed clinically and do not warrant additional investigations. When visceral haemangiomas are suspected, computed axial tomography[56], magnetic resonance imaging[52] and lung scintigraphy[32] are useful in making a diagnosis. But ultrasonography is the first line of investigation in the search for visceral haemangiomas; with its increasing use in the antenatal period haemangiomas are diagnosed antenatally[40,41,46]. Hepatic haemangiomas have been accurately diagnosed using scintigraphy with ^{99}Tc-labelled red cells[36], which is also helpful in evaluating vascularization and planning therapy. It may be used selectively for detection and follow-up of maxillofacial haemangioma[57]. Indium platelet scintigraphy has been successfully used to demonstrate platelet trapping in Kasabach–Merritt syndrome[58]. Complications in haemangiomas like

Kasabach–Merritt syndrome and congestive cardiac failure will need additional appropriate investigation.

Management of haemangioma

Four factors need to be considered in the management of haemangiomas and vascular malformations: the natural history of the lesion, the site, the likelihood of developing function-threatening or life-threatening complications, and the therapeutic options available.

Natural history of haemangioma

The tendency of haemangiomas to regress spontaneously was first emphasized by Lister[59] in 1938. Haemangiomas present at birth show a proliferative phase in the first 6–9 months, followed by a stable period of 6–12 months. Slow spontaneous involution takes place in some cases, starting at the centre, and this is completed by 1–7 years[2,19]. Involution takes place in all cases, and is perfect in 50% of patients, but residual skin changes are left in 25%. The remaining 25% undergo an alarming course, invading skin and modifying bone growth by their mass effect. They also regress; however, various skin changes and functional impairment remain, depending on the site of the lesion.

Treatment

The majority of haemangiomas completely resolve or result in such a minor degree of residual skin irregularity that no intervention is required. Parents should be reassured and the natural history of such lesions should be explained to them. In 10%–20% of cases that develop function-threatening complications and 3%–5% of cases that go on to develop life-threatening complication, this approach should be abandoned. Intervention is indicated in the following circumstances[1]:

1. Airway obstruction
2. Orbital haemangioma
3. Oral and digestive tract haemangioma
4. Bilateral auditory canal obstruction (bilateral parotid haemangioma)
5. Kasabach–Merritt syndrome (platelet trapping thrombocytopenia)
6. Congestive heart failure (visceral haemangioma)

Medical treatment

Corticosteroids

When treatment is needed for haemangiomas, oral corticosteroids should be considered as the first option. The recommended dosage is prednisolone 2–3 mg/kg per day[19]. Their mechanism of action is not fully understood. In adrenalectomized rats, corticosteroids increase vascular sensitivity to circulating vasoconstrictors[15]. They may also have an action on precapillary sphincters, causing constriction[19]. Recent experiments have shown that there are oestradiol receptors in haemangioma tissues. Steroids may occupy these sites and block the uptake of oestradiol, which may have a supporting function in haemangiomas[20]. Growing strawberry haemangiomas may be more responsive than stable haemangiomas. Therapy should be continued for 6–8 weeks; response rates have been quoted as 45%–90%[2,19]. It may be necessary to repeat the course several times in the event of rebound growth. When used in infants with alarming haemangiomas of infancy, 30% of cases had excellent results, 30% were total failures and 40% had equivocal results[7]. All the precautions usual with steroid therapy should be adhered to; side-effects are usually reversible with cessation of treatment, but early immunological damage has been reported[60].

Antifibrinolytic agents

These are not commonly used in treating haemangiomas. Regression in cavernous haemangiomas is thought to be related to local clot formation and subsequent fibrosis. Ongoing fibrinolysis may inhibit this natural resolution, and therefore administration of an antifibrinolytic should prevent fibrinolysis and promote resolution. There have been several reports of improvement in haemangioma with antifibrinolytic therapy[19,58]. Ideally, these agents (which include ε-aminocaproic acid and transexamic acid) should be used only in the presence of elevated fibrinogen degradation products in blood.

Interferon α

Although still used in only a few centres, interferon α has shown to inhibit growth of massive haemangiomas[2,61]. This may be related to its effect on endogenous cortisol secretion. Based on diurnal cortisol activity, interferon α is given at 3 million u/m^2 per day intravenously in the evenings during a 4–9 week period. Interferon α_{2a} has been successfully used to produce regression of life-threatening corticosteroid-resistant haemangiomas of infancy[62].

New drugs

New angio-inhibiting steroids have been developed, and their results in clinical trials are expected in the near future[63].

Intralesional steroid therapy

Long-acting steroids (dexamethasone and triamcinolone) have been effective as topical injections in haemangioma[10]. Short general anaesthesia is needed because multiple punctures are painful. The response is good in 50% of cases. It has been used in periorbital haemangiomas with success, but eyelid depigmentation[22], necrosis[25] and subcutaneous fat atrophy[64] have been reported when steroids are used in the upper eyelid.

Therapeutic embolization

Superselective angiography and embolization has been used as a definitive or preoperative adjunct in the treatment of cutaneous and deep haemangiomas in adults. Their use in children has been delayed because of the increased technical challenge created by the small vessels and by contrast and fluid limitations, but success in infants with this form of treatment is increasingly reported, especially in inaccessible lesions and in function- and life-threatening situations[17,65]. Various agents used for embolization include autologous blood clots or muscle, methylacrylate, steel balls and silicone spheres. Their mechanism of action apparently involves formation of thrombi around the embolic material, with propagation into the distal branches of the vessels[4]. Haemangiomas respond dramatically, with arrest of the proliferative phase and shrinking of the mass. Complications when this is used in haemangiomas of the head and neck include backflow of particles into the internal carotid artery leading to cerebrovascular accidents and into branches of the external carotid artery leading to tissue damage and skin necrosis[19]. Death following attempted embolization of arteriovenous malformations of the vein of Galen has been reported[18].

Surgery

Surgery is reserved for the few cutaneous lesions that fail to resolve or for large lesions that threaten function. There can be significant morbidity associated with resection of large lesions, depending on the location and the amount of intraoperative haemorrhage. Surgical options include arterial ligation and resection.

Arterial ligation

Circumferential ligation of afferent and efferent vessels as sole therapy for large lesions has been reported. In one series there was an 86% cure rate when arterial ligation was combined with steroid therapy in complex haemangiomas[2]. The disadvantages of arterial ligation are regrowth of haemangiomas due to development of collaterals and the inability to use the vessels for embolization if necessary[19].

Resection

The difficulty with resection of haemangiomas depends on the site and size of the lesions. The use of hypothermia and cardiopulmonary bypass for large sacral haemangioma[66], low tracheal haemangioma[67] and hepatic haemangioma[68] has been described.

Laser treatment

The increased effectiveness of the laser for the treatment of vascular lesions is due to its ability to destroy cutaneous blood vessels selectively. The degree of selectivity depends on the various laser parameters that are inherent in each type of laser.

Carbon dioxide laser

The carbon dioxide laser produces intense light in the invisible infrared spectrum that is absorbed by water, which makes up 75%–90% of most biological tissue. This water vaporizes at the focal length of the beam. The advantages of a carbon dioxide laser are that it cuts like a knife, seals small vessels and destroys small nerve endings. Scarring is similar to that obtained with conventional surgery, but pain and oedema are less. Carbon dioxide lasers are reported to be successful in the treatment of port-wine stains that fail to respond to argon or continuous-wave dye laser therapy[69].

Argon laser

Successful use of argon lasers in the treatment of port-wine stain and capillary lesions has been a significant development, but the response in children less than 10–12 years of age is poor, with markedly decreased fading and increased incidence of scarring[9]. Argon light has a wavelength of 4880–5145 Å. The haemoglobin pigment is highly absorptive in this range, and argon light is transformed into heat within the erythrocyte to produce vessel thrombosis. Skin appendages are spared and healing takes place much as with a superficial burn[4]. In many centres a "test spot" is performed to assess the response of an individual port-wine stain to argon laser therapy. The laser power that causes whitening of the spot represents the smallest effective laser power, which is used for remainder of the lesion[70]. Apart from their use in port-wine stains, argon lasers are used effectively in ulcerated anogenital haemangiomas in infants[44].

Nd-YAG laser

Nd-YAG lasers have low tissue absorption, permitting deep penetration and coagulation. The volume of radiant energy distribution is 100–1000 times greater than for a carbon dioxide laser of equal spot size. Because of the large treatment volume, one cannot judge the amount of destruction accurately: there is a greater chance of transmural injury to underlying structures. Nd-YAG lasers in combination with interluminal injection of steroid have been used successfully in treatment of periorbital haemangiomas in infants[71].

In a comparative study of the results of treatment with argon and Nd-YAG lasers, argon laser gave good results in small flat lesions, but Nd-YAG lasers were found to be superior in reducing large bulky lesions. On the basis that results of treatment are better in small lesions and because lesions are smaller when infants are only a few weeks old, a plea was made for earlier treatment of haemangiomas in infants[72].

Pulsed dye laser

There are increasing reports of successful treatment of haemangioma with flashlamp-pumped dye laser[73–75]. This method of treatment has been successfully used for treatment of periorbital port-wine stains[76] and for cutaneous haemangiomas[77]. The results are better in younger children and in superficial lesions[78,79]. This is a safe and effective method of treatment with low incidence of scarring and pigmentary alterations[78,79].

External compression

For this type of therapy to be effective, the haemangiomas have to be accessible. Circumferential pressure is desirable, and should be applied 24 h/day over the whole haemangioma. Compliance from the parents is essential[80]. It is speculated that prolonged compression of vessels might cause narrowing of their lumen, which may provoke stasis of blood flow and eventual thrombosis. Their successful use in parotid haemangiomas have been reported[81]. The advantage is that it is safe, simple and inexpensive.

Radiotherapy

Radiotherapy is no longer advocated in the treatment of haemangiomas because of the risk of development of malignancy in the long term. In a follow-up study of a cohort of 14 647 individuals less than 18 months old irradiated for skin haemangioma between 1920 and 1959, there were 56 breast cancers, 14 thyroid cancers, 16 brain tumours and eight tumours of bone and soft tissues. A statistically significant positive dose-response relationship was found in thyroid cancer and in tumours of bone and soft tissues. For breast cancer and brain tumours, no significant dose-response relationship could be found[82].

References

1. Low DW (1994) Haemangiomas and vascular malformations. Semin Pediatr Surg 3: 40–61.
2. Enjolras O, Riche MC, Merland JJ et al. (1990) Management of alarming hemangiomas in infancy: a review of 25 cases. Pediatrics 85: 491–498.
3. Weber TR, Connors RH, Tracy TF et al. (1990) Complex hemangiomas in infants and children. Individualized management in 22 cases. Arch Surg 125: 1017–1021.
4. Fonkalsrud EW (1980) Malformations of the lymphatic system and hemangiomas. In: Holder TM, Ashworth KW, eds. Pediatric surgery. WB Saunders, Philadelphia, pp 1054–1060.
5. Handley GH (1987) Hemangiomas of the head and neck. Ear Nose Throat 66: 486–490.
6. Brown DA, Smith JD (1987) Late complications of congenital hemangioma of the tongue. Head Neck Surg 9: 299–304.
7. Rosen S, Smaller BR (1987) Port-wine stains: a new hypothesis. J Am Acad Dermatol 17: 164–166.
8. Benninson J, Hurley JP (1988) Hemolymphangioma in a neonate - a therapeutic problem - case history. Angiology 39: 1043–1047.
9. Garfinkle TJ, Handlen SD (1980) Hemangiomas of the head and neck in children - a guide to management. J Otolaryngol 9: 439–450.
10. Sweetser TH (1921) Hemangioma of the larynx. Laryngoscopy 31: 797–806.
11. Bartlett JA, Riding KH, Salkfeld LJ et al. (1988) Management of hemangiomas of the head and neck in children. J Otolaryngol 17: 111–120.
12. Raffensperger JG (1990) Hemangiomas and vascular malformations. In: Raffensperger JG, ed. Swenson's pediatric surgery. Appleton and Lange, pp 157–166.
13. Lofland GK, Filston HC (1987) Giant hemangioma anaerated with axillary anteriovenous fistula causing congestive heart failure in the newborn infant. J Pediatr Surg 22: 458–460.
14. Williams HB (1980) Vascular neoplasms. Clin Pediatr Surg 7: 397–411.
15. Apfelberg DB, Smith T, White J (1989) Preliminary study of the vascular dynamics of port wine stain hemangioma with therapeutic implications for argon laser treatment. Plast Reconstr Surg 83: 820–823.
16. Mulliken JB (1991) A plea for biological approach to hemangioma. Arch Dermatol 127: 243–244.
17. Mulliken JB, Glowacki J (1982) Hemangiomas and vascular malformations in infants and children: a classification based on endothelial characteristics. Plast Reconstr Surg 69: 412–420.
18. Robinson D, Segal M, Halperin N et al. (1992) Neuropeptidergic innervation of intramuscular haemangiomas. Exp Mol Pathol 56: 186–196.
19. Burrows PE, Lasjaunias PL, Ter Brugge KG et al. (1987) Urgent and emergent embolization of lesions of head and neck in children: indications and results. Pediatrics 80: 386–394.
20. Sasaki GH, Pang CY, Wottliff JL (1984) Pathogenesis and treatment of infant skin strawberry hemangiomas: clinical and in vitro studies of hormonal effects. Plast Reconstr Surg 73: 359–367.
21. Edgerton MJ (1976) Treatment of hemangiomas: with special reference to the role of steroid therapy. Ann Surg 183: 517–532.
22. Cogen MS, Elsas FJ (1989) Eyelid depigmentation following corticosteroid injection for infantile ocular adnexal hemangioma. J Pediatr Ophthalmol Strabismus 26: 35–38.
23. George CD, Ng YY, Hull-Crags MA et al. (1991) Parotid hemangioma in infants: MR imaging at 1.5T. Pediatr Radiol 21: 483–485.
24. Totsuka Y, Fukuda H, Tomitu K (1988) Compression therapy for parotid hemangioma in infants. A report of 3 cases. J Craniomaxillofac Surg 16: 366–370.
25. Sutula FC, Glover AT (1987) Eyelid necrosis following intralesional corticosteroid injection for capillary hemangioma. Ophthalmic Surg 18: 103–105.
26. Boyd MZ, Callin JR (1991) Capillary hemangiomas: an approach to their management. Br J Ophthalmol 53: 298–300.
27 Mensell AJ, Willshaw HF (1991) Normalisation of refractive error after steroid injection for adnexal hemangiomas. Br J Ophthalmol 75: 301–305.
28. Hollinger PH, Brown WT (1967) Congenital webs, cysts, laryngoceles and other anomalies of the larynx. Ann Otol Rhinol Laryngol 26: 744–752.
29. Litter ER (1963) Asphyxia due to hemangioma of the trachea. Thorac Cardiovasc Surg 45: 552–553.
30. Meeuwi SJ, Bos CE, Hoeve LJ et al. (1990) Subglottic hemangiomas in infants: treatment with intralesional corticosteroid injection and intubation. Int J Pediatr Otorolaryngol 19: 145–150.
31. Rojiani AM, Elwott K, Dorovini-Zig K (1991) Extensive replacement of spinal cord and brainstem by hemangioblastoma in a case of Von Hippel - Lindau disease. Clin Neuropathol 10: 297–302.
32. Rush C, Langleben D, Schlesinger RD et al. (1991) Lung scintigraphy in pulmonary capillary hemangiomatosis. A rare disorder causing pulmonary hypertension. Clin Nucl Med 16: 913–917.
33. Bowyer JJ, Sheppard M (1990) Capillary hemangioma presenting as lung pseudocyst. Arch Dis Child 65: 1162–1164.
34. Paul KP, Bonner C, Muller KM et al. (1991) Capillary hemangioma of the right main bronchus treated by sleeve resection in infancy. Am Rev Resp Dis 143: 867–869.
35. Hobbs KE (1990) Hepatic hemangiomas. World J Surg 14: 468–471.
36. Miller JH (1987) Technetium-99M-labelled red blood cells in the evaluation of hemangiomas of the liver in infants and children. J Nucl Med 28: 1412–1418.
37. Hofhuis WJ, Orange A, Bouquet J et al. (1990) Blue rubber-bleb naevus syndrome: report of a case with consumption coagulopathy complicated by manifest thrombosis. Eur J Pediatr 149: 526–528.
38. Levgliton DM, Benghanem T, Mantogne JP et al. (1990) A case of rectal bleeding in infancy. Australas Radiol 34: 89–90.
39. Masterson J, Wood D, Lau G et al. (1991) Isolated colonic hemangioma in a child. Can Assoc Radiol J 42: 431–434.
40. Pollack MS, Bound LM (1989) Hemangioma of the umbilical cord. J Ultrasound Med 8: 163–166.
41. Mishriki YY, Vanyshelbaum Y, Epstein W et al. (1983)

Hemangioma of the umbilical cord. Pediatrt Pathol 7: 43–49.
42. Dombrowski MP, Budev H, Walfe HM et al. (1987) Fetal hemorrhage from umbilical cord hemangioma. Obstet Gynecol 70: 439–552.
43. Fumera-Martin AM, Graubad Z, Holloway GA et al. (1990) Placental hemangioma associated with acute fetal anemia in labour. Acta Med Port 3: 187–189.
44. Achauer BM, Vander Kam VM (1991) Ulcerated anogenital hemangioma of infancy. Plast Reconstr Surg 87: 861–866.
45. Cunrie BG, Schell D, Bowring AC (1991) Giant hemangioma of the arm associated with cardiac failure and the Kasabach–Merritt syndrome in a neonate. J Pediatr Surg 26: 734–737.
46. Malcom GP, Nicolaides K, Howard ER (1990) Giant cutaneous hemangioma with heart failure in a neonate: successful surgical treatment. Pediatr Surg Int 5: 71–73.
47. Kasabach H, Merritt K (1940) Capillary hemangioma with extensive purpura: report of a case. Am J Dis Child 59: 1063.
48. Martins A (1970) Hemangioma and thrombocytopenia. J Pediatr Surg 5: 641.
49. Stenninger E, Schollin J (1993) Diffuse neonatal hemangiomatosis in a newborn child. Acta Paediatr 82, 102–104.
50. Gozal D, Saad N, Bader D et al. (1990) Diffuse neonatal hemangiomata: successful management with high dose corticosteroids. Eur J Pediatr 149: 321–324.
51. Byard RW, Burrows PE, Izakawa T et al. (1991) Diffuse infantile hemangiomatosis: clinicopathological features and management problems in five fatal cases. Eur J Pediatr 150: 224–227.
52. Montgomery SP, Guillot AD, Burth RA (1990) MRI of disseminated neonatal hemangiomata: a case report. Pediatr Radiol 20: 204–205.
53. McShane MA, Finn JD, Hall-Craggs MA (1990) Neonatal hemangiomata presenting as infantile spasms. Neuropediatrics 21: 211–212.
54. Spiller JC, Sharma V, Woods GM et al. (1992) Diffuse neonatal haemangiomatosis treated successfully with interferon α_{2a}. J Am Acad Dermatol 27: 102–104.
55. Christofenson LA, Gustofson NB, Peterson AG (1961) Von-Hippel–Lindau's disease. JAMA 178: 280.
56. Nakasu S, Yoshida M, Nakajima M et al. (1991) Cystic carvernous angioma in an infant. J Comput Assist Tomogr 15: 163–165.
57. Fiore F, Califano L, Cortese A, Zupi A (1993) Haemangioma of the maxillofacial area. Usefulness of ^{99m}Tc-labelled red cell scintigraphy. Nucl Med Commun 14: 378–383.
58. Shulkin BL, Arqenta LC, Cho KJ (1990) Kasabach–Merritt syndrome: treatment with ε-amino caproic acid and assessment by indium III platelet scintigraphy. J Pediatr 117: 746–749.
59. Lister WA (1938) Natural history of strawberry naevi. Lancet i: 1429–1434.
60. Gunn T, Reece ER, Metrukos K et al. (1981) Depressed T cells following neonatal steroid treatment. Pediatrics 67: 61–67.
61. White CW, Walfe SJ, Koras DN (1991) Treatment of childhood angiomatous disease with recombinant interferon α-24. J Pediatr 118: 59–66.
62. Ezekowitz RA, Mulliken JB, Folkman J (1992) Interferon α_{2a} therapy for life-threatening hemangiomas of infancy. N Engl J Med 326: 1456–1463.
63. Ingben D, Fujitu T, Kishimoto S et al. (1990) Synthetic analogues of fumagillin that inhibit angiogenesis and suppress tumour growth. Nature 348: 555–557.
64. Townsend LM, Buckley EG (1990) Linear subcutaneous fat atrophy after a single corticosteroid injection for ocular adnexal hemangioma. Am J Ophthalmol 109: 102–103.
65. Sato Y, Freg EE, Kisker CT et al. (1987) Embolization therapy in the management of infantile hemangioma with Kasabach–Merritt syndrome. Pediatr Radiol 17: 503–504.
66. Milligan NS, Edwards JC, Monro JL et al. (1988) Excision of giant hemangioma in the newborn using hypothermia and cardiopulmonary bypass. Anesthesia 40: 875–878.
67. Franks R, Rothera M (1990) Cardiopulmonary bypass for resection in low tracheal hemangioma. Arch Dis Child 65: 680–682.
68. Ranse RD, Ashcraft KW, Haeden TM et al. (1988) Hepatic hemangioma: resection using hypothermic circulatory arrest in the newborn. J Pediatr Surg 23: 924–926.
69. Lannigan SW, Cotterie JA (1990) The treatment of port wine stain with carbondioxide laser. Br J Dermatol 123: 229–235.
70. Carruth JAS, Shakespeare P (1986) Towards ideal treatment for the port wine stain with the argon laser: better prediction and an "optimal" technique. Lasers Surg Med 6: 2–4.
71. Apfelberg DB, Maser MR, White DN et al. (1990) Benefits of contact and non contact YAG laser for periorbital hemangiomas. Ann Plasti Surg 24: 397–408.
72. Achaeur BM, Victoria M, Vander Kam RN (1989) Capillary hemangioma (strawberry mark) of infancy: comparison of argon and ND:YAG laser treatment. Plast Reconstr Surg 84: 60–70.
73. Garden JM, Polla LL, Tan OT (1988) The treatment of port wine stains by the pulsed dye laser. Arch Dermatol 124: 889-896.
74. Reyes BA, Geronemus R (1990) Treatment of port wine stain during childhood with the flash lamp - pumped pulsed dye laser. J Am Acad Dermatol 23: 1142–1148.
75. Achauer BM, Vander Kam VM, Miller SR (1990) Clinical experience with the pulsed-dye laser in the treatment of capillary malformations (port wine stain): a preliminary report. Ann Plast Surg 25: 344–352.
76. Holy A, Geronemus RG (1992) Treatment of periorbital port wine stains with the flashlamp-pumped dye laser. Arch Ophthalmol 110: 793–797.
77. Garden JM, Bakus AD, Paller AS (1992) Treatment of cutaneous hemangiomas with flashlamp-pumped dye laser. Prospective analysis. J Pediatr 120: 555–560.
78. Strauss RP, Resnicke SD (1993) Pulse dye laser therapy for port wine stains in children: psychosocial and ethical issues. J Pediatr 122: 505–510.
79. Goldman MP, Fitzpatrick RE, Ruiz-Esparza J (1993) Treatment of port wine stains (capillary malformation) with the flashlamp-pumped pulsed dye laser. 122: 71–77.
80. Stingel S (1987) Giant hemangioma: treatment with intermittent pneumatic compression. J Pediatr Surg 1: 7–10.
81. Totsuka Y, Fukuda H, Tomita K (1988) Compression therapy for parotid haemangioma in infants: a report of three cases. J Craniomaxillofac Surg 16: 366–370.
82. Furst CJ, Lundell M, Holm LE (1990) Tumours after radiotherapy for skin hemangioma in childhood. A case control study. Acta Oncol 29: 557–562.

Rare Tumours

Prem Puri and Rajendra Surana

14

Introduction

The commonly occurring neoplasms in newborn infants have been discussed in the preceding chapters. Some of the less common tumours are dealt with in this chapter. The rare occurrence of these tumours necessitates treatment modifications derived from management protocols for children and adults. Although rare, these tumours are encountered in paediatric surgical oncology practice from time to time.

Head and neck

Tumours of the head and neck form a heterogeneous group of neoplasms originating from different tissues. The haemangiomas and cystic hygromas are the most common lesions and are discussed in Chapters 13 and 11. Other tumours include dermoid cysts, salivary gland tumours and tumours of the oral cavity.

Diagnosis of these tumours depends largely on history and physical examination. Antenatal diagnosis helps in mobilizing resources to manage the emergency situation more effectively, decreasing the avoidable mortality rate[1,2]. After birth, ancillary studies such as plain radiography, ultrasonography, computed tomography (CT) and angiography are useful aids in diagnosis.

Subcutaneous haemangiomas, congenital goitre and ectopic thyroid may be treated conservatively. The remainder of the lesions require early surgery to avoid complications of infection[3], airway obstruction and nutritional compromise, and risk of malignant transformation[4].

Dermoid cysts

These are true congenital neoplasms and are composed of ectoderm and mesoderm[4]. Although congenital, they may not present until later in life. The common sites of occurrence are the external angular process, base of the nose, periauricular region, submental region, midline and tongue. Radiography shows a bony depression or defect. Intracranial extensions may be communicated by a narrow neck. They may be cystic or have an adipose tissue matrix, and usually contain epidermal appendages. These are inclusion cysts. Large dermoid cysts of the submental area and floor of the mouth are potentially life-threatening. If intracranial extension is suspected, CT is a useful aid. Dermoid cysts causing breathing or feeding difficulties should be excised as soon as possible. If the cysts are asymptomatic, surgery may be delayed until 6 months of age. Cysts with intracranial extension require craniotomy for complete removal.

Salivary gland tumours

These are quite uncommon in neonates and are usually benign, the majority being proliferations suggesting a tumorous arrest of maturation of salivary gland analgae[5]. Other common benign lesions include lymphangioma haemangioma and occasionally monomorphic pleomorphic adenoma[6,7]. Malignant forms include carcinoma and rhabdomyosarcoma[8,9]. Some epithelial tumours present in the perinatal period and are termed "embryomas" or "sialoblastomas". A common site of occurrence is the parotid gland. Histologically they may have hamartomatous or pleomorphic adenoma-like appearance. Approximately 25% are malignant.

They usually occur in major salivary glands, especially parotid glands. Females are more commonly affected than males. Ultrasonography is a simple non-invasive procedure that allows correct identification of benign salivary lesions in over 80% of cases. However, it has limitations such as failure to visualize the entire parotid gland and relations with the nerve plexus, and false-negative errors for malignancy of small encapsulated tumours[9]. CT with or without sialography and fine-needle aspiration biopsy will usually confirm the diagnosis.

For patients with haemangioma no treatment is necessary, as involution is the rule. Surgical removal of the tumour is recommended for benign lesions. Malignant tumours require superficial parotidectomy with facial nerve preservation. Rhabdomyosarcoma is best managed by biopsy, followed by chemotherapy and radiotherapy. The outlook for congenital malignant tumours is excellent[11].

Oral cavity

Although rare in the newborn, neoplasms can arise from the lips, jaws, cheek, palate, tongue and oropharynx. When they occur, they are usually benign. Malignant tumours are rare and often sarcomatous[12].

Lips

These are very rarely involved. Haemangiopericytoma of the lip has been reported[13].

Jaw

Epignathus is any kind of growth arising from the upper jaw that projects through the mouth. These can be polyps, hamartomas, dermoid cysts or teratomas. They are believed to arise from embryonal tissue rests in the region of Rathke's pouch[14]. The primary concern in management is to keep the airway patent. Surgical removal is usually not difficult and is curative.

Epulis means a swelling from the alveolus, but these usually arise from the overlying tissue, probably the odontogenic epithelium. They involve the maxilla more often than the mandible, and occasionally ridges of them both[15]. Clinically, they appear as smooth-surfaced pedunculated tumours, the size of which varies from a few millimetres to a few centimetres[16]. Pathologically, they are covered with squamous epithelium packed with vascular connective tissue in which many large polyhedral cells with granular cytoplasm and few spindle cells are seen[17]. Females are more commonly affected than males[15]. Lack et al.[18] have differentiated congenital gingival granular cell tumour from epulis by electron microscopic studies. All these tumours either cause difficulties in breathing and sucking or are obvious at inspection.

Treatment is surgical excision. There are no long-term complications, with normal tooth eruption and development[19].

Benign lesions of the tongue include papilloma, lipoma[20], dermoid cyst and haemangioma. Malignant tumours are exceedingly rare in the newborn. Carcinoma[21], fibrosarcoma[22], botryoid sarcoma[12] and malignant rhabdoid tumour of the tongue[23] have been reported in newborn children.

Cheek and oral cavity

Neoplasms of the cheek and oral cavity include solitary or multiple papilloma, haemangioma, lymphangioma, lipoma, neurofibroma and tumours of the minor salivary glands. Rannula is an extravasation cyst of the sublingual glands and appears as a blue cyst, which may form plunging rannula. Treatment is transoral marsupialization of the cyst. Recurrence is uncommon.

Oropharynx and neck

Teratomas arise from the totipotent cells containing all three embryonic layers – ectoderm, mesoderm and endoderm. Oropharyngeal and cervical teratomas constitute less than 5% of the teratomas[24–26], and are usually benign, but malignant tumours have been reported[27].

The usual presentation is a cervical mass that is partly cystic and partly situated close to the region of the thyroid. They are often associated with respiratory difficulties. Malignant lesions have been reported to metastasize to the liver, lung and buttock[27]. Differential diagnosis is between goitre and cystic hygroma. Ultrasonography, CT and magnetic resonance imaging are helpful in delineating the extent of the tumour and the relationship to vital structures. Antenatal diagnosis helps in organizing resources to deal with emergencies. Treatment consists of early complete surgical resection of the tumour and metastatic deposits if any. The usual cause of death is hypoxia and respiratory complications secondary to compression[28]. The mortality rate is decreasing with the advent of prenatal diagnosis. In patients with respiratory distress, tracheostomy may be necessary. The final results, both functional and cosmetic, are usually excellent[29,30].

Sternomastoid tumour is not a neoplasm, but is secondary to endomysial fibrosis. Clinically it becomes apparent at about 10–14 days after birth as an ovoid mass, and usually recedes in 4–6 months. In a few patients it persists, causing torticollis in infancy. At times it can lead to cranial, facial and thoracic asymmetry, oculomotor imbalance and infantile scoliosis. The exact cause is not known. Treatment is usually conservative, with passive manipulations, and parents are advised to place the infant to sleep on each side alternately and to avoid the supine position to prevent plagiocephaly. Surgical division of the middle third of the sternomastoid may be necessary in patients who start to develop hemihypoplasia. After operation, intensive physiotherapy is instituted.

Thyroid and parathyroid tumours are discussed under endocrinological tumours, below.

Gastrointestinal tract

Neoplasms of the gastrointestinal tract are much less common in the newborn and children than in adults[31]. Only about 5% of these tumours are malignant. The clinical presentation is non-specific and diagnosis is often delayed. The common signs and symptoms are feeding difficulties, vomiting, bleeding, mass, intestinal obstruction and occasionally meconium peritonitis[32]. The diagnosis is usually suspected after radiological investigations including plain radiography, ultra-sonography, contrast studies and CT. Endoscopy may be useful occasionally. Treatment is usually surgical.

Oesophagus

Oesophageal tumours are extremely rare in newborn infants. Benign tumours include lipoma, hamartoma, myxofibroma[33] and smooth muscle tumours like leiomyoma[34–36]. Malignant lesions of the oesophagus like carcinoma, melanoma and leukaemic infiltrates have been reported in older children. The signs and symptoms are usually feeding difficulties and non-bilious vomiting. The diagnosis is confirmed by barium swallow and upper endoscopy. Treatment is surgical excision, and resection with or without replacement.

Stomach

Gastric neoplasms are more frequently encountered than oesophageal, but are still rare. Benign tumours include polyps (e.g. in Peutz–Jeghers syndrome or juvenile polyposis[37]), adenoma, carcinoids, leiomyoma and haemangiopericytoma[38].

Gastric teratomas have also been reported in neonates[39–41]. Malignant lymphoma, neuroblastoma and leukaemic infiltrates can involve the stomach. Carcinoma of the stomach has been reported in an infant[42–43]. Leiomyosarcoma and malignant leiomyoblastoma with pulmonary chondrohamartomas have been noted in children[44–46].

The usual signs and symptoms of gastric tumours are vomiting, haematemesis, malaena, respiratory difficulties and abdominal mass. These tumours can be large enough to cause premature labour or dystocia. Immunodeficiency states and ataxia–telangiectasia are associated with increased frequency of adenocarcinoma of the stomach[47].

Radiographs of the abdomen may show calcification in teratoma. Contrast studies are often undertaken. Abdominal ultrasonography and CT with contrast are useful. Endoscopy and biopsies will confirm the diagnosis.

Treatment of gastric neoplasms is primarily surgical: either extirpation of the tumour, or partial or subtotal gastrectomy for benign tumours. Total gastrectomy with or without adjunctive chemotherapy is practised for malignant tumours according to the guidelines established for adults.

Small intestine

Neoplasms of the small intestine are rare in adults and children and much rarer in newborn infants. Benign tumours of the small intestine include adenoma, haemangioma, lymphangioma, leiomyoma and neurofibroma. Juvenile polyps are encountered mainly in the jejunum and are seen in patients with Peutz–Jeghers syndrome[48,49], which is characterized by circumoral and buccal pigmentation. These polyps are hamartomatous lesions. Half of these patients will have a positive family history with autosomal dominant inheritance. Malignant change is rare. These present with gastrointestinal bleeding or intussusception. Excision or resection of the segment of the small bowel is indicated in symptomatic patients. Carcinoids are more common in the appendix but can occur in the ileum and infrequently in the jejunum, Meckel's diverticulum and stomach. These are discussed under appendiceal tumours, below.

The commonest malignant lesions of the small intestine are the non-Hodgkin's lymphoma; other malignant tumours are rare. Leiomyosarcoma and angiosarcoma have been reported in newborn infants[50]. Other lesions include rhabdomyosarcoma and fibrosarcoma, usually involving the duodenum, and have good prognosis following pancreaticoduodenectomy[51,52].

Colon, appendix and anorectum

The commonest tumours of the gastrointestinal tract in children are juvenile polyps, 90% of which occur in the rectum or sigmoid colon[53]. Usual presentation is painless rectal bleeding, infrequently intussusception and, rarely, prolapse of the polyp through the anus. The polyps within the reach of a sigmoidoscope may be easily removed. Treatment of other symptomatic polyps is polypectomy by colonoscopy or surgical colotomy. Asymptomatic polyps can be watched because of their benign clinical course, excellent prognosis and possibility of autoamputation. However, there are other types of polyp which have a dissimilar course.

Familial polyposis coli is an autosomal dominant disorder. Its incidence has been estimated to be around one in 8300 births[54]. It can also affect a child who has no positive family history because of a new mutation, incomplete penetrance in which a generation is skipped, or inadequate evaluation of seemingly unaffected persons[55]. Commonly these are limited to colon and rectum, but occasionally the stomach is involved[56,57]. Although the disease has been seen in early infancy and childhood, it becomes more symptomatic in the late teens. Patients may be asymptomatic and undergoing investigation because of a positive family history, or may present with a history of diarrhoea, rectal bleeding, abdominal pain, tenderness and anaemia. Diagnosis is made by positive family history, rectal examination, proctosigmoidocolonoscopy and barium enema. Once diagnosed patients should be examined carefully every 2 years up to 20 years of age. If no polyps are detected at 20 years, 5 yearly follow-up will suffice until 50 years of age. High levels of cholesterol and low levels of coprostanol and coprostanone in the stools, or cultured fibroblasts showing abnormalities, have been suggested as screening techniques[58,59]. These patients have inherited predisposition of the colonic mucosa to undergo malignant transformation at an early age. If untreated, all these patients will eventually develop malignancy. Treatment is total colectomy at any age if the patient is symptomatic; otherwise surgery should be undertaken between 10 and 15 years of age, as it is unlikely to develop malignancy before then. The Ravitch–Soave type of pull-through ileoproctostomy removes all the colon and rectal mucosa, thus removing the danger of malignancy. Other options involve total proctocolectomy with permanent ileostomy (which has the disadvantage of social inconvenience) or subtotal colectomy with fulguration of rectal polyps and ileoproctostomy (which requires careful follow-up and has a danger of developing malignancy in the rectal mucosa). Whatever the surgical approach, genetic counselling is important.

Gardner's syndrome is a condition of multiple intestinal polyposis with soft tissue and bony abnormalities, namely lipomas, dermoid tumours, leiomyomas and multiple sebacious cysts, and osteomas of the skull and facial bones. This is also an autosomal dominant disorder, with an estimated incidence of one in 14 025 births[60]. The natural history of this syndrome is the same as that of familial polyposis coli, and the treatment strategy is similar.

Diffuse gastrointestinal juvenile polyposis is a non-sex-linked recessive disorder involving the rectum, colon and whole gastrointestinal tract. It is characterized by gastrointestinal bleeding, protein-losing enteropathy, malnutrition, anasarca and severe anaemia. Although histologically benign, clinically it is a fatal condition[61].

Other benign tumours of the large intestine and anorectum include haemangioma, lymphangioma, lipoma, leiomyoma and neurofibroma. Malignancy is rare in the newborn, but leiomyosarcoma has been reported. Local resection has been advocated, with good prognosis[62,63]. Adenocarcinoma of the colon, although common in adults, is rare in infants, but a case of adenocarcinoma in a 9-month-old infant has been described[64].

Appendiceal tumours are extremely rare. Carcinoids arising from Kulchitsky cells are commonly found in the appendix and occasionally in the jejunum, Meckel's diverticulum and stomach. These metastasize to the liver more frequently than appendiceal carcinoids and produce carcinoid syndrome, which includes patchy cyanosis, transient vasodilatation of the skin with flushing attacks, diarrhoea, borborygmi, tachycardia and eventually pulmonary and tricuspid stenosis. This is believed to be secondary to 5-hydroxytryptamine (serotonin) secreted by the tumour. Elevated levels of serotonin in blood and of 5-hydroxyindoleacetic acid in urine are found during the attack. Appendiceal tumours are usually cured by appendicectomy. The remainder need radical operation. In cases with metastasis, excision of local lesions and if feasible partial hepatectomy is undertaken. Chemotherapy may be given for inoperable metastasis but its efficacy is not yet established. Medical measures like use of serotonin antagonists, long-acting antihistamines and α-methyldopa are useful to reduce the frequency and severity of attacks.

Biliary tract

Tumours of the biliary tract are extremely rare. Rhabdomyosarcoma can occur at this site. Choledochal cysts cause obstructive jaundice in the neonatal period, and total excision of the cyst and mucosa-to-mucosa anastomosis by Roux-en-Y choledochojejunostomy is the treatment of choice. Leaving mucosa of the cyst behind is thought to predispose to malignancy[65].

Pancreas

Pancreatic tumours can be exocrine, endocrine or mesenchymal in origin. Benign tumours include islet cell adenoma, which has been reported in neonates[66]. Diffuse islet cell dysplasia is seen in the form of nesidioblastosis. All these patients present with severe neonatal hypoglycaemia with relatively high levels of insulin. Prompt diagnosis and treatment is recommended to prevent mental retardation[67]. Ultrasonography, CT and selective angiography may be useful as adjuncts to diagnosis[68]. Maintenance of glucose levels is vital in the preoperative period. Near-total (95%) pancreatectomy is advocated for nesidioblastosis[67], with good results and no need for medication following surgery. Solitary adenomas can be treated by extirpation of the tumour; partial or subtotal pancreatectomy is undertaken for multiple adenomas.

Mesenchymal tumours like haemangioendothelioma are rare and usually present with obstructive jaundice and platelet consumption coagulopathy. Near-total pancreatectomy is the treatment of choice.

Pancreatoblastomas are infantile carcinomas of the pancreas that behave like benign lesions. They usually arise from the head of the pancreas and are postulated as a developmental anomaly from ventral pancreas that has been isolated due to lack of communication with the duct of Wirsung[69]. Clinically, they usually present with abdominal mass and infrequently with hypoglycaemia and haemorrhage. A strong relationship of these tumours with Beckwith–Wiedemann syndrome has been suggested[70]. The prognosis is excellent with surgical removal of these tumours[69], and they therefore need to be differentiated from carcinoma. Rarely, sarcomas have been reported[71].

Spleen

These tumours are rare. Haemangioma[72,73] and hamartomas have been described in the newborn. Haemangioma can cause thrombocytopenia, haemolytic anaemia and disseminated intravascular coagulation. CT is useful in diagnosis. These patients can be treated with splenectomy with or without autotransplantation. Those who undergo splenectomy will need vaccines and prompt treatment of infection.

Peritoneum

Primary peritoneal tumours are rare. Mesothelioma and leiomyomatosis[74] have been reported, and a case of malignant mesothelioma in a 16-day-old boy is on record[75].

Respiratory system

These are extremely rare with the exception of nasopharyngeal rhabdomyosarcoma, which is discussed in Chapter 7. The rarity of these tumours may be due to less exposure to causal agents such as cigarette smoke and asbestos. The common symptoms are stridor, breathing difficulties and cough. Chest radiography and CT are usually used as diagnostic aids. A careful search should be made for the tumour at another site. Isolated primary lesions and metastatic lesions after the primary tumour has been dealt with are best treated by surgery. Prognosis is variable and depends on the type of tumour.

Nasopharynx

Benign nasopharyngeal tumours in newborns have been reported[76], including hamartoma, simple hairy polyps, dermoid cysts and teratoma. Juvenile angiofibromas are usually encountered in bigger children. The usual symptoms are stridor, and breathing and feeding difficulties. Treatment is surgical excision. Malignant forms include rhabdomyosarcoma and nasopharyngeal carcinoma. Nasopharyngeal carcinoma has been reported in young infants[77,78], and seems to have a genetic predisposition as it is indicated by familial tendency and a predilection for the Chinese race with certain human leucocyte antigens (HLA) types. Association of Epstein–Barr virus is well established. The symptoms and signs are enlarged tender cervical lymph nodes, nasal obstruction, epistaxis, weight loss, severe trismus, earache, headache, aching throat, hearing loss and chronic otitis media. Local, regional and distant metastases are common. Diagnosis is usually established by cervical lymph node and/or nasopharyngeal biopsies. CT of the nasopharynx, lungs and abdomen are required. The World Health Organization has classified these tumours into three histological groups: squamous carcinoma, non-keratinizing carcinoma and undifferentiated carcinoma. Treatment is radiotherapy. Chemotherapy may be required before radiation for bulky tumours or as an adjunct. The disease-free survival rate is 50%–60%.

Larynx

Benign laryngeal tumours include haemangioma, lymphangioma, haemangioendothelioma, papilloma and neurofibroma. Congenital laryngeal papillomatosis may be caused by human papovavirus from the mothers but not become symptomatic until 1–5 years of age. Malignant transformation has been reported in 1%–2% of cases[79]. Fibrosarcoma of the larynx has been reported[80]. Stridor, abnormal cry, hoarseness and breathing difficulties are the presenting features. Diagnosis is established by laryngoscopy and biopsy. Treatment involves surgical removal of the lesion or laser debulking to maintain a patent airway and preserve the voice. Haemangiomas may be treated with steroids.

Lower respiratory tract

Congenital malformations such as congenital cystic adenomatoid malformation, pulmonary sequestration, congenital lobar emphysema and bronchogenic cysts often present as congenital pulmonary cystic lesions. Lymphangioma[81] and hamartoma[82] have been described in neonates; bronchial adenoma usually occurs in older children. Primary malignant tumours in newborns include bronchogenic carcinoma[83], fibrosarcoma[84] and pulmonary blastoma[85].

Pulmonary blastomas originate from mesenchymal pulmonary blastema analogous to nephroblastoma. Histologically, it may resemble metastasis from nephroblastoma. Therefore appropriate investigations should be carried out to rule out nephroblastoma. The lung is also a site of metastatic deposits from a variety of tumours, especially Wilms' tumour and osteogenic sarcoma.

Pulmonary blastoma usually presents with persistent cough, haemoptysis, pneumonia and atelectasis. Persistence of radiographic abnormalities in spite of adequate treatment raises the possibility of neoplasia. Bronchoscopy, CT and pulmonary tomography may be useful aids. The diagnosis is established by bronchial aspirates or biopsy of the lesion. Treatment involves excision of the tumour, lobectomy or pneumonectomy. Adjunctive chemotherapy may be necessary.

Genitourinary tumours

The most common tumours of the urinary tract are congenital mesoblastic nephroma, Wilms' tumour and rhabdomyosarcoma. Other tumours are rare and usually presented as isolated case reports. The common presentation is abdominal mass, urinary tract infection and haematuria. Occasionally they are diagnosed prenatally. Investigations used to evaluate these masses are abdominal ultrasonography, radionucleid scans (diethylnetriamine, dimercaptosuccinate), CT and occasionally micturating cystourethrogram, intravenous urography and renal angiography[86].

Kidneys

Although Wilms' tumour contributes 95% of the renal tumours in childhood[87], congenital mesoblastic nephromas are common in neonates[88]. Other tumours include lymphangioma, haemangioma, teratoma and ossifying tumours of the kidney[89]. Diagnosis is based on radiological investigations and biopsy. Benign tumours are dealt with by conservative surgery if indicated; malignant lesions are best dealt with by radical nephroureterectomy. The overall survival rates for malignant tumours in children are better than those in adults.

Pelvis and ureter

Tumours of the pelvis and ureter are very rare. Benign lesions are usually fibrous polyps. Transitional cell carcinoma of the renal pelvis has been described in an infant[90]. Treatment for benign lesions includes excision; malignant lesions are best dealt with by nephroureterectomy.

Bladder and urethra

Various benign tumours of the bladder have been reported, and include papilloma, dermoid cyst and phaeochromocytoma. Haemangiomas usually present with gross haematuria, and may be associated with similar lesions elsewhere. Diagnosis is established by cystoscopy. Cystoscopic resection is contraindicated because of the risk of haemorrhage. Fulguration or laser therapy can be used, but partial cystectomy is a safe and effective method.

Neurofibromas of the bladder and urethra are extremely rare: most patients also have other neurofibromas and cafe-au-lait pigmentation with a strong family history. They present with urinary infection, obstruction or abdominal mass. Sarcomatous degeneration can occur. Small lesions can be excised transurethrally; big lesions will require an open procedure[91].

Fibrous polyps and papillomas can occur in the bladder and prostatic urethra. Transurethral excision is adequate[92,93].

Malignant tumours apart from rhabdomyosarcoma are rare. Transition-cell carcinoma and leiomyosarcoma have been reported[94]. Transition-cell carcinomas are usually non-invasive, whereas leiomyosarcomas tend to infiltrate locally. Treatment is surgical with partial cystectomy. Chemotherapy and radiation may be used in unresectable lesions[95].

Genital tract

Ovarian tumours are discussed in Chapter 8. Tumours involving the penis, uterus, cervix, fallopian tube, vagina and vulva are rare.

The commonest penile tumours in the newborn are haemangiomas, most of which need no treatment. A small proportion of patients may require intervention[96]. Primary sarcoma of the penis involving the corpora cavernosa has been reported in infants[97].

Vaginal hamartoma and polyps have been reported in newborn infants and should be considered malignant until proved otherwise[98,99]. Adenocarcinoma or endodermal sinus tumour of infant vagina is usually located in the posterior vaginal wall or fornices. These probably arise from mesonephric remnants of diverticula of yolk sac endoderm[100]. They are highly malignant tumours with very poor prognosis[101,102]. Diagnosis is based on characteristic histological findings[103]. Treatment is conservative surgery with adjuvant chemotherapy, which has better results than radical surgery[103,104]. Monitoring of α_1-fetoproteins in the serum is useful to establish the response and to detect recurrence.

Clear-cell adenocarcinoma occurs later in life, usually after 2 years of age and most frequently after menarche.

Endocrine tumours

These tumours are rare. They may secrete excessive amounts of hormones or intermediate products of hormone synthesis. They constitute about 5% of paediatric neoplasms[105]. Most are benign or low-grade malignant.

Adrenal cortex

Adrenal cortex secretes three major classes of hormone derived from cholesterol, namely glucocorticoids, mineralocorticoids and sex steroids. Tumours of the adrenal cortex may secrete excessive amounts of one or more hormones, producing associated syndromes. In decreasing frequency, these are virilization syndrome, Cushing's syndrome, feminization syndrome and hyperaldosteronism. These syndromes can be produced by other disease processes involving adrenal or other gonads. Tumours of the adrenal cortex can be benign adenoma or carcinoma. Non-functional adrenal tumours are rare.

Virilization syndrome

The commonest cause of virilization at birth is congenital adrenal hyperplasia, but occasionally adrenal tumours can be responsible. This syndrome is caused by excessive secretions of dehydroepiandrosterone, which is a weak androgen.

Symptoms and signs include hypertrophy of the clitoris, hirsutism, increased facial hair, acne, accelerated growth in height, and muscular hypertrophy with or without palpable abdominal mass. Sometimes these are incidentally found on abdominal ultrasound or CT. Malignant lesions can metastasize to the liver, lungs and skin.

Laboratory investigations measuring high levels of urinary 17-ketosteroids and serum dehydroepiandrosterone suggest adrenal source of androgens. Failure to suppress these excessive secretions indicates an ovarian or autonomous adrenal source. Skeletal radiographs show a marked advance in osseous maturation. Localizing studies include abdominal ultrasonography or CT. Adrenal scintigraphy using [^{131}I]iodocholesterol may be helpful in some cases[106]. Intravenous pyelography may be helpful in demonstrating adrenal tumours but is not as useful as ultrasonography or CT. Selective arteriography or venous sampling may be required occasionally.

Cushing's syndrome

Cushing's syndrome is caused by overproduction of glucocorticoids, and causes diversion of amino acids from protein synthesis to gluconeogenesis and lipogenesis, which results in muscle wasting, growth retardation and osteoporosis. Usually there is an element of associated virilization or feminization.

Obesity and short stature are the commonest features of Cushing's syndrome in infants. Deposition of fat is characteristic – truncal obesity with thin legs, buffalo-hump neck and moon-shaped face. Striae are rare in infants. Increased hair growth is commonly seen over the trunk, forearms and face. Infants may exhibit irritability.

Sustained hypersecretion of cortisol causes Cushing's syndrome. This is shown by 24 h urinary measurements of free cortisol or by repeatedly elevated levels of cortisol. Demonstration of persistently elevated cortisol secretions despite administration of supraphysiological doses of potent glucocorticoid cortisol confirms the diagnosis of Cushing's syndrome and differentiates tumours from hyperplasia, where cortisol secretion will decrease[107,108]. ACTH levels are low in Cushing's syndrome as opposed to pituitary tumours. Abdominal ultrasonography and CT are useful in localizing the tumour and in detecting metastasis. Adrenal scintigraphy may be of use where other investigations are not diagnostic[109].

Feminizing tumours and aldosterone-secreting tumours are extremely rare in children. Feminizing tumours are more common in boys than in girls. The usual features are enlargement of the breast and accelerated growth. Skeletal age is usually advanced, and girls may experience precocious vaginal bleeding whereas puberty is delayed in males due to excessive secretions of oestrogen. Aldosterone-secreting tumours cause hyperkalaemia and hypertension with its secondary effects.

Tumours of the adrenal cortex include adenoma and carcinoma; non-functional tumours are usually hamartomas. The distinction between adenoma and carcinoma is difficult. The size, weight and mitotic activity of the tumour are considered to predict its behaviour[110–112]. However, some reports contradict this[113]. Quantitative analysis of DNA has been applied to these tumours in an effort to measure the biological potential. DNA aneuploidy has been associated with metastasizing tumour[114]. Adrenal adenomas are generally small and encapsulated, with characteristically increased smooth endoplasmic reticulum and lipid droplets inside the cells. Carcinomas are divided into two groups: "anaplastic" if 50% or more of the tumour is composed of large pleomorphic cells, and "differentiated" if only a few pleomorphic cells are detected[115]. Adrenal hyperplasia is characterized by the presence of small nodules dispersed in both glands with hypertrophy of the internodular parenchyma.

Treatment of adrenal tumours is surgical. Preoperative preparation is vital, as excessive glucocorticoid secretion suppresses response of the hypothalamo–pituitary–adrenal axis to stress and can precipitate adrenal crisis. These patients should receive perioperative supplemental methylprednisolone. Antihypertensive therapy may be required for patients with aldesterone-producing tumours.

Benign adrenal tumours can be excised by a posterior approach; malignant tumours or large bilateral tumours are removed by an anterior approach.

Patients should be continued on exogenous methylprednisolone in gradually decreasing doses. Laboratory abnormalities should be monitored after operation. Where surgical treatment is not curative for a malignant disease, mitotane has been tried with response in 20%–50% of cases[116–118].

Prognosis of patients with adrenal adenoma and adrenal hyperplasia is excellent. The outcome in patients with anaplastic carcinoma is dismal, with a median survival time of 5 months, whereas those with differentiated carcinoma have longer survival. Sagrocco et al. have suggested the possibility of an adrenal tumour with properties similar to those of stage IV-S neuroblastoma[119].

Adrenal medulla

Phaeochromocytomas are rare tumours arising from chromaffin cells, mostly from the adrenal medulla. Other sites include the organ of Zuckerkandl, sympathetic ganglia, nerve plexuses and nerves. About 90% of these tumours are benign, and 10% malignant. These tumours secrete adrenaline, noradrenaline or dopamine. Although noted in the newborn, the common age is between 6 and 14 years. Paroxysmal hypertension is the presenting feature of these tumours. About 1% of patients with hypertension will have phaeochromocytoma.

Approximately 10% of these tumours are familial, and 10% of patients will have associated familial conditions like neuroectodermal disorders and multiple endocrine disorders (MEN syndromes)[120]. Elevation of urinary metanephrine and vanillylmandelic acid levels are good screening tests. Further confirmation can be achieved by fractionated plasma and urinary free catecholamine determinations. Abdominal ultrasonography and CT are helpful in localizing the tumours.

Metaiodobenzylguanidine scan is a more accurate method of diagnosis, localizing the tumour and metastases. Treatment is surgical: the transabdominal approach is advocated because of the high incidence of bilaterality. Total adrenalectomy is preferred, as it reduces the risk of recurrence and seeding of the tumour. Biopsy of the ipsilateral adrenal is undertaken if bilateral disease is suspected. Perioperative mortality rates are decreased considerably with proper control of hypertension. Patients with unresectable malignant tumours or metastases are managed with phenoxybenzamine. The prognosis following surgery is excellent.

Thyroid

Thyroid gland masses in neonates are uncommon, and apart from neoplasms may be caused by congenital goitre, which is caused by inability to secrete thyroid hormones, causing increased secretion of thyroid-stimulating hormone and hypertrophy of the thyroid gland. This is caused by a number of inborn errors of metabolism, which are specific and involve different genetic defects[121]. Occasionally thyroid hormone secretion is adequate, but there is peripheral resistance because of receptor inadequacies. These patients usually exhibit hypothyroidism or euthyroidism. Diagnosis is based on family history, clinical examination, and low or normal levels of thyroid hormones with elevated levels of thyroid-stimulating hormone. Tissue cultures will indicate specific defects. Thyroid hormone replacement is the treatment of choice and will correct metabolic abnormalities. Thyroidectomy is occasionally required for cosmetic reasons or to relieve compression.

Benign thyroid nodules are much less common. About 50%–75% of these are malignant, and so a solitary nodule in neonates and children should be considered malignant until proved otherwise. Benign lesions are usually adenomas; of the malignant lesions, papillary carcinomas have been reported in neonates[122], and other malignancies include follicular carcinoma and anaplastic carcinoma. Medullary carcinoma of the thyroid is usually familial and associated with MEN syndrome. Females are more commonly affected than males. Lymph-node metastasis is more common with papillary carcinoma and is the initial finding in 60%–75% of patients. A palpable thyroid nodule is present in one-third of children. Distant metastasis is common with follicular carcinoma. ^{99}Tc scans are useful in delineating "hot" nodules, but are not specific. ^{131}I has the disadvantage of exposing the patient to more radiation, so in patients with equivocal results from ^{99}Tc scan, ^{123}I scans are used. Usually malignant lesions will not scan hot nodules. Diagnosis is confirmed by needle aspiration biopsy. Treatment is total thyroidectomy with frozen section histological examination, if diagnosis cannot be established before operation. Total thyroidectomy with bilateral regional lymph node dissection is undertaken for papillary carcinoma. Because of the excellent prognosis, some surgeons do not advocate radical surgery for these papillary carcinomas. Subsequent to surgery, all thyroid hormone replacements are withheld for 6 weeks and then ^{131}I scan is performed. If this shows evidence of the disease, a therapeutic dose of radioactive iodine is administered. Prognosis of patients with papillary carcinoma is excellent, the mortality rate being 5%–10%. Patients with recurrent disease who are unresponsive to radioactive iodine have a less favourable prognosis. Prognosis in patients with follicular carcinoma and anaplastic carcinoma is poor, but prognosis in all malignant carcinoma of the thyroid is related to the extent of disease at the initial operation: if the disease is localized, a cure is possible and can be determined by postoperative calcitonin testing. The prognosis is guarded for patients whose disease involves the jugular or lateral lymph nodes or is associated with MEN IIB.

Parathyroid

These are exceedingly rare but can occur at any age from birth to young adulthood. Adenomas constitute 80% of cases, carcinoma 10% and hyperplasia 10%. They secrete parathormone, causing primary hyperparathyroidism, which is characterized by polydipsia, polyuria, mental confusion, pruritus, headache, band keratitis, bone pains, skeletal deformities and fractures. Resorption cysts of the phalanges are also seen. Nephrolithiasis, nephrocalcinosis, gastric ulcer and pancreatitis may develop. Asymptomatic patients are found to have these tumours on routine electrolyte checks. The diagnosis is established by demonstrating high levels of calcium and alkaline phosphatase and non-suppressible high concentrations of parathormone. Electrocardiography shows shortening of Q–T interval. Skeletal radiography shows changes of rickets. Localizing techniques include abdominal ultrasonography, CT and selective venous sampling. Adenomas are removed surgically and a second gland located and excised. If the second gland is normal, further exploration is not necessary. If hyperplasia or multiple adenoma is found, all but one gland should be removed. Some advocate transplant of parathyroid into the forearm to avoid hypoparathyroidism. Parathyroid carcinomas are best dealt with by surgery. Complications include hypoparathyroidism and recurrent laryngeal nerve injury. In the postoperative period, transient hypocalcaemia needs treatment with calcium and vitamin D if there is any bone involvement.

Multiple endocrine tumours

These involve more than one endocrine gland. These neoplastic changes include hyperplasia, adenomas and carcinomas. These are divided into three groups:

- MEN I (Werner's syndrome) comprises parathyroid tumour, islet-cell tumour or other gastrointestinal endocrine tumour, such as lipoma, glucanoma, ppomas or somatotrophinoma. In addition to adrenal carcinoma or adenoma and hyperplasia, the thymus and bronchus may be involved.
- MEN II (Sipple syndrome) is characterized by combinations of medullary thyroid carcinoma, phaeochromocytoma and parathyroid hyperplasia.
- MEN IIb is represented by multiple mucosal ganglioneuromas, medullary thyroid carcinoma and phaeochromocytoma.

Diagnosis is based on the characteristic of each tumour. Involvement of one gland should suggest the possibility of other gland involvement. Treatment is directed towards the individual tumour. The prognosis in MEN is generally good, and the risk of recurrence is lessened by early and complete removal.

Most of MEN I and MEN II, and half of MEN IIb cases have autosomal dominant transmission with variable penetrance and expression.

Skin

Congenital skin tumours are rare in newborn infants and are usually benign. Malignant tumours may be present at birth, but usually appear later in life. These tumours can arise from any of the constituents of skin or ectopic tissue.

Hamartoma is defined as a malformed growth of normal tissues normally situated at the site. These can be surgically excised for cosmetic reasons. Despite local recurrence, prognosis is excellent[123].

Epithelial tissue tumours can be benign or malignant. Benign tumours include dermoid cysts (discussed previously), papillomas and sweat gland tumours like spiradenoma, which present as superficial dermal nodules. Treatment is complete local excision to prevent recurrence. Malignant epithelial tumours are rare. Basal-cell carcinoma, squamous-cell carcinoma and malignant sweat gland tumour have been reported in neonates[124,125].

Dermatofibroma is a hard tumour of the fibrous tissue of Corinn; dermatofibrosarcoma is a malignant form.

Benign adipose tissue tumours are lipomas, and malignant lesions are liposarcomas. These are extremely rare in newborn infants.

Neoplasms of the breast in neonates are a medical curiosity. A breast carcinoma in a neonate has been reported in the literature[125].

Pigmented tissue

Naevi, pigmented spots anywhere in the body, are the commonest lesions. These are discussed in Chapter 13. Up to 5% of giant naevi will undergo malignant transformation[126]. However, other malignant tumours, such as liposarcoma and rhabdomyosarcoma, have been reported to arise in congenital giant naevi[127,128].

Malignant melanoma can occur prenatally[129,130], acquired transplacentally or arising de novo or in a previous congenital melanocyte naevus or xeroderma pigmentation[131,132].

Some of these patients have a hereditary, autosomal dominant form. These melanomas arise from melanocytes. They can occur anywhere (apart from the orbit and leptomeninges), but are commonly found in a limb or the head and neck area or on the trunk. The pattern of spread of melanoma in children is similar to that in adults, with satellitosis and regional lymph node metastasis followed by involvement of the viscera, lungs, bone or brain[133]. Boys and girls are equally affected, but it is rarer in dark-skinned races[134,135]. Melanomas are classified according to clinical presentation, cutaneous invasion, histological type, and thickness of the primary melanoma[135,136]. Clinically they are staged in three stages: stage I, localized disease; stage 2, metastasis to regional lymph nodes; and stage 3, distant metastasis[137]. Depth of invasion has been indicated to correlate with survival and recurrence. Melanoma is divided into four stages according to depth of invasion[138].

- Level I: confined to the epidermis with no invasion through the basement membrane
- Level II: tumour cells penetrate through the basement membrane into the papillary dermis but do not extend to the reticular dermis
- Level III: extension into the reticular dermis
- Level IV: invasion into subcutaneous tissue

Complete surgical excision is the primary form of therapy for stage I disease. Radical lymph-node discussion has been advocated for stage II disease or tumours 0.75–4.0 mm thick. Treatment for metastatic lesion is still controversial and response poor. Radiotherapy is of no value. Chemotherapy, immunotherapy and surgical resection of isolated metastases have been attempted.

References

1. Holinger LD, Birnholz JC (1987) Management of infants with prenatal ultrasound diagnosis of airway obstruction by teratoma. Ann Otol Rhinol Laryngol 96: 61–64.
2. Zarella JT, Finbery FJ (1990) Obstruction of the neonatal airway from teratomas. Surg Gynecol Obstet 170: 126–131.
3. Wisewell TE, Miller JA (1986) Infection of congenital cervical neck masses associated with bacteremia. J Pediatr Surg 21: 173–174.
4. Avarisco JL (1991) Congenital head and neck masses in infants and children. Part II. Ear Nose Throat J 70: 75–82.
5. Batsakis JG, Makkay B, Ryka AF, Scifert RW (1988) Perinatal salivary gland tumours (embryomas). J Laryngol Otol 102: 1007–1011.
6. Casas LA, Gonzales Crussi F, Pensler JM (1989) Monomorphic adenoma of the parotid in a premature neonate. Ann Plast Surg 211: 47–49.
7. Luna MA, Batsakis JG, el Naggar AK (1991) Salivary gland tumours in children. Ann Otol Rhinol Laryngol 100: 869–871.
8. Satage D, Phillippe E, Ruppe M et al. (1988) Neonatal carcinoma. Review of the literature. A propos of a case. Bull Cancer (Paris) 75: 373–384.
9. Rogers DA, Rao BN, Bowman L et al. (1994) Primary malignancy of the salivary gland in children. J Pediatr Surg 29: 44–47.
10. Ferreiro JA, Weiland LH (1994) Pediatric surgical pathology of the head and neck. Semin Pediatr Surg 3: 169–181.
11. Gale GB, D'Angio GJ, Vri A et al. (1982) Cancer in neonates. The experience in the Children's Hospital of Philadelphia. Pediatrics 70: 409–413.
12. Telleschi S (1970) Unusual pathology of cytological peculiarities of the so called botryoid sarcoma (congenital botryoid sarcoma) of the tongue and infantile uterine botryoid sarcoma with rupture of the organ of hemoperitoneum. Arch Vecchi Anat Pathol 56: 671–705.
13. Van Buavlen J, Orogtrop AP, Box NM (1988) Congenital hemangiopericytoma: report of a case. Pediatr Pathol 8: 109–115.
14. Pavlin JE, O'Gorman A, Williams MB et al. (1984) Epignathus. A report of two cases. Ann Plast Surg 13: 452–456.
15. Blair AE, Edwards DM (1977) Congenital epulis of the newborn. Oral Surg 43: 687–691.
16. Henefer ZP, Abaza NA, Anderson SP (1979) Congenital granular epulis. Oral Surg Oral Med Oral Pathol 47: 515–518.
17. Langley FA, Davson J (1950) Epulis in the newborn. Arch Dis Child 25: 89.
18. Lack FE, Perez-Atayde AR, McGill JJ et al. (1982) Gingival granular cell tumour of the newborn (congenital epulis). Ultrastructural observations relating to histogenesis. Hum Pathol 13: 686.
19. Charni RA, Wong HS (1986) Large congenital epulis of the newborn. J Pediatr Surg 21: 929–930.
20. Dimitrokapoulos I, Zoulomis L, Trigonidis G (1990) Congenital lipoma of the tongue. Report of a case. Int J Maxillofa Surg 19: 208.
21. Frank LW, Enfield CD, Miller AJ (1936) Carcinoma of the tongue in a newborn child. Report of a case. Am J Cancer 26: 775–777.
22. Zanetti B, Signovi E, Consolavo G et al. (1982) Congenital fibroma of the tongue, Z Kinderchirurgie 35: 7–8.
23. Patron M, Palacios J, Rodriguez-Peralfo JL et al. (1988) Malignant rhabdoid tumours of the tongue. A case report with immunohistochemical and ultrastructural findings. Oral Surg Oral Med Oral Pathol 65: 67–70.
24. Gundry SR, Wesley JR Jr, Klien MN et al. (1983) Cervical teratomas in the newborn. J Pediatr Surg 18: 282–286.
25. Gonzales Crussi F (1982) Extragonadal teratomas. Armed Forces Institute of Pathology, Washington DC, pp 118–129.
26. Tapper D, Leck E (1983) Teratomas in infancy and childhood. Ann Surg 198: 398–410.
27. Touran T, Applebaum H, Frost DB et al. (1989) Congenital metastatic cervical teratoma: diagnostic and management considerations. Pediatr Surg 24: 21–23.
28. Filston HC (1994) Hemangiomas, cystic hygromas and teratomas of the head and neck. Semin Pediatr Surg 3: 147–159.
29. Devens K, Holzmann K, Spier J (1980) Teratoma in the cervical region . Z Kinderchirurgie, 30: 119–121.
30. Byard RW, Ziemenez CL, Carpenter BF et al. (1990) Congenital teratomas of the neck and nasopharynx – a clinical and pathological study of 18 cases. J Pediatr Child Health 26: 12–16.
31. Miller RW (1969) Fifty-two forms of childhood cancer: United States mortality experience 1960–1966. J Pediatr Surg 79: 80–88.

32. Nagaya M, Tsuda M, Ischiguro Y (1989) Leiomyosarcoma of the transverse colon in a neonate and rare cause of meconium peritonitis. J Pediatr Surg 24: 1177–1180.
33. Gryboskin J (1975) Gastrointestinal problems in the infant. WB Saunders, Philadelphia, p 97.
34. Nahamal M, Clatworthy HW Jr (1973) Leiomyoma of the entire esophagus. J Pediatr Surg 8: 829.
35. Yannopoulos K, Stout AP (1962) Smooth muscle tumours in children. Cancer 15: 1958.
36. Cohen SR, Thompson JW, Sherman NJ (1988) Congenital stenosis of the lower oesophagus associated with leiomyoma and leiomyosarcoma of the gastrointestinal tract. Ann Otol Rhinol Laryngol 97: 454–459.
37. Archord JL, Proctor HF (1963) Malignant degeneration and metastasis in Peutz–Jeghers syndrome. Arch Intern Med 111: 498–502.
38. Quinn FM, Brown S, O'Hara D (1991) Hemangiopericytoma of the stomach in a neonate. J Pediatr Surg 26: 101–102.
39. Esposito G, Cigliano B, Paludetto R (1983) Abdominothoracic gastric teratoma in a female newborn infant. J Pediatr Surg 18: 304–305.
40. Atwell JD, Claireaux AE, Nixon HH (1967) Teratoma of the stomach in the newborn. J Pediatr Surg 2: 197–204.
41. Stage B, Ange B, Phillipe E et al. (1990) Gastric teratoma in newborn children. Ann Pediatr 37: 235–241.
42. Cullingworth CJ (1877) Case of cancer of the stomach in an infant five weeks old. Br Med J ii: 253.
43. Siegel SE, Hays DM, Romansky S et al. (1976) Carcinoma of the stomach in childhood. Cancer 38: 1781–1784.
44. Tissel SE, Angervall L, Dahl J et al. (1978) Recurrent and metastasizing gastric leiomyoblastoma (epithelioid leiomyosarcoma) associated with multiple pulmonary chondrohamartomas. Cancer 41: 259–265.
45. Wierlitzer FR, Maires AJ, Issacs H Jr et al. (1973) Smooth muscle tumors of the stomach in childhood and adolescence. J Pediatr Surg 8: 421.
46. Appleman HD, Helwig EB (1926) Gastric epithelioid leiomyoma and leiomyosarcoma (leiomyoblastoma). Cancer 38: 708–728.
47. Stagel H, Romansky R, Shackerford GD et al. (1975) Primary immunodeficiency diseases and malignancy. Am J Roentgenol Radiat Ther Nucl Med 123: 144.
48. Ruyman FB (1969) Juvenile polyps with cachexia. Report of an infant and comparison with Cronkhite–Canada syndrome in adults. Gastroenterology 57: 431–438.
49. Yosowitz P, Hobson R, Ruyman F (1974) Sporadic Peutz–Jeghers syndrome in early childhood. Am J Dis Child 128: 709–712.
50. El Shafie M, Spitz L, Ikeda S (1971) Malignant tumors of the small bowel in neonates presenting with perforation. J Pediatr Surg 6: 62–64.
51. Sherburn FW, Teja K, Botero LM et al. (1975) Pancreaticoduodenectomy in the treatment of congenital fibrosarcoma of the duodenum. J Pediatr Surg 10: 801–806.
52. Isaacson C (1978) Embryonal rhabdomyosarcoma of the ampulla of Vater. Cancer 41: 365–368.
53. Knox WG, Miller RE, Begg CF et al. (1960) Juvenile polyps of the colon – a clinicopathological analysis of 75 polyps in 43 patients. Surgery 48: 201–210.
54. Reed TE, Neel JV (1955) A genetic study of multiple polyposis of the colon (with an appendix deriving a method of estimating relative fitness). Am J Hum Genet 7: 236–263.
55. Erbe RW (1976) Inherited gastrointestinal polyposis syndromes. N Engl J Med 294: 1101–1104.
56. Halstead JA, Harris EJ, Barret ML (1950) Involvement of the stomach in familial polyposis of the gastrointestinal tract. Gastroenterology 15: 763–770.
57. Utsunomiya J, Maki T, Twama T et al. (1974) Gastric lesions of familial polyposis coli. Cancer 34: 745.
58. Reddy BS, Mastromarino A, Gustasfson C et al. (1976) Fecal bile acids and neural sterols in patients with familial polyposis. Cancer 38: 1694.
59. Kopelorich L, Sielin S (1980) Human skin fibroblasts from individuals genetically predisposed to cancer are sensitive to an SV40 induced T antigen display of transformation. Cancer 45: 1108.
60. Pierce ER (1972) Pleomorphism and heterogeneity in hereditary intestinal polyposis. Birth Defects 8: 52.
61. Kucukaydin M, Patinglu TE, Okur H (1992) Infantile Cronkhite–Canada syndrome? – case report. Eur J Pediatr Surg 2: 295–297.
62. Ein SH, Robert Beck A, Allen JE (1979) Colon sarcoma in the newborn. J Pediatr Surg 14: 455–457.
63. Nagaya M, Tsuda M, Ishigoro Y (1989) Leiomyosarcoma of the transverse colon in a neonate. A rare cause of meconium peritonitis. J Pediatr Surg 24: 1177–1180.
64. Kern WH, White WC (1958) Adenocarcinoma of the colon in a 9 month old infant. Cancer 11: 855–857.
65. Flanigan DP (1975) Biliary cysts. Ann Surg 182: 535.
66. Garcies LY, Drash A, Kenny FM (1968) Islet cell tumours in the neonate. Pediatrics 41: 789.
67. Wardon MJ, German JC, Buckingham BA (1988) The surgical management of hyperinsulinism in infancy due to nesidioblastosis. J Pediatr Surg 23: 462–465.
68. Kirkland J, Ben-Menachen Y, Akhtar M et al. (1978) Islet cell tumours in a neonate: diagnosis by selective angiography and histological findings. Pediatrics 61: 790–791.
69. Horie A, Yano Y, Kottoo Y, Miwa A (1977) Morphogenesis of pancreatoblastoma, infantile carcinoma of the pancreas, report of two cases. Cancer 39: 247–254.
70. Amt R, Jones MC (1988) Congenital pancreatoblastoma in Beckwith–Wiedemann syndrome – an emerging association. Pediatr Pathol 8: 331–339.
71. Grosfield JG, Clatworthy HW Jr, Hammoudi AB (1970) Pancreatic malignancies in children. Arch Surg 101: 370.
72. Bravo M, Aldunate A, Les Heras J, Pumario G (1989) Hemangioma of the spleen in a newborn infant. Postsplenectomy course and splenic autotransplantation. Rev Chil Pediatr 60: 40–43.
73. Spencer S, Coulter-Knoff A, Day D et al. (1987) Splenic hemangioma with thrombocytopenia in a newborn. Pediatrics 79: 960–966.
74. Hiabourska M, Kadylak B (1989) Leiomyomatosis peritonealis disseminata in a fetus. Zentrabl Allg Pathol 135: 685–689.
75. Nishioka H, Furusho K, Yajunga T et al. (1988) Congenital malignant mesothelioma: a case report and electron microscope study. Eur J Pediatr 147: 428–430.
76. Loeb WJ, Smith EE (1967) Airway obstruction in a newborn by a pedunculated pharyngeal dermoid. Pediatrics 40: 20.
77. Pick T, Maurer HM, McWilliams NB (1974) Lymphoepithelioma in childhood. J Pediatr 84: 96.
78. Jenkin ROT, Anderson JR, Terds B et al. (1981) Nasopharyngeal carcinoma – a retrospective review of patients less than 30 years of age. A report from Children's Cancer Study Group. Cancer 47: 360.
79. Cotton RT, Richardson MA (1981) Advances in head and neck surgery in children. Head Neck Surg 3: 424–437.
80. Simpson AT, McGill T, Healy GB et al. (1979) Benign tumors and lesions of the larynx in children. Ann Otol Rhinol Laryngol 88: 479.
81. Zimmermann H, Habenricht R (1989) Congenital lymphangioma of the lung. Z Kinderchir 44: 111–114.
82. Graham JM Jr, Boyle W, Oxell J et al. (1987) Cystic hamartoma of lung and kidney: a spectrum of developmental abnormalities. Am J Med Genet 27: 45–49.
83. Cayley CK, Caez JH, Mersheimer W (1951) Primary bronchogenic carcinoma of the lung in children. Am J Dis Child

82: 49.

84. Desrousseaux B, Gourdin C, Atat T et al. (1989) Neonatal pulmonary fibrosarcoma. Chir Pediatr 30: 295–296.
85. Tetley NK, Bhatnagar V, Krishna A et al. (1988) Pulmonary blastoma in a neonate. J Pediatr Surg 23: 1009–1010.
86. Fernbach SC (1991) Imaging of neonatal renal masses. Urol Radiol 12: 214–219.
87. Young JL, Miller RW (1975) Incidence of malignant tumors in US children. J Pediatr 86: 254.
88. Angulo Cuesta J, Ereno Z, Arate C et al. (1991) Congenital mesoblastic nephroma in childhood. Our experience apropos of 3 cases. Prenivos Espanoles de Urologica 44: 59–62.
89. Chatten J, Cromie WJ, Duckett JW (1986) Ossifying tumor of infantile kidney. Report of two cases. Cancer 45: 609.
90. Kyanagi T, Sarakik, Arikodo K et al. (1975) Transitional cell carcinoma of the renal pelvis in an infant. J Urol 113: 113–114.
91. Rathburn NP (1937) Primary bladder tumors in infants and young children with report of a case of hemangioma in a male child 27 months of age. Surg Gynecol Obstet 64: 914–918.
92. DeWolf WC, Fraley EE (1973) Congenital urethral polyp in the infant and review of the literature. J Urol 109: 515–516.
93. Lorentzen M, Rohr N (1979) Urinary bladder tumours in children. cases of inverted papilloma. Scand J Urol Nephrol 13: 323.
94. McGuire EJ, Weiss RM, Barkin AM (1973) Neoplasms of transitional cell origin in first twenty years of life. Urology 1: 57.
95. Ray B, Grabstald H, Exelby GR et al. (1973) Bladder tumors in children. Urology 2: 426.
96. Casale AJ, Manashe DS (1989) Massive strawberry hemangioma of the male genitalia. J Urol 141: 593–594.
97. Jodson JJ (1924) Primary sarcoma of the penis. Surg Gynecol Obstet 38: 150–158.
98. Pul M, Xilmaz N, Guisser N, Fozoran Y (1990) Vaginal polyp in a newborn – a case report and review of the literature. Clin Pediatr 29: 1346.
99. McHenry CR, Reynolds M, Raffensperger JG (1988) Vaginal neoplasms in infancy. The combined role of chemotherapy and conservative surgical resection. J Pediatr Surg 23: 842–845.
100. Hinman F, Perez-Mis C (1958) Infantile adenocarcinoma: a clinicopathological study and classification of 39 cases. Cancer 11: 181–199.
101. Norris HJ, Bagley UV, Taylor HB (1970) Carcinoma of infant vagina. A distinctive turnout. Arch Pathol 10: 473–479.
102. Allyn DL, Silverberg SA et al. (1971) Endodermal sinus tumour of the vagina. Report of a case with seven year survival and literature review of so called mesonephroma. Cancer 27: 1291.
103. Copeland LJ, Shiege N, Ordonez NA et al. (1985) Endodermal sinus tumour of vagina and cervix. Cancer 55: 2558–2565.
104. Anderson WA, Sabio H et al. (1985) Endodermal sinus tumour of the vagina. The role of primary chemotherapy. Cancer 56: 1025–1027.
105. Young JL, Heisc HO, Silverberg E et al. (1978) Cancer incidence, survival and mortality for the children under 15 years of age. American Cancer Society, New York.
106. Schteingart DF, Seabold JE, Gross MD et al. (1981) Iodocholesterol adrenal tissue uptake and imaging in adrenal neoplasms. J Clin Endocrinol Metab 52: 1156.
107. Liddie AW (1963) Tests of pituitary–adrenal suppressibility in the diagnosis of Cushing's syndrome. Arch Intern Med 111: 471.
108. Linn JE Jr, Bondoin B, Farmer TA, Meador CK (1967) Observations and comments on failure of dexamethasone suppression. N Engl J Med 277: 403.
109. Abrams HL, Siegelman SS, Adams DF et al. (1982) Computed tomography versus ultrasound of the adrenal gland: a prospective study. Radiology 143: 121.
110. Riebero RL, Sandrini RS, Schell MS et al. (1990) Adrenocortical carcinoma in children: a study of 40 cases. J Clin Oncol 8: 67–74.
111. Cagle PT, Hough AJ, Pysher TJ et al. (1986) Comparison of adrenocortical tumors in children and adults. Cancer 57: 2235–2237.
112. van Slooten H, Schaberg A, Smenck D et al. (1985) Morphological characteristics of benign and malignant adrenocortical tumors. Cancer 55: 766–773.
113. Glandour MJ, Grizzle WE (1986) A small adrenocortical carcinoma with aggressive behaviour. An evaluation of criteria for malignancy. Arch Pathol Lab Med 110: 1076–1079.
114. Taylor SR, Murphy RF, Roederer M (1987) Flow cytometric DNA analysis of adrenocortical tumors in children. Cancer 59: 2059–2061.
115. Hogan TF, Gilchrist KW, Westring DW et al. (1980) A clinical and pathological study of adrenocortical carcinoma. Therapeutic implications. Cancer 45: 2880–2883.
116. Hajjar RA, Hickey RC, Samaan NA (1975) Adrenal cortical carcinoma: a study of 32 patients. Cancer 31: 549.
117. Hutter AM Jr, Kayhoe DE (1966) Adrenal cortical carcinoma: results of treatment with opDDD in 138 patients. Am J Med 41: 581.
118. Lubitz JA, Freeman L, Okun R (1973) Mitotane use in inoperable adrenal carcinoma. JAMA 223: 1109.
119. Sagrocco S, Abramowsky C, Taylor S et al. (1988) Spontaneously regressing adrenocortical carcinoma in a newborn. A case report with DNA ploidy analysis. Cancer 62: 507–511.
120. Caty MA, Coran AG, Geogen M et al. (1990) Current diagnosis and treatment of pheochromocytoma in children. Experience with 22 consecutive tumors in 14 children. Arch Surg 125: 978–981.
121. Suder H (1984) Pathogenesis of goitre. A unifying hypothesis. Thyroid Today 7: 1–7.
122. Dehner LP (1975) Pediatric surgical pathology. CV Mosby, St Louis.
123. Lee JT, Girwan DP, Armstrong RF (1988) Fibrous hamartoma of infancy. J Pediatr Surg 23: 759–761.
124. Figuerva Tovar MI, Laterza AM, Tamayo L et al. (1989) Incidence of malignant, primary and metastatic solid skin tumors at a pediatric dermatology service. Med Cutan Iber Lat Am 17: 52–57.
125. Satge D, Phillipe E, Ruppe M et al. (1988) Neonatal carcinoma. Review of the literature. A propos of a case. Bull Cancer 75: 373–384.
126. Hori Y, Nakayama J, Okamato M et al. (1989) Giant congenital naevus and malignant melanoma. J Invest Dermatol 92 (Suppl): 3105–3145.
127. Hendrickson MR, Ross JC (1981) Neoplasms arising in congenital giant naevi: morphologic study of seven cases and a review of the literature. Am J Surg Pathol 5: 109–135.
128. Sergio-Zuniga R, Horas JL, Benveniste S (1987) Rhabdomyosarcoma arising in a congenital giant nevus associated with neurocutaneous melanosis in a neonate. J Pediatr Surg 22: 1036–1038.
129. Sweet LK, Connerty HV (1941) Congenital melanoma. Report of a case in which antenatal metastasis occurred. Am J Dis Child 62: 1029–1040.
130. Schneidermann H, Yu-Yuan Wu A, Campbell WA et al. (1987) Congenital melanoma with multiple prenatal metastasis. Cancer 60: 1371–1377.
131. Proje NS, Laude TA, Heilman ER et al. (1987). Congenital malignant melanoma. Pediatrics 79: 967–970.
132. Takebe H, Nishigori C, Tatsumi K (1989) Melanoma and

other skin cancers in xeroderma pigmentosum patients and mutation of their cells. J Invest Dermatol 92 (Suppl): 2365–2385.
133. Trozak DJ, Rowland HVF (1975) Metastatic malignant melanoma in prepubertal children. Pediatrics 55: 191–204.
134. Pratt GB, Paloner MK, Thatcher N et al. (1981) Malignant melanoma in children and adolescents. Cancer 47: 392–397.
135. Bader JL, Li RW, Miller R et al. (1979) Malignant melanoma in persons under 20 years of age. An epidemiologic study. Proc Am Assoc Cancer Res 20: 316.
136. Day CL, Sober AJ, Fitzpatrick TB et al. (1980) Prognosis in malignant melanoma. J Am Acad Dermatol 5: 525.
137. Goldsmith HS, Shab JP, Kim DK (1970) Prognostic significance of lymph node dissection in the treatment of malignant melanoma. Cancer 26: 606.
138. Clark WH Jr, Ainsworth AM, Bernandino EA et al. (1975) The developmental biology of primary human malignant melanomas. Semin Oncol 2: 83–103.

Index

MIX
Papier aus verantwortungsvollen Quellen
Paper from responsible sources
FSC® C105338

If you have any concerns about our products,
you can contact us on
ProductSafety@springernature.com

In case Publisher is established outside the EU,
the EU authorized representative is:
Springer Nature Customer Service Center GmbH
Europaplatz 3, 69115 Heidelberg, Germany

Printed by Libri Plureos GmbH
in Hamburg, Germany